ADVANCES IN

Pharmacology and Chemotherapy

VOLUME 9

ADVISORY BOARD

ADVANCES IN

Pharmacology and Chemotherapy

EDITED BY

Silvio Garattini

Istituto di Ricerche Farmacologiche "Mario Negri" Milano, Italy

A. Goldin

National Cancer Institute Bethesda, Maryland

F. Hawking

Delta Primate Research Center Covington, Louisiana

I. J. Kopin

National Institute of Mental Health Bethesda, Maryland

Consulting Editor

R. J. Schnitzer

Mount Sinai School of Medicine New York, New York

VOLUME 9

ACADEMIC PRESS New York and London 1971

ACADEMIC PRESS, INC.
111 Fifth Avenue, New York, New York 10003

United Kingdom Edition published by
ACADEMIC PRESS, INC. (LONDON) LTD.
24/28 Oval Road, London NW1 7DD

LIBRARY OF CONGRESS CATALOG CARD NUMBER: 61-18298

PRINTED IN THE UNITED STATES OF AMERICA

CONTENTS

Drug Effects and Learning and Memory Processes

Walter B. Essman

CONTRIBUTORS TO THIS VOLUME

Numbers in parentheses indicate the pages on which the authors' contributions begin.

RICHARD P. BOBBIN (93), *Department of Pharmacology, Tulane University, New Orleans, Louisiana*

WALTER B. ESSMAN (241), *Departments of Psychology and Biochemistry, Queens College of the City University of New York, Flushing, New York*

PAUL S. GUTH (93), *Department of Pharmacology, Tulane University, New Orleans, Louisiana*

CARL D. KING* (1), *Department of Pharmacology, Emory University, Atlanta, Georgia*

B. J. LUDWIG (173), *Wallace Laboratories, Division of Carter-Wallace, Inc., Cranbury, New Jersey*

J. R. POTTERFIELD (173), *Wallace Laboratories, Division of Carter-Wallace, Inc., Cranbury, New Jersey*

WILLIAM V. SHAW (131), *Departments of Medicine and Biochemisty, University of Miami School of Medicine, Miami, Florida*

* Present address: Department of Medicine, University of California, San Diego, La Jolla, California 92037.

ADVANCES IN

Pharmacology and Chemotherapy

VOLUME 9

The Pharmacology of Rapid Eye Movement Sleep

CARL D. KING*

Department of Pharmacology, Emory University, Atlanta, Georgia

I. Sleep

In our rhythm of earthly life we tire of light. We are glad when the day ends,
when the play ends; and ectasy is too much pain.
We are children quickly tired: children who are up in the night and fall asleep
as the rocket is fired; and the day is long for work or play.
We tire of distraction or concentration, we sleep and are glad to sleep,
Controlled by the rhythm of blood and the day and the night and the seasons.

T. S. Eliot

* Present address: Department of Medicine, University of California, San Diego, La Jolla, California 92037.

A. Definitions

Everyone intuitively knows what sleep is and what it is for. Sleep is rest, quiescence, a time when bodily functions subside to a low point. Its purpose is surcease and restoration.

Unfortunately, intuition is a bad instructor; so, too, is subjective experience. A person will complain that he has tossed and turned all night—objective observation will show that he tossed and turned for only 5 minutes out of a total of 500. Another will claim that he never dreams—objective observation will show that he dreams 4 or 5 times every night. Intuition will say that sleep is a nadir, a "kinsman of death"—objective observation will show that some functions reach their zenith only in the depths of sleep.

Given, then, the wealth of intuitive and anecdotal observation, and the relative lack of objective observation, any definition of sleep and any statement of its purpose is, at this time, hazardous. As Kleitman (1963) has pointed out, what the poet has said concerning sleep is just as apt to be right—or wrong—as what many a scientist has said. Shakespeare was more attuned to the real nature of sleep than were all the physiologists of the nineteenth century put together. But both—poet and physiologist alike—have suffered from insufficient evidence.

Despite the hazards of relative ignorance, some working definition of sleep should be attempted, realizing all the while that what we state today as fact may, 5 years from now, prove only to have been fancy.

This working definition will not be very much like one of the classic views of sleep—a view which Hess (1929) termed the "negative" view of sleep. This negative outlook was the one which dominated physiology in the last century and, indeed, was the one which dominated the thought of philosophers for thousands of years. It stated that sleep is simply an extinction of functional potencies; as such, it is, in the general scheme of things, undesirable (though unavoidable). Aristotle (noted in Kleitman, 1963) arrived at such a formulation: in his system of dichotomies (strength–weakness; health–sickness) he saw sleep simply as the opposite of wakefulness, and therefore, since health is good and sickness bad, sleep was "bad." This led to the view that sleep is a form of weakness: Kleitman (1963) quotes A.P.W. Philip, who wrote in 1834: "We can perceive no final cause of the alternation of watchfulness and sleep, but such as has its origin in the imperfection of our nature." Sleep, owing to our mortal weakness, is a disturber of the "natural" waking state. Sleep is the kinsman of the negative half of the ultimate dichotomy: life–death.

Not everyone has thought of sleep in this way. Many, notably the poets, have expressed what Hess (1929) termed (and advocated) the "positive" view of sleep—sleep is an integral part of our makeup, no less positive than wakefulness; it is a process that promotes renewal and has a restorative function. Sleep, wrote Shakespeare, is a boon; and therefore he advised us to "enjoy the honey-heavy dew of slumber," and he had the weary Henry IV, suffering from insomnia, complaining:

> How many thousand of my poorest subjects
> Are at this hour asleep! O sleep, O gentle sleep!
> Nature's soft nurse, how have I frighted thee,
> That thou no more wilt weigh my eyelids down
> And steep my senses in forgetfulness?

The conversion of physiology to the positive view of sleep has been complete in the present century. This conversion was signaled by Sir Frederick Mott (1924), who (with a distinct dash of sinophobia) wrote:

> Since sleep occupies a large part of our life it must be physiological function and one of great importance. In fact, it requires no great consideration to make it obvious that without the repetition of sleep, healthy mental and bodily life is impossible... . It is known that a person can live a few minutes without air, a few days without water, and a few weeks without food, but, although he can live several weeks without food, he cannot live a week without sleep. How do we know this? In China, where refined modes of death by torture have been long practiced, death by prevention of sleep is one of the methods employed. The victims do not live more than five to seven days.

So we now recognize and appreciate sleep's necessity and value. It is, as Kleitman (1963) wrote, the "complement to the waking state, the two (states) constituting alternate phases of a cycle, the one related to the other as the trough of a wave is related to the crest." Sleep is as characteristic a manifestation of life as is wakefulness. The two go together and form the basic rhythm of the existence of all the higher forms of life. Death is not simply the termination of wakefulness—it is also the termination of sleep.

Sleep can be defined, then (and I here slightly modify the definition of Kleitman, 1963) as a rhythmical and temporary interruption of wakefulness, induced by internal, not external, factors, in which consciousness of environmental features subsides to a minimum; in which movement of the body is almost completely absent; in which there is an increase in the thresholds of reactivity and of reflex irritability; in which there occurs a continuum which leads from light sleep to deep sleep; in which there occurs, also, a rhythmical alternation of this light sleep–deep sleep cycle; in which at the peak of each of these cycles, certain functions become accelerated and, at least in the human, there occurs the phenomenon of dreaming; and in which there exists a built-in mechanism which after a time produces the phenomenon of arousal.

Thus coma is not, by this cumbersome definition, sleep; nor is anesthesia; nor is the somnolence which follows the use of certain drugs.

Lacking, in this definition, is a statement of sleep's purpose. A real definition of sleep will perhaps come someday and will say that sleep is a function which accomplishes certain ends for the organism. We think that sleep accomplishes certain ends, but we do not know what those ends are.

B. Phylogeny

Who sleeps? I said that sleep is a hallmark of all the higher forms of life. This implies that somewhere there is a dividing line, separating the "higher" forms (who sleep) from the "lower" forms (who do not). Does a virus sleep? A bacterium? A protozoan? Does a hydra have a rest–activity cycle? and sleep? Does the grass, exposed to the same astronomical rhythm that dictates the human pattern of rest and activity, sleep? Does the morning glory sleep? It furls at night, then opens again as the sun comes up. Do trees sleep, perhaps with a rhythm measured by months instead of by hours? The answer, by our weak present definition of sleep, is No. Despite this, rest–activity cycles are all around us. Life processes wax, then wane, and then wax again. When we finally understand sleep's purpose, when we really know the thing for the first time, on a molecular basis, then maybe our definition of sleep will be at once more concise than it is now, and at the same time more all-inclusive; and we will be able to say that a hydra sleeps, and that, yes, the morning glory, with a rhythm like our own, also sleeps.

Given our present definition of sleep, however, Who sleeps? The answer is that probably most mammals sleep. If the definition of sleep is slightly amended, to exclude the statement concerning a light sleep–deep sleep cycle, then it is probably accurate to say that all vertebrates sleep. [There is some controversy concerning the frog, though. In 1913 Pieron (cited in Hobson, 1967), stated that frogs sleep; this was on the basis of their nocturnal immobility. Hobson (1967), however, concludes differently. He admits that frogs rest, but, because he could not demonstrate any hyporeactivity, he concluded that this rest was not sleep. This little controversy simply further demonstrates the weakness of our present definition of sleep.]

Fish sleep, and electro-oculographic signs of this have been found in at least two species of Bermuda reef fish (Tauber and Weitzman, 1969). Fish, however, have certain problems (Hediger, 1969)—with a few exceptions, they cannot close their eyes or even constrict their pupils. They, and many other forms, have developed a special ability to filter out innocuous environmental factors, to shut off, as it were, the optic nerve for everything except potentially dangerous situations. For this reason, a sudden light flashed upon sleeping fish can produce panic, and the animals may dash themselves to death against rocks or aquarium walls. This is a well-known fact to zookeepers, who use special precautions when they make nocturnal visits to their aquaria (Hediger, 1969).

The diversity of nature is a truism. Given this, it is only to be expected that sleep habits will be as diverse as the animal kingdom itself.

Steinhart (cited in Kleitman, 1963) in an heroic study of the sleep of 600 army horses, found what any farm boy might have been able to relate, i.e., horses sleep while standing upright. In addition, however, the horse has three other sleeping postures, which, in order of declining frequency, are standing, but with its head resting limply upon some support such as a stall partition; lying down upon its belly; and (in the deepest stage) lying down upon its side.

Perhaps the most spectacular example of sleep in the upright position is the flamingo, who draws up one of its limbs and sleeps entirely supported by a single, spindly leg.

There are other odd forms of sleep to be found among animals. Hediger (1969) claims that bats and flying foxes can only sleep when their heads hang down and they are suspended by their feet. In the laboratory, however, bats occasionally sleep on the floor of their cage (Brebbia and Paul, 1969). Hediger notes that dolphins have a most peculiar pattern of sleep behavior. These mammals awaken for every respiration and rise to the surface for each breath. Even more odd, they habitually sleep with one eye closed and the other eye open. Each eye (or visual cortex) is allowed to "sleep" several hours each day.

As Hediger notes, however, the sleep habits of animals are chiefly determined by the degree of threat to which the animal is exposed. This determines both the location the animal seeks out in which to sleep and the length of sleep which the animal can enjoy.

Many animals have a "territory," and in this territory there are fixed points for such activities as eating, drinking, and toilet functions. The most important fixed point is the home proper, the area of maximum safety—the den, the hole, the lair. It is at this place of greatest safety that two functions, as a rule, occur—the birth and care of the young, and sleep. Thus the mole and the echidna sleep in holes dug in the ground. The hippopotamus is most safe in the water, and so it is there, writes Hediger, that it sleeps (and there that it gives birth, under the water).

Hediger notes that birds, in general, behave a bit differently. Only a few actually sleep in the nest where the young are cared for; most sleep on nearby branches. The peacock carries this habit to an odd extreme—each peacock selects for itself a "sleeping tree"; this tree is chosen carefully and is occupied regularly for decades, night after night, in every season and weather. The peacock's nest, by contrast, is on the ground.

Anthropoids, Hediger relates, even those that spend their waking hours on the ground, revert to their ancestral arboreal origins when they sleep. Such behavior is generally dictated by the demands for safety. Even the gorilla is prey to the big carnivores; this is especially true for the gorilla's young, and, hence, refuge is sought out for sleep.

If a species has nothing to fear from other forms, it tends to sleep out in the open (Hediger, 1969). The lion is an example; the Indian sloth bear (*Melursus ursinus*), whom even the tiger keeps well clear of, is another, and is noted for its very long, sound naps.

But what do animals do if they are unable to dig or climb, or if they are not at home in the water? Many species are unable to find places of security, and are out in the open, exposed to danger, all of the time. Examples are the antelope, the hare, the zebra, the giraffe, and the ostrich. Hediger finds that such species have evolved two solutions to the problem of sleep. One solution is the drastic elimination of sleep to a bare minimum. In fact, according to Hediger, the antelope has never been seen asleep in the wild. Deer and other ruminants, on the other hand, have been seen asleep in their natural environments, and even have a special sort of very deep sleep in which they can be approached and even touched. Such episodes are very brief, however (1–10 minutes), and when awakened from this state, the animal will dart off in a flash. This state of sleep, as judged by the presence of muscular twitchings, is probably, says Hediger, a form of rapid eye movement sleep.

Hediger writes that the second solution to the problem of sleep which animals in constant peril have evolved is a social solution. This is exemplified by the zebra, which lives its whole life in a large herd. A few members of the herd sleep while the majority remain vigilant; the members of the herd take turns, so that in the long run each animal receives a quota of sleep.

Thus sleep habits, as one could only expect, show a great lack of catholicity. Security and survival do much to determine any given species' mode of rest.

C. Sleep Concomitants

What are the concomitants of sleep? To answer this question we must leave the broad animal kingdom, and consider only a very few species, most notably man and the cat. The reason for narrowing our view so markedly and suddenly is the simple lack of data from any other species.

(A few remarks, however, can be made concerning the phylogeny of rapid eye movement sleep, and these will be mentioned in the next chapter.)

The phenomena of sleep have been extensively described by Kleitman (1963), upon whom I will extensively rely for the next few paragraphs; where another author is not indicated, my source is Kleitman.

1. The Central Nervous System (CNS)

The most pronounced changes in sleep occur in the CNS. A general decline of excitability appears; reflexes become attenuated, and may vanish; the knee-jerk, for example, is not elicitable in the deeper stages of sleep. Reflexes which do not disappear altogether, wane considerably, and the reflex time is lengthened. A very peculiar phenomenon which, in the normal adult, occurs only in deep sleep is the appearance of a positive Babinski sign, i.e., toe-extension provoked by scratching the sole of the foot. This "sleep reflex," in fact, was noted a full 16 years before Babinski described the sign as a diagnostic clue indicative of an interruption of the pyramidal pathways from the cerebral cortex to the lower part of the spinal cord. Aside from such lesions and sleep, the positive Babinski sign appears only in the newborn and in anesthesia. That it occurs in deep sleep tends to indicate that there is some kind of functional interruption of the connection between the cortex and the lower segments of the CNS.

Several investigators, notably Bremer (1935), have said that sleep is a functional deafferentation of the cortex. The positive Babinski sign indicates, perhaps, a functional deefferentation as well. Other data give the same indications. Thus the tremor of Parkinsonism dramatically declines in sleep; most often it is absent altogether; it may return at times, but these instances are rare and are associated with gross body movements and, more rarely, with the bursts of rapid eye movements seen in rapid eye movement sleep (Stern *et al.*, 1968). Another indication of functional deefferentation was noted by Gibbs and Gibbs (1947) who found that, unexpectedly, seizure discharges in the electroencephalogram increase sharply with the onset of sleep. This was especially true of patients with grand mal and psychomotor epilepsy, less often the case with petit mal. Yet, despite the frequent seizure discharges, there were no seizures. If, however, a patient were aroused while a grand mal seizure discharge was taking place, then a full-blown fit would occur. The localization and mechanism of this functional disconnection of the cortex in sleep is not known. The inhibitory influence apparently does not arise within the cortex itself, else the seizure discharges would subside in sleep instead of increase. Further, as Kleitman (1963) notes, the cortex is not required for the occurrence of sleep—in decorticated dogs, there still occur periods of sleep and cryptoarousal, and in the episodes of sleep there still occurs a marked loss of reactivity to the environment and inhibition of peripheral reflexes.

The electroencephalogram (EEG) was developed by the German psychiatrist, Berger. As noted by Gloor (1969), Berger's work was motivated by a desire to find an objective physiological method with which to study the ancient problem of the relationship between mind and brain. Although Berger's aims have not been fully realized, the EEG has proven to be of great value, and had become central to the study of sleep. The first description of the sleep EEG in man was made by Loomis *et al.* (1935a) Their recordings were made upon paper which was wrapped around a huge (8-ft long, 44 in. in circumference) metal drum; the drum revolved once a minute. Onto the paper went tracings of the heart beat, respirations, and bed movements (all in red ink) and a tracing of brain potentials (in green ink). Loomis and his co-workers proved that these brain potentials were cortical in origin, and were quite distinct from muscle potentials and movement artifacts. They also discovered the first sleep waves, which they described as "very regular bursts lasting 1 to $1\frac{1}{2}$ seconds of 14 per second frequency. The amplitude builds regularly to a maximum and then falls regularly so that we have designated these 'spindles,' because of their appearance in the record." We still call them spindles today.

In later publications (Loomis *et al.*, 1935b; Harvey *et al.*, 1937) the same group described the existence of slow waves, and classified the different phases of sleep into five different stages. This classification was standard for many years, but was modified, out of necessity, by Dement and Kleitman (1957); the modification was necessary because, despite their outstanding efforts, the Loomis group had missed one of the stages of sleep altogether. Today, the human sleep EEG fairly much follows the Dement and Kleitman modification of the Loomis classification, and briefly, is as follows:

Stage 1—an absolute lack of spindle activity; predominant low voltage, fast activity

Stage 2—spindles, with a low-voltage background

Stage 3—high-voltage slow waves with spindles

Stage 4—at least half or more of the record is dominated by waves of 100 uV or more, in the 1–2-Hz range or slower.

Stage REM (also called "emergent state 1")—rapid eye movement sleep

Derbyshire *et al.* (1936) were among the first to record the sleep EEG of an animal. These workers, using cats, observed spindles and "large waves, larger than those recorded in the waking state." The sleep EEG of the cat has not yielded to as fine an analysis as has that of the human, and, indeed, most workers subdivide the cat's sleep only into two stages: rapid eye movement sleep and nonrapid eye movement sleep. This is an over-simplification. At least three different stages of cat sleep can easily be identified (Jewett, 1968; Ursin, 1968): spindle sleep (similar to the human stage 2); slow-wave sleep (human stage 4); and rapid eye movement sleep (human stage REM).

The EEG has proven to be an excellent tool for the study of sleep, but not an infallible one. There can be dissociations between the EEG and the behavior of the test subject or animal. Atropine, as Kleitman notes, can produce a sleeplike EEG in the conscious animal; with any drug study of sleep, therefore, one must be careful to check for such possible dissociations. As Kleitman states:

> ...it is clear that the EEG by itself not only fails to gauge the depth of sleep but the very presence of behavioral sleep. It does not mean that the EEG is not a useful tool when coupled with other concomitants of sleep..., (but) where there is a conflict between the different indices, behavioral signs must be given preference over EEG patterns.

It is not always clear, either, just what an EEG pattern means when one asks what individual neurons in the cortex are doing. It was long held, largely due to the influence of Pavlov, that in sleep the majority of cortical neurons were doing nothing; they were "sleeping." This certainly is not the case, however. Evarts *et al.* (1962) studied the activities of single units in the cat's visual cortex, middle suprasylvian association cortex, and brainstem, in various stages of arousal and sleep. They found that the rate of spontaneous discharge from these single neurons is actually higher in sleep than in wakefulness. In waking, there is a greater variability of discharge from these cells and a greater differentiation of discharge rates from one cell to another, but the overall discharge rate is lower than in sleep.

2. Musculature

Muscle tone is, in general, diminished in sleep. Some muscles, however, work harder in sleep than in wakefulness; these include the muscles which cause closure of the eyes, the sphincter of the pupil (miosis is the tonic state of the pupil in sleep), and the muscles of the anal and vesicular sphincters.

3. Composition of the Blood

The composition of the blood in sleep is a controversial topic. Glucose concentrations, for example, are claimed to rise by some, to fall by others, and to remain unchanged by still others. Various changes in blood pH, pCO_2, pO_2, cholesterol, catecholamines, etc., have been claimed—and disputed.

4. Cardiovascular System

There is general agreement that in sleep, the heart rate and mean blood pressure fall somewhat (Khatri and Freis, 1967). Variations in each occur, however; these are generally restricted to stage REM.

An unexpected finding is the change in cerebral blood flow which occurs with sleep. It was held by many for a very long time that cerebral blood flow declined in sleep. It does not. Kety and associates (Mongold *et al.*, 1955) studied cerebral blood flow in a group of 50 young men during quiet arousal and in natural sleep (i.e., no drugs were used). They found that in sleep, the cerebral blood flow increased from a mean of 59 to 65 cc/100 gm/minute; the change was statistically significant. Despite this increased flow, the mean arterial blood pressure declined from 94 to 90 mm Hg—another statistically significant change. Thus cerebral vascular resistance must fall in sleep. The mechanism is unknown (and the full magnitude of the effect was not really appreciated until 1967, as will be mentioned in the next chapter). Sleep, concluded Kety and his co-workers, is a "puzzling phenomenon."

5. Respiratory System

Respiratory changes occur in sleep, but, as Kleitman notes, there is wide disagreement both as to the magnitude of the change and even to the direction of the change. Most observers claim a general decline of the respiratory rate, but the variability of the change is marked.

6. Body Temperature

The body temperature falls in sleep, but probably not as a direct result of sleep itself. As Kleitman notes in an extensive discussion, there is a circadian rhythm of the body temperature, which crests in the afternoon and falls to its low point in the hours before dawn; this rhythm persists in sleepless individuals.

7. Metabolic Changes

Various metabolic changes have been described to occur in sleep. Most of these, Kleitman feels, are due to such concomitants of sleep as horizontal posture, relaxation, fasting, and darkness. The picture really is not that simple. Reich *et al.* (1967) have found that in sleep there is a two to threefold increase in the incorporation of inorganic phosphate into the substance of the brain. Some of this may be due to incorporation into phosphoproteins. Some is also due to incorporation into brain nucleotides and glycolytic intermediates, as shown by Van den Noort and Brine (1970). These authors found that there is an increased concentration of adenosine triphosphate (ATP), creatine phosphate, and fructose diphosphate in the brains of sleeping rats. Brain glucose levels are increased. These changes occurred without any alteration of the metabolic rate. In sleep, then, some special mechanism may be operative which allows an increased formation of brain labile phosphates without any concomitant fall of the brain's metabolic rate. In a different area, it has been clearly demonstrated by several groups (Takahashi *et al.*, 1968; Honda *et al.*, 1969; Parker *et al.*, 1969; Sassin *et al.*, 1969) that there is in man a large increase in the release of growth hormone during sleep. The onset of sleep seems to trigger this secretion of growth hormone. Thus the increase does not occur in individuals who remain awake through the night. Further, the secretion of the hormone is inhibited during episodes of rapid eye movement sleep. Honda *et al.* (1969) suggest that neocortical activation inhibits the secretion of growth hormone and that cortical synchronization induces the secretion of growth hormone-releasing factor in the hypothalamus. Beyond this, little is known. The study of the metabolic changes which occur in the brain with sleep is virgin, and critically important, territory.

8. Duration of Sleep

Sleep's duration is another topic which Kleitman discusses at length. The length of sleep decreases rapidly with age, then plateaus. The newborn child sleeps most of its time; it awakens at fairly regular intervals regardless of the time of day or night. But the infant soon learns that night is the time for sleep, and by the twelfth month of extrauterine life, a pattern of night-long sleep, plus a morning nap and an afternoon nap, has been established. By the twenty-fourth month, the morning nap usually has been given up. The afternoon nap then begins to shrink, and finally is also given up. This occurs usually by the child's fifth year. Following the fifth year, night sleep itself begins to shrink, until the adult pattern—the plateau—is reached in adolescence. The normal range of sleep for the adult is, according to Kleitman, 5–10 hours.

D. Why Do We Sleep?

Why? This is still the *arcanum arcanorum*. It is now generally agreed that sleep confers something upon the sleeper, but what? Why are those 5–10 hours necessary?

Sleep Deprivation

Investigators have attempted to answer the question by removing the phenomemon, i.e., as Kleitman (1963) puts it:

> Organ extirpation, as a means of determining its function through the ensuing deficiency symptoms, has long been a recognized method in physiological research. Depriving the organism of a certain activity is the functional counterpart. Fasting and prolonged sleeplessness have been used to study the effects of lack of food and of sleep.

The general aim of sleep-deprivation studies is to answer the "why" question. All such studies have shown at least that the previous citation from Mott (Section I, A) which indicates that sleep deprivation can cause death in a week was misinformed—people do survive 5–7 days of sleeplessness. Kleitman himself writes that he has remained awake for as long as 100 continuous hours and on one occasion pushed this, with the aid of amphetamine, to 180 hours. Such a trial is no fun, however. It is unpleasant but not fatal.

The results of sleep-deprivation experiments have a peculiar monotony—they all tend to give similar data. Kleitman (1963) reviewed a group of earlier studies; a more recent study by Pasnau *et al.* (1968) involved the continuous deprivation of sleep in 4 young men for 205 hours (the longest controlled study on record). The results of Pasnau *et al.* mirror earlier results and so may be taken as a typical experiment. The experimental subjects felt, of course, a gradual onset of fatigue, and a gradual falling off of mental capabilities. Fatigue came and went in waves at first; it was always worse in the late night hours. During the first days of deprivation, the subjects could muster themselves with fairly good efficiency to perform various tasks, but this fell progressively. On the fifth day of deprivation there was a turning point, and things deteriorated at a more rapid rate than before. This is the so-called "fifth-day effect." The subjects became very irritable and hostile. They began to have pronounced weakness of the skeletal musculature. Illusions were common; hallucinations began. And there occurred the onset of "lapses." These phenomena seemed to be brief intrusions of sleep into the waking state—the subjects, with their eyes remaining open, abruptly lapsed into a state of disorientation and nonresponsiveness to the environment. The lapse would end as abruptly as it began. Often, amnesia for the events just antecedent to the lapse would be found. As the deprivation period lengthened, the lapses increased both in number and duration. The subjects' emotions became extremely labile. One subject, after 165 hours of wakefulness, went suddenly "beserk"—he began to scream, fell to the floor, sobbed and yelled incoherently. A gorilla was threatening him. It was, the authors state, like a child's night terror.

And that was all. After a recovery sleep, the subjects showed no lasting effects. Nor were there any deteriorations, during the period of deprivation or after, of any visceral activities. The effects of sleeplessness refer to the skeletal musculature, and, more emphatically, refer to the CNS. By inference, the level of the CNS most affected is the level responsible for the higher mental functions, i.e., the cerebral cortex.

Is that the answer, then? We sleep in order to allow our musculature and our brain to rest. Such an answer "fits" insofar as the musculature is concerned; it truly does "rest" in sleep. But the brain is hard at work in sleep, harder at work than we have previously realized. If part of the brain rests in sleep, which part? What does "rest" mean, anyway? How can an organ that, at least in part, is more active than usual and is receiving more blood than is usual, be considered to be at rest? In short, why do we sleep? Sleep-deprivation studies have not answered the question, they have only made the mystery more mysterious.

E. How Is Sleep Generated?

If the "why" of sleep is the *arcanum arcanorum*, the "how" of sleep is not far behind. How do we pass from wakefulness into sleep? from sleep back into wakefulness? Kleitman (1963) rightly points out that, in a way, these are not fair questions, they tend to oversimplify. The questions assume two states, awake and asleep, and imply that the passage from the one to the other is an all-or-none thing. Actually, as Kleitman notes, there is a continuum of awareness, leading from coma to mania. Even with this assumption, we still may ask legitimately how it is that sleep begins (and ends).

In the days when the negative view of sleep was popular, several theories of sleep were in vogue, and, expectedly, they had a negative "coloration" about them. The two most discussed such theories were the theory of cerebral anemia and the dendritic theory.

The theory of cerebral anemia dated back to the ancient Greeks. And even Mott, while championing the "positive" view of sleep, could not escape this widespread notion. "It is . . .probable," he wrote (Mott, 1924), "that during sleep there is a partial anaemia of the brain, and that the blood is determined away to other organs and tissues." Where does the blood go? Probably into the splanchnic and cutaneous vessels. What does this accomplish? Central hypoxia. Which leads to? Sleep, naturally. Awakening occurs as the blood flow to the brain picks up once more. This theory has had a long life and has died a hard death. As late as 1952 (Doust and Schneider, 1952), data were being presented to prove the notion. Kety and his associates finally laid the idea into its too long empty grave.

Another early theory of sleep, and a most ingenious one, was the dendritic theory of Duval (1895). Duval saw in the CNS histological findings of Golgi and Ramon y Cajal hope for understanding the histological basis of memory, the association of ideas, imagination, habit, and education; and, of course, sleep. Suppose, Duval suggested, that the dendrites of CNS neurons are mobile, are like little pseudopodia, can extend and make contacts with dendrites from other cells, and can contract, breaking those contacts. Then might not sleep be a result of a pulling-back of the dendrites, and awakening a process attendant upon the restoration of the broken contacts? The idea, Kleitman (1963) tells us, gained considerable popularity, so much so that another worker, Lepine, claimed that he had really thought up the idea before Duval and that history should so remember.

Pavlov's theory of sleep was one of the most influential; even Hess (1932b) was impressed. Pavlov (as summarized in Hess, 1932b; Kleitman, 1963) noted in his work with the conditioned reflex that dogs trained to respond to a stimulus, such as a bell, by salivating, often, when the food was not presented, would fall asleep. Why? Omission of the food, said Pavlov, causes an inhibition of the flow from the salivary glands. This inhibition quickly spreads out from the areas of the brain controlling the digestive secretory glands. A wave of inhibition moves out from this localized zone of the brain, by "irradiation," to create a state of inactivity in nearby nuclei, and, eventually, within the entire cortex. The result: sleep. Sleep is, thus, a conditioned inhibitory reflex. What sets off the conditioned reflex in man? Darkness, the bedroom, and so on—these, through habit, have become the conditioned stimuli.

Despite much contradictory data, this theory was in vogue for many years and was the center, Kleitman (1963) writes, of a personality cult, which defended the theory from attack with chauvinistic zeal. Kleitman (1963) quotes a Russian named Bogorad who wrote in 1954 that non-Pavlovian theories of sleep are all the inventions of "foreign bourgeois scientists." The discovery of rapid eye movement sleep has been the undoing of Pavlov's theory.

There have been, Kleitman (1963) notes, numerous humoral theories of sleep. People have blamed sleep on lactic acid, cholesterol, carbon dioxide, "toxins", calcium, pituitary hormones (and, I might add, serotonin, norepinephrine, and acetylcholine). Two of these humoral theories bear special mention. One is an old theory now being reexamined. The other is quite new and still only tentatively formulated.

Legendre and Pieron (1910, 1911, 1912a,b) found that when dogs are deprived of sleep for a few days, there appears in their cerebrospinal fluid a substance which, upon injection into the fourth ventricle of a non-deprived dog, will promptly induce sleep. The injection of cerebrospinal fluid from dogs who had not been deprived of sleep caused no effect in the recipient animal. The investigators called the principle a "hypnotoxin." The substance could not be dialyzed, was destroyed by heating the cerebrospinal fluid to 65°C, and was inactivated by oxidizing agents. The hypnotoxin caused no changes when injected intravascularly; it only worked by the intraventricular route.

This work has now been repeated by Pappenheimer and his associates (1967). These workers, in their studies of the physiology of the cerebrospinal fluid, devised a method for the atraumatic collection of large volumes of cerebrospinal fluid from goats. They decided to reinvestigate what they called the "Pieron phenomenon." Cerebrospinal fluid from control goats produced no changes either in cats or rats but that from goats deprived of sleep for 72 hours caused a profound "sleep or torpor" which in the cat lasted for 12 to 24 hours. The sleep (if that is what it was) seemed to be much like natural sleep, since the cats could be aroused; when left undisturbed, the animals would go back to sleep. The same sort of effect was seen in rats. Again, the principle had to be administered directly into the ventricular system. Upon partial purification, the substance seemed to be a peptide with a molecular weight of between 1000 and 2000. Work is now being done further to clarify the nature of Pappenheimer's peptide.

In the meantime, Axelrod and associates have been studying the indole, melatonin (5-methoxy-*N*-acetylserotonin). The enzyme which forms this compound from *N*-acetylserotonin is apparently restricted in mammals to the pineal gland and is directly influenced by environmental lighting (R. Y. Moore *et al.*, 1967). Light inhibits the enzyme; darkness induces it. In an elegant study, R. Y. Moore *et al.* (1967) elucidated the pathway leading from the retina to the pineal gland. The pathway involves first the optic nerve; at the chiasm, the path leaves the primary optic system and descends by way of the inferior accessory optic tract to the midbrain nucleus of the inferior tract, then through the brainstem into the intermediolateral cell column of the spinal cord; from there the pathway passes out with the sympathetic outflow and rises to the superior cervical ganglia; from the ganglia, sympathetic nerves pass upward and end directly upon pineal parenchymal cells. Environmental light activates the pathway and inhibits melatonin's synthesis; darkness does the opposite. Melatonin, once synthesized, can then enter the bloodstream and might be, suggest Wurtman and co-workers (Anton-Tay *et al.*, 1968), an endocrine signal which influences various circadian rhythms. One of the effects of melatonin is an acute elevation of brain serotonin levels, especially in the midbrain. Anton-Tay *et al.* suggest tentatively that this effect may have a role in the induction of sleep.

If so, would this mean that the pineal body is a sleep center?

Is there a sleep center? Is there an area in the brain that actively generates sleep? Pavlov (cited in Kleitman, 1963) thought the idea preposterous. For once, Kleitman agreed with Pavlov.

Many have regarded sleep as the "natural" state of life—the primal condition is the absence of consciousness, and cortical neurons are made to function only by the stimulatory effects of afferent impulses. Such a view was given a boost by the classic experiments of Bremer. This investigator (Bremer, 1935) found that if the brainstem is sectioned at the level of the rostral midbrain, then the isolated cortex, deprived of all input save for that of the first two cranial nerves, shows an EEG pattern indistinguishable from sleep. The state persists indefinitely, or at least as long as this cerveau isole preparation can be kept alive. Bremer (1936) further showed that if the section is through the base of the medulla, then the preparation, an encephale isole, can show regular rhythms of wakefulness and sleep. Bremer concluded that sleep is the consequence of a functional deafferentation of the cortex. Such a view implies that the natural state of the cortex is, after all, sleep. It also implies that somehow the brainstem acts as a kind of "waking center."

That this may be so is now well known from the classic experiments of Moruzzi and Magoun (1949). These workers produced EEG changes seemingly identical to those of physiological arousal by direct stimulation of the brainstem's reticular formation. The effect was not mediated by any of the then known ascending or descending pathways. Instead, it was suggested that the collaterals of afferent pathways terminate diffusely in the brainstem reticular formation and are relayed from there by way of the thalamus diffusely to the cortex, producing arousal. And, indeed, Lindsley *et al.* (1950) showed that lesions which interrupt the ascending reticular activating system are followed by chronic somnolence and EEG synchronization.

So there may be an arousal center. Sleep may simply be the result of inactivity of this center. That is, sleep may be an entirely passive phenomenon. Such is Kleitman's view. But what Kleitman and others who favor a passive theory of sleep never satisfactorily explain is how the mesodiencephalic "wakefulness center" is turned off. They imply that when sleep begins, afferent stimuli are so weak and sporadic that the reticular activating system becomes deactivated, thus allowing the cortex to revert to its primal state of slow waves and spindling. But is afferent stimulation ever really that low? Descending inhibitory impulses have been demonstrated, which can mute afferent nerve traffic. But can these really turn off the arousal system? It has been shown that many hypnotic and anesthetic drugs can act by decreasing the activity of the reticular formation (Killam, 1962). Is natural sleep induced in a similar fashion? Is sleep passive?

Again I ask the question stated before and left answerless; Is there a "sleep center?" The work of Hess (1929, 1932a,b, 1949, 1965) seemed so to indicate. Hess was able to produce sleep in cats by the direct stimulation (at a critical frequency rate) of various centers in the brainstem. Especially likely to produce sleep was stimulation of the periventricular gray matter. The sleep was indistinguishable from natural sleep—even to the extent that if the floor of the cage were wet, the cats would refuse to lie down despite the presence of the electrical stimulation. When sleep was induced, it could readily be interrupted; this was not electroanesthesia. "These findings," wrote Hess (1929), "show us that sleep is the consequence of a *state of excitation* of certain portions of the central nervous system." (The italics are Hess's.) Such a notion is clearly not consonant with a passive view of sleep. Rather, sleep is an active process, of which the function is the promotion of restorative events within the organism.

Magni *et al.* (1959) found an interesting phenomenon with the encephale isole preparation. These workers ligated the communicating vessels between the internal carotid and the vertebral arteries at the base of the brain; when a barbiturate was injected into the vertebral artery of a "sleeping" preparation it produced arousal—the drug, apparently acting in the brainstem upon some tonically active sleep center, inhibited that center and "woke up" the preparation. More recently, McGinty and Sterman (1968) have found that certain lesions in the cat's brain can cause chronic (and finally fatal) insomnia.

Is there a sleep center? Current evidence suggests that there is. Where is it? Probably in the brainstem. The controversy, however, has only begun.

II. Rapid Eye Movement Sleep

Why, Jenny, you're asleep at last!—
Asleep, poor Jenny, hard and fast,—
So young and soft and tired; so fair,
With chin thus nestled in your hair,
Mouth quiet, eyelids almost blue
As if some sky of dreams shone through!

Dante Gabriel Rossetti

A. Historical Background

I once asked a class of students if they had ever seen their pet cat or dog in rapid eye movement sleep; I mentioned, too, that this phase of sleep was known by a number of synonyms (paradoxical sleep, activated sleep, fast sleep, deep sleep, rhombencephalic phase, D-sleep, the D-state)—no one raised a hand. I then asked them if they had ever seen their pet in a peculiar sort of sleep—sprawled flat on the floor, with eyes often half open, and with little spasms of the paws and eyes and vibrissae. Now almost all of the students raised a hand. They had seen it many times; so had I. Yet in a sense none of us had really seen a thing.

Lucretius had seen it in the first century B.C. In "De Rerum Natura" he wrote of how men in their dreams often move spasmodically and cry out. This was a special kind of sleep. And not just in humans:

> Have you not seen strong steeds even when their limbs are reposing
> Panting unceasing and sweating in sleep as they strain to the utmost
> As for a prize or as if their doors of a sudden were opened?
> Often again in the stillness of sleep do the dogs of the huntsmen
> Suddenly jerk out their legs and utter spasmodical barkings:
> Over and over again they sniff the air with their nostrils
> As 'twere in hot pursuit of the new-found tracks of their quarry

Derbyshire *et al.* (1936), in their pioneer study of the cat's sleeping EEG, saw it. Usually the animals' sleep EEG was dominated by spindles and slow waves, but " . . .at other times when sleep was apparently less less tranquil, judging by twitching of the vibrissae, there were only small rapid waves, as in the alert waking state." They saw it but did not recognize it.

R. Hess, Jr., *et al.* (1953) noted that apparently sleeping cats could have an "awake" pattern in their EEG's, but the authors attributed the effect to arousals by stimuli which could be detected by the cats but not by the experimenters.

It remained, in the end, for Aserinsky and Kleitman (1953) to both look and, finally, see. And even then, it was an accidental finding. (The history of science has been dotted with such "accidents." It requires real scientific vision—the ability to look at nature free of preconception and prejudice—in order to see anything at all when such an accident occurs.)

Kleitman, in 1963, wrote:

> In our laboratory we literally stumbled on an objective method of studying dreaming while exploring eye motility in adults, after we found that in infants eye movements persisted for a time when all discernible body motility ceased. Instead of direct inspection, as was done for infant eye movements, those of adult sleepers were recorded indirectly, to insure undisturbed sleep in the

> dark... . By this technique, pendular, often bilaterally asymmetrical, slow eye movements..., each completed in 3 to 4 seconds, were found to be related to general body motility. In addition, jerky rapid eye movements (REMs), executed in only a fraction of a second and binocularly symmetrical, tended to occur in clusters for 5 to 60 minutes several times during a single night's sleep... . It was soon apparent that the REMs were associated with a typical low-voltage EEG pattern and statistically significant increases in the heart and respiratory rates... . These changes suggested some sort of emotional disturbance, such as might be caused by dreaming. To test this supposition, sleepers were aroused and interrogated during, or shortly after the termination of, REMs, and they almost invariably reported having dreamed. If awakened in the absence of REMs, or when questioned after a night of undisturbed sleep, they seldom recalled dreaming.

In their brief paper in *Science* (1953), Aserinsky and Kleitman described in definitive fashion many of the phenomena of rapid eye movement (REM) sleep.

Dement, working with Kleitman, established, as noted in the first section, the signs by which the various stages of sleep could be identified. He also (Dement, 1958) established conclusively that cats, like humans, have periods of REM sleep, and that these periods come in regularly recurring cycles; in the cat, as in the human, Dement noted the cortical EEG reverted from a pattern of slow waves and spindles to a pattern like that seen in alert arousal—low-voltage, fast, desychronized activity. External manifestations of REM sleep were twitchings of the limbs and ears and vibrissae; these did not occur in non-REM sleep. These findings were quickly confirmed by Jouvet *et al.* (1959b).

B. Phylogeny

Who has REM sleep? Humans, yes; the cat, yes. Do all sleepers have it? The answer is no.

It is present in the rabbit, but only in minute amounts; in the female rabbit, though, an episode of REM sleep always follows copulation (Sawyer and Kawakmi, 1959). Rats have REM sleep (Michel *et al.*, 1961), as do mice (Weiss and Roldan, 1964), sheep (Ruckenbusch, 1963a), donkeys (Ruckenbusch, 1963b), monkeys (Weitzman, 1961), and chimpanzees (Adey *et al.*, 1963); as might be expected from the observations of Lucretius, dogs have episodes of REM sleep (Shimazono *et al.*, cited in Hartmann, 1967a). So, too, do pigs (Ruckenbusch and Morel, 1968), whales (Shurley *et al.*, 1969), bats (Brebbia and Paul, 1969), moles (Allison and vanTwyver, 1970), and ground squirrels, hamsters, and the chinchilla (vanTwyver and Webb, 1968). Mammals, then, in general, all exhibit this phase of sleep. There is at least one exception, e.g., the echidna—

this very primitive monotreme has no REM sleep at all (Allison and Goff, 1968). Among the mammals there are marked variations. As noted, the rabbit has very little REM sleep; the same is true of sheep, and, it will be recalled, the same is probably true of deer (Hediger, 1969). Further, the "cycle length," the amount of time between two adjacent REM sleep periods, varies considerably. It is long in man, quite short in mice; in fact, Hartmann (1967a) has shown that the cycle length varies inversely with the metabolic rate. Further, as Hartmann notes, there is a correlation between the amount of REM sleep and the mammal's vulnerability. Animals who need not fear sleeping out in the open or who can find secure holes or lairs in which to sleep, often have more REM sleep than species which are exposed to perpetual danger. This makes evolutionary sense, as Hartmann notes, owing to the relatively high insensitivity to the environment which is a hallmark of REM sleep.

Nonmammalian vertebrates have little or no REM sleep. Birds, in general, do have REM sleep, but only in tiny episodes, measured not in minutes but in seconds (Klein *et al.*, 1964). The situation is possibly quite different in the newly hatched bird (Greenberg *et al.*, 1969)—brand new chicks spend almost all of their sleep time in REM sleep. In fact, slow-wave sleep does not appear at all until about 24 hours after hatching.

What about other vertebrates? In general, they do not seem to have much, it any, REM sleep. This is true of most reptiles and fish (Hartmann, 1967a), though the caiman (*Caiman latirostris*) does have just a touch (1% of its total sleep) (Peyrethon and Dusan-Peyrethon, 1968).

C. Signs of Rapid Eye Movement Sleep

1. *Dreaming*

What are the signs of REM sleep? Dreaming is one, as already mentioned. Do animals dream? Kleitman (1963) wrote that dogs do, since they have all the signs of REM sleep that humans have, but that cats do not, since their mean heart rate goes down in REM sleep instead of up. Such reasoning is less than secure. We shall probably never know if mammals other than man dream. As for now, I would trust Lucretius and say that animals probably dream, in their own fashion.

Does mentation in human sleep occur only during REM sleep? No, mentation may be present in all the stages of sleep. Foulkes (1962), however, showed that there is a distinct difference between mentation in REM sleep and mentation in slow-wave sleep. He studied 8 subjects for a total of 57 nights. The subjects were awakened by a bell while they were in various stages of sleep. In each case, Foulkes asked the subject if he had been dreaming. If the subject said yes, the content of the dream was described. If the answer was no, then Foulkes asked the subject if he had been thinking or whether anything had been going through his mind. Foulkes found that reportable mental activity was always present in sleep. But the mentation in REM sleep was always more elaborate than that found in slow-wave sleep, was always more visual, more "muscular," more vivid, more emotional, and importantly, had less correspondence to the subject's waking life. By contrast, mentation in slow-wave sleep was more akin to thinking than it was to an elaborate hallucination and was tied to the subjects' waking activities and memory processes. Thus the kind of mentation which we call "dream" occurs in REM sleep; the mentation of the others stages of sleep does not have the special characteristics of dreaming.

Whitman *et al.* (1963) noted again what Aserinsky and Kleitman (1953) had noted—the memory trace left by a dream is very ephemeral. This, of course, has implications concerning the validity of the analysis of dreams in psychoanalysis. Whitman and co-workers noted that what a patient dreams and what he later tells his analyst are quite often two distinctly different things. The patient often elaborates upon what he has dreamt, coloring some aspects, suppressing others, so that by the time he reaches the analyst's couch, the dream has been altered in various ways—usually in ways designed to curry the analyst's favor.

What do dreams mean? Need they mean anything at all? As will be mentioned in the next section, many have claimed that the dream is a form of psychosis, very much like schizophrenia. And the idea is not altogether unattractive. The dreamer is hallucinating; his ideas skip from one subject to another with no apparent continuity or organization; the dreamer is, as it were, out of himself watching things that are not a part of himself, and yet the whole process is one which he himself is generating; the dreamer's mind is, in short, out of willful control. The similarity of all this to schizophrenia is obvious.

Is schizophrenia the dreaming process extended from sleep into wakefulness? Many so believe. Nevertheless, it is possible that the dream has no innate meaning or purpose. It may just be, as Kleitman (1963) suggested, the consequence of the cortical activation which occurs in REM sleep.

I must mention, however, that there are many who would vehemently disagree. As I have said, Dement and others with a psychiatric orientation entered the area of REM sleep research at an early stage. This has had a profound effect upon the direction which such research has taken. This basic psychiatric orientation, plus the psychiatrist's proverbial preoccupation with dreams, has meant that the whole field of sleep research has been colored with a neo-Freudian tint. This coloration is reflected even in the name of the association to which sleep researchers belong: the Association for the Psychophysiological Study of Sleep. Notice that "psycho" comes before "physiological." Thus for many, the dream remains as important an object for study as it was to Freud. Hartmann (1965) expressed what many sleep investigators feel, i.e., the study of sleep, and especially of REM sleep will at last shed light upon the "shaky bridge between mind and body," and will lead to basic discoveries concerning mental disease. However, in all too many instances, researchers have been, simply, hell-bent on proving that there is a connection between REM sleep and schizophrenia. The results have not been very encouraging. And, along the way, the orientation of sleep research has meant that studies into the basic physiology of sleep have had often to wait in the sidelines.

2. *Electroencephalogram Characteristics*

The activated cortical EEG of REM sleep has been mentioned; by this criterion, the sleeper appears to be awake. Despite this, REM sleep is the soundest stage of sleep. It is more difficult to arouse a human or an animal with sensory stimuli, or even with direct electrical stimulation of the reticular activating system, when the human or animal is in REM sleep than when he is in one of the other stages of sleep. Thus, REM sleep is "deep" (Jouvet *et al.*, 1959b; Candia *et al.*, 1962; Roldan *et al.*, 1963; Williams *et al.*, 1964; Siegel and Langley, 1965). It is because of the discrepancy between EEG arousal and behavioral inertia that Jouvet *et al.* (1960) coined the name "paradoxical" sleep. But yesterday's paradox is today's commonplace, and the semiofficial name for dreaming sleep (as adopted by the Association for the Psychophysiological Study of Sleep) is "REM sleep" or "stage REM"; such is the terminology use in this report; an attractive alternative terminology, however is that used by Hartmann and his co-workers, "D-sleep" and the "D-state." Hartmann's "D" refers both to desynchronization of the EEG and to dreaming.

Waves with a sawtooth configuration frequently (though not always) appear in the cortical EEG of humans in REM sleep; these sawtooth waves usually appear in conjunction with rapid eye movements (Jouvet *et al.*, 1960). Similar waves appear in the cortical EEG of the chimpanzee (Freeman *et al.*, 1969). Sawtooth waves may be the human analogy of the PGO spikes of the cat, which are discussed below.

Another EEG characteristic of REM sleep is a pattern found in the cat's hippocampus. In wakefulness, there is a rough theta rhythm (4–6 Hz, low voltage) in this area of the brain; it returns in REM sleep, and its rhythm is much more regular than is the case in wakefulness (Jouvet *et al.*, 1959a). In the rat, a regular theta rhythm is the EEG hallmark of REM sleep. Primates, in contrast, do not have a hippocampal theta rhythm in REM sleep (Rhodes *et al.*, 1965).

A final EEG characteristic of REM sleep—and one which has generated a great deal of hubbub—is the presence in the cat of high-voltage, monophasic spikes. These spikes can be recorded in the pons, the lateral geniculate nucleus, and the occipital cortex. They are linked—apparently they are generated by the pons, travel from there to the lateral geniculate, and then to the occipital cortex (Mouret *et al.*, 1963; Bizzi and Brooks, 1963). These pontine–geniculate–occipital (PGO) spikes occur only infrequently in non-REM sleep and wakefulness. As a cat passes from slow-wave sleep into REM sleep, PGO spikes herald the approaching REM sleep episode. They are the first sign of REM sleep; they precede the full-blown picture of REM sleep by a minute or less; then, with the cat frankly in the REM episode, the PGO spikes continue until the end of the episode; finally, along with all the other signs of REM sleep, they terminate abruptly, and the cat returns to a stage of slow-wave sleep, or awakens. The voltage of the PGO spikes is highest in the pre-REM seconds of slow-wave sleep and at the beginning of the REM episode; the voltage gradually declines during the course of the episode, but the spikes never subside altogether. In addition, the spikes have another quality—they occur in bursts. They are one of the phasic signs of REM sleep. The bursts coincide rather well with the bursts of rapid eye movements, though not perfectly. The PGO spikes are not affected by orbital enucleation or by severance of the optic nerve. They can be recorded in waking cats as well as in sleeping animals, in association with sudden movements of the eyes; in wakefulness, however, the spikes' amplitude is sometimes small, and the spikes are far less profuse than they are in REM sleep (Brooks, 1968).

Why the hubbub over the spikes? To answer, one may ask, where does the visual imagery of dreams originate? This imagery does not, it is assumed, come from the retina; but it must come from somewhere. Could it be the pons? It is claimed that the pons gives rise to all the signs of REM sleep. One of these is PGO spiking, and PGO spiking equals the images of dreaming. Is this true? It really is more an assumption than a fact. If it is true, then if profuse PGO spiking could be induced in the waking animal, the animal should hallucinate each time a train of PGO spikes appears in the EEG. As will be mentioned in the next section, Dement and his associates claim to have demonstrated this.

Jouvet and his co-workers (Dusan-Peyrethon *et al.*, 1967) have claimed that a cat will generate a constant, fixed number of PGO spikes every day.

The number is 14,000, with a standard deviation of 3000. The idea has arisen that cats have a quota of PGO spikes that must be filled each day. As will be discussed shortly, if a subject is deprived of REM sleep, he will, when allowed to sleep undisturbed, have a postdeprivation rebound, as though making up for that which had been lost. What element of REM sleep is so important to the organism that a rebound will always follow deprivation? Perhaps the PGO spikes. Ferguson and Dement (1968) subjected cats to deprivation of REM sleep, and then subjected them to deprivation of PGO spikes as well. The first end was accomplished by awakening the cats when the full picture of REM sleep appeared. The second end, spike deprivation, was accomplished by awakening the animals at the first PGO spike, which occurs, as mentioned above, as much as a full minute before the onset of REM sleep per se. The rebound was greater after spike deprivation than after deprivation of REM sleep alone. The conclusion was that it is the phasic events of REM sleep that are the important events. They are responsible for a postdeprivation rebound; loss of phasic events creates the deficit that must be made up for; and deprivation of the tonic signs of REM sleep, cortical activation, for example, is said to be totally irrelevant. This is all probably nonsence. The data are unconvincing, and the whole concept of the rebound has been challenged, as will be mentioned in the next section.

One final remark about the EEG of REM sleep. In the cat, most investigators simply distinguish between REM sleep and all the other stages of sleep, which are lumped together as non-REM sleep. This has led to the notion of the "duality" of sleep—sleep (in the cat) is either REM or not. But non-REM sleep of the cat, as mentioned already, is clearly divisible into at least two stages: spindle sleep and slow-wave sleep. Ursin (1968) has demonstrated, in the cat, a significant positive correlation between slow-wave sleep and REM sleep; she also found a tendency toward a negative correlation between spindle sleep and REM sleep—but this second trend was not statistically significant. Nevertheless, Ursin has challenged the REM–non-REM dichotomy. The real dichotomy, she feels, is one between spindle sleep, on the one hand, and slow-wave plus REM sleep, on the other. If Ursin is correct, then there could follow some important implications. As mentioned below, it is said that REM sleep is generated by the pons and non-REM sleep by the midbrain; Ursin's data would challenge this probably oversimplified anatomical formulation.

3. *Other Signs*

At the level of the single CNS unit, there is in most areas an increase of activity with REM sleep, both over the quiet awake state and non-REM sleep. In the rat the average firing rate of CNS neurons peaks in REM sleep; in the hypothalamus the firing rate rises by more than 200% (over the wakeful rate); elsewhere the increases are smaller; and in the hippocampus there is a consistent decrease in the firing rate of single units (Mink *et al.*, 1967). Thus, on the whole, the brain is quite busy during REM sleep.

The rapid eye movement of REM sleep are, as Aserinsky and Kleitman (1953) first noted, phasic—they occur in bursts. The muscles of the middle ear also show phasic bursts of activity in REM sleep (Dement, 1968). Also phasic are the sudden twitches of the limbs and facial musculature and the sudden bursts of mydriasis which alter the tonic miosis of sleep (Jouvet, 1967).

The respiratory rate becomes irregular in REM sleep; so, too, do the blood pressure and the heart rate. Even in the cat this is true. Although the cat's heart rate response to the onset of REM sleep is a tonic fall, phasic bursts of tachycardia are characteristic and may be due to phasic inhibitions of vagal activity (Baust and Bohnert, 1969). In man, there is a significant correlation between the bursts of rapid eye movements and the phasic changes of the respiratory and pulse rates (Spreng *et al.*, 1968). In humans, there occurs a peripheral vasoconstriction, suggestive of increased activity in the sympathetic nervous system (Khatri and Freis, 1967). The peripheral correlates of REM sleep have been called an "autonomic storm" (Hobson, 1969a). They can lead to attacks of angina (Nowlin, *et al.*, 1965), asthma (Ravenscroft and Hartmann, 1968), and emphysematous anoxia (Trask and Cree, 1962), and may precipitate fatal cerebrovascular accidents and myocardial infarctions (Hobson, 1969a). Thus, as Hobson (1969a) notes, the patient with a predisposition to these diseases may be potentially at great risk during times when prompt medical care is likely to be least available; sleep, that is, may be "killing the patient and drugging the doctor."

In man and cat, REM sleep is characterized by a profound tonic hypotonia of the skeletal musculature; this inhibition of muscular tonus is supposedly generated by the locus coeruleus of the pons (Jouvet, 1967; Henley and Morrison, 1969).

Reite and Pegram (1968) suggested that cerebral blood flow may increase in REM sleep; this was on the basis of data collected from thermistors implanted subdurally in monkeys. Kety and his associates (Reivich *et al.*, 1967, 1968) studied cerebral blood flow in cats using a radioautographic technique. The results showed that in slow-wave sleep, there occurs an increased blood flow in thirteen of twenty-five different areas of the brain. These changes varied from a 29% increase in the thalamus to an 84%

increase in the superior olive. Some areas exhibited no change, but none of the areas showed a decreased blood flow. These results, of couse, confirm and extend the findings which had been made earlier in humans. The startling new findings concerned cerebral blood flow in REM sleep. In contrast to slow-wave sleep, the flow of blood increased in all twenty-five of the areas examined. These increases varied from a 58% increase in the cerebellar white matter to a 188% increase in the cochlear nuclei. The greatest increases (up 100% or more) were in the brainstem and the diencephalon. The smallest increases were in the white matter and in the sensory and motor areas of the cerebral cortex. The authors weighted the twenty five regions according to their relative size and calculated that, in the cat's brain as a whole, there occurs in slow-wave sleep an overall 20% increase of blood flow, whereas in REM sleep, the overall increase is about 80%. There is only one other known condition which is accompanied by so large an increase of the cerebral blood flow and that is a full-blown grand mal convulsion.

Thus REM sleep is characterized by a number of distinct phenomena; some of these are tonic, others phasic. They are listed in Table I, for summary; the list, of course, is incomplete, and much doubtless remains to be found.

TABLE I

SIGNS OF REM SLEEP

Tonic	Phasic
Low voltage, desynchronized cortical EEG[a]	PGO[c] spikes
Hippocampal theta rhythm	—
Suppression of skeletal muscle tone	Sudden muscular twitchings (limbs, face)
High arousal threshold	—
Increased CNS[b] neuronal activity	Rapid eye movements
Miosis	Bursts of mydriasis
—	Bursts of middle ear muscle activity
—	Respiratory rate variability
Blood pressure rise (man); fall (cat)	Blood pressure variability
High flow of blood to the brain	Heart rate variability

[a] Electroencephalogram.

[b] Central nervous system.

[c] Potine–geniculate–occipital.

D. Normal and Abnormal Rapid Eye Movement Sleep

As is mentioned in Section III, REM sleep is "fragile"—it is easily disrupted; the stages of slow-wave sleep show no such fragility (Hartmann, 1968a). Despite its fragility, REM sleep is an integral part of normal mammalian sleep (always excepting the echidna). In man, it accounts for about 20 to 25% of total sleep time (Dement, 1960). In cats, on a 23- or 24-hour time basis, it accounts for about 20 to 28% of total sleep, and about 14 to 16% of the total elapsed time. Total sleep of a cat in an experimental chamber such as is used in sleep studies accounts for about 58 to 65% of the total elapsed time (23–24 hours); the mean duration of a REM sleep episode in the cat is about 5 to 6 minutes (Sterman *et al.*, 1965; Delorme, 1966; Jouvet, 1967). In man, the mean duration of a REM sleep episode is about 20 minutes (Dement, 1960)—and so the old supposition that dreams, even long ones, are over in a flash is incorrect (Kleitman, 1963).

The values given above are for adults. The picture is quite different for infants (and for the young of various other species). The human neonate spends as much as 80% of its total sleep in REM sleep (Hartmann, 1967a). This relatively huge amount declines fairly quickly so that by the second year, the percentage is between 25 and 40. The decline then levels off so that the normal adult figure is reached in adolescence. Hartmann (1967a), by extrapolating the curve backward, speculated that the fetus *in utero* spends all of its time in REM sleep; Hartmann admits, however, the need for intrauterine EEG studies.

Going in the other direction—from young adulthood to old age—there is a decline in the amount of REM sleep. Aged individuals often have not only disturbed sleep in general, but also less REM sleep, as a percentage of their total sleep, than they had in their younger years (Hartmann, 1967a). This decline of REM sleep with age is variable and only slight until the individual reaches his eighty-fifth year or thereabouts; thereafter the decline becomes marked, and the individual enjoys greatly reduced amounts of REM sleep (Kahn and Fisher, 1969). "Enjoys" may be the proper verb to use here, too, because there appears to be a strong correlation between the amount of REM sleep one has experienced and how refreshed one feels upon awakening; there is no strong correlation, on the other hand, between the total length of sleep and the feeling of morning well-being (Hartmann, 1968a).

Rapid eye movement sleep can be a sign of abnormality. In the normal individual, it never occurs without there being a preceding period of slow-wave sleep. As a rule, the shortest duration of this pre-REM slow-wave sleep is 45 minutes; i.e., from the onset of sleep to the first REM episode, the shortest normal time is about 45 minutes. Generally, this parameter, which is called "REM latency," is even longer, between 60 and 90 minutes in humans (Oswald, 1968). Yet, as Vogel (1960) first noted, narcoleptic patients have a very brief REM latency—very often, they pass directly from wakefulness into REM sleep. Vogel interpreted his finding in a neo-Freudian fashion—the sudden attack of "dreaming" serves a useful psychodynamic purpose, i.e., "the narcoleptic patient makes use of his sleep for the projection of fantasy which is gratified in a dream in a way unacceptable during waking life." Such an interpretation is no longer held, and narcolepsy is thought to be a sudden attack of sleep, most of it REM sleep (Dement *et al.*, 1964). How this occurs is unknown.

It has been claimed that psychiatric patients have abnormal sleep patterns, but no consistently convincing picture has been developed. Cohen and Dement (1966) found that electroconvulsive shock can inhibit the cat's REM sleep. Cohen *et al.* (1967) speculated that this effect could mean that electroconvulsive therapy can satisfy some of the daily need for REM sleep. Such an interpretation is, at best, metaphysical. Electroconvulsive shock remains a valuable therapy for psychotic depression, but why it is valuable is still unknown.

Three areas now remain for discussion: the deprivation of REM sleep; the anatomy of REM sleep; and theories of REM sleep. The last two areas will largely be discussed in the next section.

E. Deprivation of Rapid Eye Movement Sleep

Kleitman (1963) noted that there is a large amount of REM sleep in the sleep which follows total sleep deprivation; it was this, he writes, which led Dement to conduct the first REM deprivation experiment. The classic paper which resulted climaxed the series of memorable papers which issued forth from the Chicago sleep laboratory in the 1950s.

Dement (1960) at first tried selectively to inhibit REM sleep in his human subjects with depressant drugs, but this, for some reason, failed. He then adopted the rather drastic procedure of awakening the sleepers each time they entered into a REM period. After a series of undisturbed, base line nights, the drastic procedure was instituted and continued for a number of nights. Then a series of recovery nights was allowed. For a control, the subjects were later awakened in various stages of non-REM sleep. The results of this experiment were that 1 subject left the experiment after three nights of deprivation with a "flurry of excuses;" 2 subjects insisted on stopping after four nights of deprivation, but did go on into the recovery period; 4 subjects were deprived for five nights; and 1 was "pushed" to seven. As the nights of REM deprivation progressed, the number of forced awakenings needed to inhibit REM sleep steadily increased to as many as thirty per night. [In cats, the number of awakenings can increase to several hundred in an 8- hour period (Dewson *et al.*, 1967).] In the recovery period, there was a "rebound" of REM sleep, i.e., an increase over baseline, especially marked on the first recovery night, but lasting as long as five. No rebound of any sort occurred after the series of forced awakenings from non-REM sleep. During the period of REM deprivation—but not during non-REM awakenings—the subjects exhibited certain daytime behavioral changes: anxiety, irritability, difficulty in concentrating, a markedly increased appetite. One subject became seriously agitated; another (the subject who quit the project) left "in an apparent panic"; the 2 who stopped after four nights did so "presumably because the stress was too great." All of these psychological changes disappeared "as soon as the subjects were allowed to dream."

The interpretation of the results was entirely psychological—REM sleep deprivation shows that dreaming is a necessity. If dreaming is prevented, a "serious disruption of the personality" may follow. Such a conclusion is no longer generally held, as will be mentioned in the next section.

The experiments have been repeated many times; in humans, these repetitions have reproduced the psychological changes in some instances (Agnew *et al.*, 1967; Clemes and Dement, 1967) but failed to do so in others (Kales *et al.*, 1964). Psychic change or not, the rebound always occurred. As Ferguson and Dement (1968) have noted, the compensatory rebound after REM sleep deprivation is one of the most clearly established phenomena of neurobiology. The interpretation placed upon the rebound, however, has been convincingly challenged, as will be mentioned in the section.

The stress of REM sleep deprivation provokes several measurable biochemical changes. The absolute levels of brain norepinephrine and serotonin are not changed (Hartmann and Freedman, 1966), but there is an increased turnover of norepinephrine (Pujol *et al.*, 1968) and serotonin (Glowinski *et al.*, 1969). Other changes include a drop in the rat's telencephalic acetylcholine (Bowers *et al.*, 1966); an increase in cats of the concentration of γ-aminobutyric acid in the reticular formation, the thalamus, and the frontal cortex, and a decrease of the same amino acid in the colliculi and the caudate nucleus; also, an increase of the aspartic acid content of the thalamus, frontal cortex, and the reticular formation, with a decrease of aspartate in the caudate nucleus; and a slight increase of glutamic acid in the thalamus (Micic *et al.*, 1967). It has also been claimed that in the rat, REM deprivation causes a considerable fall of the total glycogen content of the subcortex and the caudal brainstem (Karadzic and Mrsulja, 1968). Functional changes may also occur; in cats, for example, increased cortical excitability (Dewson *et al.*, 1967). In the rat, REM deprivation can decrease the potassium concentrations of the brain and blood, and this may lead to heightened neural excitability (Heiner *et al.*, 1968).

It is difficult to evaluate such experiments—most have been poorly controlled. Indeed, there is really no control for REM deprivation. Non-REM awakenings do not constitute a suitable control, i.e., non-REM awakening does not equal REM awakening. Nor has it ever been shown satisfactorily that the changes seen after REM sleep deprivation are in any way specific—other kinds of chronic stress might produce the same sort of changes.

However, it is clear that increased amounts of REM sleep will follow upon the inhibition of REM sleep; this is true for almost every known method of REM sleep inhibition.

F. Theories of Rapid Eye Movement Sleep

If sleep is active instead of passive, then there may be a REM center; there also may be a slow-wave sleep center. Jouvet claims to have found both.

Jouvet and Jouvet (1963) examined several possibilities in cats. Removal of the cerebellum had no effect on the stages of sleep. Decortication neither modified the signs of REM sleep in the lower brain areas nor did it prevent the cardiovascular irregularities of REM sleep and the rapid eye movements themselves. A section through the brainstem at the midbrain–pontine junction removed the signs of REM sleep from the areas rostral to the section, but the signs of REM sleep below the section (muscle atony, cardiovascular irregularities) continued. A section at the caudal end of the pons stopped the occurrence of the cardiovascular irregularities and the muscle atony; in contrast, the signs of REM sleep rostral to this section continued. Hence, REM sleep is generated by the pons, which sends out both ascending and descending fibers to produce all of the signs of this state of sleep.

The locus coeruleus is a small, bilateral nucleus located near the floor of the fourth ventricle in the rostral pons. In the past, the locus has been regarded as a part of the pneumotaxic center (Johnson and Russell, 1952). Jouvet disagrees; he maintains that the locus and nearby pontine nuclei constitute the REM center, and further, the midline raphe system of the midbrain is the non-REM sleep center. Further discussion of the anatomy of sleep will be deferred to the next section.

Why REM sleep? A number of theories have been evolved; most of these rely heavily, or, in some cases, completely, upon pharmacological data; so discussion of these, too, will be largely deferred to the next section.

Dewan and his associates have evolved a "P-theory" of REM sleep—REM sleep is the function which "programs" (thus the "P") the brain, a function which, in short, sorts out and discards irrelevant data, and files away relevant data into the stores of memory. The evidence in support of the P-theory is circumstantial and, as yet, unconvincing. An example is seen in Greenberg and Dewan (1969). The P–theory would predict that an animal or human engaged in the vigorous learning of new material would exhibit large amounts of REM sleep. A patient recovering from aphasia should fit into such a category. Greenberg and Dewan studied the sleep of a group of patients recovering from aphasia. They scored the EEG records "blindly," i.e., they did not know the clinical history of the patients until after all of the sleep data had been tabulated. The results showed a clear distinction—patients successfully relearning how to talk had more REM sleep than patients whose progress was retarded or absent. In the first (improving) group, REM sleep constituted 20.1% of the total sleep time; in the second (nonimproving) group, it constituted 12.7%. The difference is statistically significant. It should be pointed out at once that the improving patients had not an increased amount of REM sleep—they had a "normal" amount (as already mentioned, 20% is approximately the usual figure for the adult human). The data show only that the nonimproving patients had less REM sleep than is normal for adults. Thus the data do not really support the predictions of the P-theory.

This theory, like all theories of REM sleep, has serious gaps in its supporting evidence. To date, no single theory of REM sleep is entirely satisfactory. Oswald's, to be discussed at length in the next section, has the fewest gaps, but it is also the newest, and, hence, has had the fewest opportunities of testing.

I can only conclude that there is at present no convincing theory either of REM sleep or of sleep in general. We sleep. We also dream, and dreaming is a part of a complex stage of sleep marked by (and named for) rapid eye movements. That much we know. There, however, our knowledge stops. We do not know why we sleep; we do not know why we dream. All we firmly know is that we do.

III. The Pharmacology of Rapid Eye Movement Sleep

> In the summer of the year 1797, the author, then in ill health, had retired to a lonely farmhouse between Porlock and Lynton, on the Exmoor confines of Somerset and Devonshire. In consequence of a slight indisposition, an anodyne had been prescribed, from the effects of which he fell asleep in his chair at the moment he was reading the following sentence, or words of the same substance, in *Purchas's Pilgrimage*: "Here the Khan Kubla commanded a palace to be

built, and a stately garden thereunto. And thus ten miles of fertile ground were inclosed with a wall". The author continued for about three hours in a profound sleep, at least of the external senses, during which time he has the most vivid confidence that he could not have composed less than from two to three hundred lines; if that indeed can be called composition in which all the images rose up before him as *things*, with a parallel production of the correspondent expressions, without any sensation or consciousness of effort. On awaking he appeared to himself to have a distinct recollection of the whole, and taking his pen, ink and paper, instantly and eagerly wrote down the lines that are here preserved. At this moment he was unfortunately called out by a person on business from Porlock, and detained by him above an hour, and on his return to his room, found, to his no small surprise and mortification, that though he still retained some vague and dim recollection of the general purport of the vision, yet, with the exception of some eight or ten scattered lines and images, all the rest had passed away like the images on the surface of a stream into which a stone had been cast, but, alas! without the after restoration of the latter!

Samuel Taylor Coleridge

It has been known for thousands of years that various potions, extracts, and brews can exert profound effects upon consciousness. The consumption of such agents for the production of sleep has always been heavy. This is no less true today than it was in past times. As Oswald (1968) has pointed out, the consumption of barbiturates is on the increase, and the use of sedatives and tranquilizers has, in recent years, increased dramatically in the United States and Europe.

As knowledge began to accumulate concerning the stages of sleep, it was noted that certain drugs rather selectively inhibited (or altogether abolished) REM sleep; these agents at the same time either did not change the stages of slow-wave sleep or else increased these phases of nondreaming sleep. Such findings were unexpected and were at first a source of surprise (Gresham *et al.*, 1963; Norton and Jewett, 1965).

In the past few years the pharmacological investigation of sleep has mushroomed, and what was at first a surprise has now become well-known—a great number of drugs, of a wide diversity of classification, inhibit REM sleep. Further, the rebound effect has been noted to occur after such pharmacological REM deprivation (Rechtschaffen and Maron, 1964). Drugs, then, can markedly upset a natural rhythmic function. Such effects might be harmful; it was postulated (Hartmann, 1965) that the condition of psychiatric patients could be worsened. It has thus become important to discover what drugs can do to REM sleep. In addition, as will be seen, a few drugs can elevate REM sleep; a few others seem to leave this stage of sleep unaffected. It is not altogether clear what such actions might mean (if anything) for the patient's well-being.

Two words of caution need to be injected here. The first is that pharmacological studies of REM sleep must be conducted with a great deal of care, and the results of such studies interpreted with caution. This is so, as has been emphasized by Hartmann (1968a), because of the fragility of REM sleep. As was noted in the foregoing section, REM sleep, unlike the stages of slow-wave sleep, is easily disrupted by a variety of "nonspecific" factors. This is seen in the "first night effect", i.e., subjects regularly have decreased REM sleep on the first night they spend in a sleep laboratory, owing, perhaps, to the strangeness of the environment (Rechtschaffen and Verdone, 1964). Other factors can also add to the variability. Monroe (1969) studied 28 married sleepers in a laboratory situation for three consecutive nights. The subjects were studied under two conditions—sleep with spouse and sleep alone. The sleep-alone condition caused a significant inhibition of REM sleep and an elevation of stage 4 sleep. In addition, as noted by Hartmann (1968a), nausea, pain, psychological upset, fever, diseases of many sorts, and even the menstrual cycle, can influence REM sleep in a profound fashion. Thus when an investigator says that such and such a drug inhibits REM sleep in a selective manner we need to ask if this is truly a specific CNS effect or whether it is some nonspecific effect due to side effects of the drug or to the drug's toxicity. If the REM sleep of a man with gout is suppressed by a drug which also makes his big toe ache, then the effect is just as likely to be "mediated" at the bottom end of the body as it is by some would-be neurohumor at the body's top end.

The second word of caution concerns the interpretation investigators make concerning the effects of drugs upon sleep. This whole area of pharmacology is not only new but is also, as might be expected, in a state of flux. What was accepted a year ago is under question today and will likely be subject to reinterpretation a year or so hence.

With all this in mind, I would like to describe what I can concerning the pharmacology of REM sleep.

The topic has received several recent reviews (Jouvet, 1968; Oswald, 1968). The review by Jouvet concerns chiefly drugs that affect CNS amines; the review by Oswald is more comprehensive. The present review will, at appropriate spots, attempt to explore some general theories of REM sleep currently under discussion—the protein synthesis theory; the unitary theory; the drive-serotonin theory; and the dualistic theory. All these notions are young, and all have been insufficiently tested. The most widely discussed of the four is the dualistic theory; the most sweeping and promising is the protein synthesis theory; the unitary theory is all but forgotten (and its originator is dead prematurely); and the drive-serotonin theory is notable for its showmanship, if nothing else. There will be more hypotheses of REM sleep in the years to come. This is healthy. It is a sign of vitality. One can only hope, however, that as ideas become disproved, they will be abandoned as quickly as possible. There is no room in this or any area of science for dead wood and tattered notions.

A. Fatty Acids

Various short-chain fatty acids can induce sleep; the pattern consists of an initial period of slow-wave sleep followed by an episode of REM sleep (Jouvet, 1967). Sodium *n*-butyrate, for example, in a dose of 1.5 mmole/kg, administered intravenously to an awake cat, brings on within a minute an EEG pattern of slow waves with spindles; after 2 or 3 minutes, there appears a typical episode of REM sleep (REM latency is thus quite short); then, after 4 to 15 minutes, the animal awakens (Matsuzaki *et al.*, 1964). Dose is critical—smaller doses cause a brief period of slow-wave sleep only; larger doses lead to extended periods of REM-less slow-wave sleep. The following compounds were found by Matsuzaki *et al.* (1964) to have similar effects: the sodium salts of isobutyrate, isovalerate, *n*-caproate, γ-hydroxybutyrate, and α-hydroxyisobutyrate. However, the sodium salts of γ-butyrolactone, propionate, acetoacetate, and β-hydroxybutyrate did not induce sleep. Atropine did not interfere with the REM sleep-inducing effects of γ-hydroxybutryate, but nialamide did (Delorme *et al.*, 1966).

The naturally occurring constituent of brain, γ-aminobutyrate, does not induce sleep (Hernandez-Peon and Sterman, 1966). In man, γ-hydroxybutyrate (30 mg/kg intravenously) induces in the waking subject cortical slow waves. The same dose given at bed time seems to induce sleep, but neither increases nor decreases REM sleep (Yamada *et al.*, 1967). It is clear, then, that this agent may induce a dissociation between behavior and the EEG—an all-important point which is too often neglected in pharmacological studies of sleep.

It is hard to see any meaning in these results at the present time. It is thought that γ-hydroxybutyrate may be a product, via transamination and dehydrogenation, of γ-aminobutyrate. The other compounds listed above as successful sleep inducers, however, are either abnormal, or usually insignificant, metabolites of fatty acids (Mandell and Mandell, 1965); it is doubtful that they have a natural role. They remain of interest, however, because, unlike most CNS depressants, they do not inhibit REM sleep (if the dose is just right, that is).

Prostaglandins are longer (C_{20}) fatty acids than the compounds mentioned above. There are fourteen different prostaglandins now known. A variety of these occur naturally in brain; peripheral, afferent stimuli evoke a release of prostaglandins from various CNS sites (Ramwell and Shaw, 1966). In rats, prostaglandins E_1 and E_2 antagonize the effects of norepinephrine on cerebellar Purkinje cells (Hoffer *et al.*, 1969). Horton (1964) found that prostaglandins E_1 and E_2 induced in the cat, after a 20-minute latent period, first sedation and then stupor, or, as Horton called it, "catatonia." The animals sat still, in shadows, avoiding sunlight; they would remain motionless for hours, with their eyes closed. Yet their coordinated movements were unimpaired and if picked up and moved, they would walk back to their dark corner and sit motionless again. The righting reflex was intact. But, in a few animals, the stupor was so profound that the cats could be suspended in an odd, precarious position, such as across the rungs of an inverted stool, and they would maintain that position for several hours. The deep CNS depression lasted for up to 24 hours, and the animals showed decreased activity for several days. It should be mentioned that the effect was seen only after the injection of the agents directly into the lateral ventricle; in young chicks, the effect could be obtained after intravenous injection. I know of no EEG studies of this peculiar syndrome. I would imagine, however, from all the evidence of persisting skeletal muscle tone, that REM sleep was probably inhibited.

The roles, if any, of the fatty acids and of various other active principles found in brain, such as substance P, remain unknown. [The distribution of substance P in the brain is similar to the distribution of serotonin and norepinephrine (Amin *et al.*, 1954).] It is well, however, in the present enthusiasm over the monoamines, not to forget that such substances do exist. The same certainly also applies to Pappenheimer's peptide.

B. Steroid and Pituitary Hormones

Seyle (1942) first demonstrated that certain steroid hormones could exert hypnotic effects. Of the hormones investigated, progesterone was the most potent. It was later found that a metabolite of progesterone, pregnanolone, was an even more potent hypnotic than progesterone, and, unlike the parent steroid, had no "hormonal" effects. Gyermek (1967) compared pregnanolone to thiopental in a variety of species, including cats, and found that it was at least as potent as the thiobarbiturate. It was equally short-acting. Its margin of safety, however, was even less than thiopental's. Gyermek made no comments on any effects the drug might have upon REM sleep; he was working with pregnanolone chiefly as an anesthetic agent. Thus the possible effect of pregnanolone on the sleep–wakefulness cycle remains unexamined.

Progesterone itself, either injected intravenously in cats or applied topically to the preoptic area, can bring on the quick onset of sleep; this sleep lasts for 5 or 6 hours and contains several periods of REM sleep (Heuser *et al.*, 1967).

As was briefly mentioned in Section II, the female rabbit shows a stereotyped EEG "after-reaction" to copulation or vaginal stimulation—first a period of slow-wave sleep, then an episode of REM sleep; after that, the animal awakens (Sawyer and Kawakmi, 1959). Faure (1964) was able to elicit to the slow-wave sleep–REM sleep sequence in rabbits (both male and female) by the administration of several hormones: luteotropic hormone, lactogenic hormone, human chorionic gonadotropin, and, sometimes, testosterone. In humans, the amount of REM sleep has been reported to vary with the menstrual cycle, being the greatest during the late progestational stage (Hartmann, 1967a). Thus tentative data suggest possible hypnogenic activities for a number of hormones.

The posterior pituitary and the anterior pituitary adrenal axis appear to become activated during REM sleep. Changes in the volume and osmolality of the urine suggest the secretion of vasopressin during REM sleep (Mandell *et al.*, 1966). Vasopressin itself can induce REM sleep in rabbits (Faure, 1964) and cats (Domino and Yamamoto, 1965). In line with these observations, it was found that osmotic variations can influence REM sleep. Injections into cats of hypertonic saline solutions can lead to a 100–300% increase of REM sleep; hypotonic saline, however, suppresses REM sleep for several hours; acetazolamide suppresses REM sleep in cats (Delorme, 1966). In addition, REM sleep is also accompanied by an increase in the total urinary excretion of 17-hydroxycorticosteroids (Mandell and Mandell, 1965). Mandell and Mandell suggest that the activation of the hypothalamic–pituitary–adrenal system may be a central "reason" for REM sleep. Triggered by low circulating levels of necessary metabolites, such as glucose or fatty acids, REM sleep could be a means of stimulating gluconeogenesis and maintaining the animal's energy-producing mechanism throughout the long fast of sleep. This perhaps is an oversimplification. Although undoubtedly involved in REM sleep, the pituitary is not necessary for its occurrence—hypophysectomized cats still show regular periods of REM sleep (Jouvet, 1967).

In summary, the pituitary, adrenocortical, and gonadal hormones may have a role in the modulation of REM sleep and in the expression of some of its physiological manifestations, but the data are still fragmentary.

C. Central Nervous System Stimulants

Inhibitors of monoamine oxidase will be mentioned in a later section.

Amphetamine causes a decided inhibition of REM sleep. This acute suppression has been noted both in animals (Shimizu and Himwich, 1968) and in humans (Rechtschaffen and Maron, 1964; Baekland, 1967). In cats, amphetamine causes such acute excitation that wakefulness is increased at the expense of all stages of sleep; slow-wave sleep is reduced and REM sleep tends to be extinguished altogether (Jewett and Norton, 1966). Methamphetamine causes similar effects in cats (Wallach, *et al.*, 1969b). When amphetamine is given to humans along with pentobarbital, the suppression of REM sleep is greater than with the barbiturate alone (Baekland, 1967).

The study of amphetamine's effects on REM sleep constitutes an excellent example of how pharmacology changed some of the basic notions concerning this stage of sleep. The particular phenomenon which has been subjected to reinterpretation is the rebound of REM sleep which follows deprivation.

Dement (1960), as already noted, at first interpreted the rebound to mean that humans have an innate need to dream. If one prevents a subject from dreaming, the subject when allowed to sleep in peace, will make up for lost dreams. The consequences of dream deprivation could be psychiatric disorders.

This if-you-don't-dream-you'll-go-crazy theory of REM sleep has long since been abondoned by most investigators (though it is still with us in a greatly altered form, as will be seen later). It was followed by a more physiological, less psychological, interpretation (see Hartmann, 1965). Rapid eye movement sleep is a basic physiological function. If a subject is deprived of water, he becomes thirsty; he drinks, and the thirst subsides. The same applies to hunger, and, in its own fashion, to REM sleep. If one deprives a subject of REM sleep then a "need" for that which has been taken away arises, a kind of thirst or hunger for the missing physiological function. Thus, after a period of REM deprivation, a subject will promptly enter into a REM sleep rebound. He will make up for that which had been lost, and the rebound will continue until the need has been mollified. This, of course, is simply a restatement of Dement's original formulation. Only the semantics are different.

All along, however, a basic factor may have been overlooked. When one deprives a subject or a test animal of REM sleep, one must adopt fairly drastic measures. As Dement (1960) was the first to point out, as deprivation continues, the subject or animal will attempt to enter into the REM state in an increasingly persistent manner. This is because of the pressure which builds up during the course of deprivation—a pressure driving the subject toward the REM state. Waking a subject 30 times in the course of a single night is a drastic procedure. So, too, are the methods used to deprive laboratory animals of REM sleep. Cats, commonly, are deprived by having them live (say for 16 hours a day) on a continuously moving treadmill; while riding the treadmill the cats can snatch a few moments of slow-wave sleep, but are never able to sleep long enough to enter into the REM state. After 16 hours on the treadmill, the animal is allowed to sleep in an experimental chamber, but is allowed to experience only non-REM sleep; he is aroused manually as each REM episode begins (Dewson *et al.*, 1967). Rats commonly are deprived of REM sleep by placing them upon everted flower pots in a lake of water (Jouvet, 1967). The circumference of the flower pot's bottom is such that the rat can enter into slow-wave sleep, because this stage of sleep is characterized by a maintenance of skeletal muscle tonus and a crouching, curled-up sort of posture. But when the rat enters into REM sleep, he loses his tonic muscle support and eases into a thoroughly relaxed, sprawled sort of posture; the surface of the flower pot is no longer large enough to support the animal, and he falls into the lake. This, of course, wakes the animal up, and he crawls back to his perch, wet and deprived of his REM sleep. Again, the method is drastic.

As has already been mentioned, such procedures can provoke several measurable biochemical changes. What has gone unquestioned is whether or not such drastic measures might be actually injurious to the subject or animal. Physically injurious. Might not the stress involved in these approaches actually lead to physical damage of the CNS? Then, if so, might not the rebound be a manifestation of injury and subsequent repair? Might not, in other words, the rebound be, not a making-up for that which had been lost, but, instead, a sign of the healing of that which had been hurt? Oswald (1969), on the basis of pharmacological studies, has reached such a conclusion.

The observations which led Oswald to answer yes to the questions posed above involve a basic discrepancy between REM deprivation achieved by physical means (awakenings, flower pots) and REM deprivation achieved pharmacologically. When a subject is deprived by one of the physical methods, the rebound never is so large that all of the REM sleep that had been lost is made up for. At best, the rebound gives back to the animal only 30–50% of the REM sleep which had been taken away. It is on the basis of such results that people have stated that in the rebound, subjects and animals behave as though they were making up for that which had been lost.

Quite a different rebound was found by Oswald and Thacore (1963) in patients addicted to amphetamine and phenmetrazine. Amphetamine, as already noted, acutely suppresses REM sleep, but humans chronically addicted to the drug may have entirely normal sleep. Rapid eye movement sleep may be suppressed at the start of addiction, but within a short time it comes back to preaddiction levels. Patients addicted for years show normal amounts of REM sleep. Upon withdrawal of the drug, however, there occurs a huge rebound increase, with a reduction of REM latency from a normal value of about 60 to 90 minutes to as low a value as 4 minutes; this spectacular "withdrawal syndrome" lasts for the spectacular duration of 3 to 8 weeks. This can hardly be called a rebound in the sense that a rebound is a making up for that which had been lost; instead, this rebound gives the patient more REM sleep than he otherwise ever would have experienced. He most certainly is not making up; he has had, over the months or years of his addiction, essentially no loss of REM sleep. Therefore, the concept of making up just will not work. How can one be considered as making up for something if that something has never been lost?

Similar reactions have since been found with various drugs other than amphetamine and phenmetrazine, as will be mentioned below. In each case, chronic drug administration led first to a brief period of inhibition of REM sleep, then to a more prolonged period of normal sleep patterns, and then, on withdrawal, a huge, protracted increase of REM sleep. Such recovery curves in animal brains, are not, as Oswald (1969) points out, new. The recovery of brain acetylcholinesterase, after inactivation with organophosphates, follows a very prolonged course. So, too, do recoveries of brain tissue from various sorts of physical trauma. Oswald thus proposes that the REM sleep rebound after drug withdrawal may reflect protein synthesis and neuronal repair. Physical methods of REM sleep deprivation might entail less extensive damage, and thus less extensive REM rebound. Oswald (1969) writes, in *Nature:*

> ...I suggest that REM sleep rebound betrays increased protein synthesis in the brain. I would go further and propose that REM sleep is a non-specific indication of many forms of synthesis within cerebral neurones, which would explain the "strange" finding that streptomycin (an inhibitor of protein synthesis capable of damaging human neurones) reduces REM sleep. The proposal is consistent with the uniquely high proportion of REM sleep in the 2 months both before and after birth in animals such as the human in which the central nervous system is not mature at birth. During these months the finer differentiation of the brain occurs. It is also consistent with the increased brain blood flow and temperature during REM sleep. NREM (nonrapid eye movement) sleep is especially enhanced after strenuous physical exercise and, in contrast to REM sleep, is accompanied by a high concentration of growth hormone in the blood, suggesting that its chief function is for bodily restitution, while REM sleep may be chiefly for brain repair. I could also predict that conditions associated

with massive learning would cause high percentages of REM sleep, for example, when an "enriched" environment for growing rats leads to a heavier brain cortex and greater development of glial cells. Human mental retardates, it may be noted, have REM sleep reduced both in amount and intensity.

Finally, it seems to me that, in the study of brain and behaviour, we shall be compelled increasingly to think in terms of slow shifts of function mediated by protein synthesis. So far the latter has scarcely entered the psychiatrist's conceptual framework, but it seems as probable that it underlies personality modification through psychotherapy as that it underlies drug tolerance or REM sleep rebound. The healing of hurt minds proceeds by processes equally as slow as the healing of hurt brain cells.

This sweeping theory of REM sleep has, in my opinion, much promise. The hypothesis may not be entirely correct, however, as will be mentioned. Even so, Oswald has, I feel, tellingly challenged earlier concepts of the rebound which follows the deprivation of REM sleep.

Caffeine has no discernible effect upon REM sleep in humans (Gresham *et al.*, 1963). Oswald (1968), however, thinks that the effects of caffeine are not yet fully understood, and that what evidence there is suggests that the alkaloid leads to some sort of "deficiency" in the quality of sleep.

The tricyclic antidepressants cause a very severe inhibition of REM sleep in cats and man. This is true of imipramine and demethylimipramine (Hishikawa *et al.*, 1965; Whitman *et al.*, 1966; Ritvo *et al.*, 1967) and of amitriptyline (Hartmann, 1968b). These drugs tend also to increase total sleep time by promoting an augmentation of slow-wave sleep. In the cat, however, some of this increased slow-wave activity occurs during wakefulness. There is, in other words, some dissociation between the EEG and behavior (Wallach *et al.*, 1969a). The suppression of REM sleep in the cat after amitriptyline, demethylimipramine, and imipramine (10–15 mg/kg intraperitoneally) is total on the day following the drugs' administration; predrug baselines are reached only after 3 days (Wallach *et al.*, 1969b).

How the effects are produced is unknown; some (Mandell and Mandell, 1965; Delorme, 1966) feel that imipramine's anticholinergic effects may be involved (anticholinergics tend to inhibit REM sleep) but, of course, altered metabolism of brain amines could also be a factor (see Glowinski and Axelrod, 1964). Despite these findings, the sleep patterns of depressed patients—who may show abnormally low amounts of REM sleep (Gresham *et al.*, 1965; Hawkins and Mendels, 1966)— tend to revert toward normal after imipramine therapy (Gresham *et al.*, 1965). This reversion toward normal may be the kind of effect noted above for amphetamine and phenmetrazine. Lewis and Oswald (1969) report that following an overdose of imipramine (1000 mg), there is in humans initially a supression of REM sleep, with augmented slow-wave sleep. Rapid eye movement sleep then gradually rises to abnoramlly high levels, and there are frequent nightmares;

this trend peaks at about 2 weeks after the overdosage, then subsides very slowly back to normal. The full process takes a month to run its course.

In view of the wide variety of drugs which can produce the Oswald effect, i.e., an acute inhibition of REM sleep, with a return of REM sleep to baseline on chronic drug administration, and then a massive postdrug rebound, I would like to suggest that all future drug studies of sleep should examine the effects both of the acute and the chronic administrations of the drug and should look for any possible postdrug changes. Studies that neglect to examine these three areas will have to be considered incomplete.

D. Minor Tranquilizers

Tissot (1965) claimed that diazepam and nitrazepam can increase the length and frequency of REM sleep episodes in man. His data have not been confirmed by others. Hartmann (1968b) found that in humans chlordiaepoxide increases slightly total sleep time without inhibiting REM sleep. The dose of chlordiazepoxide was high (100 mg); the data are from 10 human subjects. Oswald (1968) has criticized these results—there were apparent changes in the sleep of the subjects given chlordiazepoxide, and these were in the same direction as the changes caused in the same subjects by pentobarbital, namely suppression of REM sleep. The data were statistically significant with pentobarbital, but not with chlordiazepoxide. Oswald suggests that a more thorough study, perhaps with larger doses, would have shown a statistically significant effect for chlordiazepoxide. I think that Oswald may be belaboring the point—100 mg of chlordiazepoxide is at the high end of the clinical dose spectrum, and, if this dose fails to inhibit REM sleep, then it is probably safe to say, as Hartmann does, that chlordiazepoxide is among the few CNS depressants used by humans which does not suppress REM sleep. Of course, though, it is possible that an overdose of the drug might have different effects.

However, nitrazepam (Oswald and Priest, 1965) does seem to inhibit REM sleep in humans, and withdrawal leads to a rebound increase which can last as long as 4 weeks. Lanoir and Killam (1968) studied nitrazepam and diazepam in cats and found a dose-dependent reduction of REM sleep; both drugs also caused long periods of restlessness, with unusual fast waves in the cortical EEG, so that, in effect, total sleep was also inhibited. What sleep there was tended to be slow-wave sleep. When REM sleep finally reappeared, it tended to manifest itself with few or any rapid eye movements; the other correlates of REM sleep were unchanged.

Meprobamate in humans significantly enhances slow-wave sleep at the expense of REM sleep (Freeman *et al.*, 1965). Withdrawal of meprobamate produces a prolonged REM rebound (Oswald, 1968).

Promethazine is a phenothiazine, but lacks the molecular structure and the antipsychotic effects of the phenothiazines which are used as major tranquilizers. It is classified as an antihistaminic but also has anticholinergic effects. It is widely used as a sedative or minor tranquilizer. Jewett (1968) found that this agent in cats increases total sleep and slow-wave sleep in a dose–response fashion; at the highest of the doses used (2.0 mg/kg), minutes of REM sleep were significantly suppressed. Rapid eye movement sleep as a percent of total sleep was suppressed by several doses. There was a suggestion of a rebound increase on the day after the drug was given. The inhibition of REM sleep caused by promethazine came about chiefly because the REM periods were further apart from one another than in placebo experiments and because REM latency was likewise increased. There was no change in the mean duration of the REM episodes. Promethazine also inhibits REM sleep in man (Brannen and Jewett, 1969).

The study by Jewett of promethazine in the cat followed a procedure too often ignored in pharmacological studies of sleep: the examination of dose-response effects. This basic strategem should, where possible, always be observed.

E. Major Tranquilizers

Mention of reserpine will be deferred to a later section.

The phenothiazines with antipsychotic activity are generally stated to inhibit REM sleep. Thus chlorpromazine reduces REM sleep and enhances slow wave sleep in cats (Jewett and Norton, 1966) and rabbits (Khazan and Sawyer, 1964). Wallach *et al.* (1969b) note that the suppression of REM sleep in the cat after a single dose of chlorpromazine (15 mg/kg intraperitoneally) lasts for 2 days. In humans, Lewis and Evans (1969) found that 100 mg of chlorpromazine inhibits REM sleep; but 25 mg of the drug in these same subjects seemed to enhance both slow-wave sleep and REM sleep. Oswald (1968) points out that the effects of chlorpromazine are probably dose-related, with lower doses enhancing REM sleep and higher ones suppressing it. Even if this is so, the effects of this important drug on REM sleep in the human are still unclear, and if these effects are dose-related, and biphasic according to dose, no one has yet demonstrated the fact convincingly.

Perphenazine (4 mg/kg, intraperitoneally) inhibits REM sleep in cats; the effect is not marked, however, and lasts but a day (Wallach *et al.*, 1969b).

Trifluoperazine in cats causes a dose-related inhibition of REM sleep (Jewett, 1971). On the other hand, Brannen and Jewett (1969) found that trifluoperazine can enhance REM sleep in the same schizophrenic patients in whom promethazine had caused an inhibition.

Haloperidol in the cat acutely suppresses REM sleep (Monti, 1968). It delays the onset of the first REM period, decreases the number of REM periods, and decreases REM sleep as a percentage of total sleep. These effects are dose-related.

It is not at all clear what any of the major tranquilizers do to REM sleep on chronic administration. Does the Oswald effect occur with these agents? The answer hopefully will be forthcoming in the future.

F. Hypnotic Agents (Including Alcohol)

Do hypnotic agents do the job for which they are prescribed? In other words, do sleeping pills cause sleep? The answer, of course, depends upon the definition of sleep. If this definition includes a statement about normal amounts of REM sleep, then the answer for many hypnotics—and for the human, at least—is probably no.

Barbiturates are the most widely prescribed hypnotics. In the cat, thiopental (Jewett and Norton, 1966) and pentobarbital (Jouvet and Delorme, 1965) fail to inhibit REM sleep unless given in anesthetic doses (Jouvet, 1968). Subanesthetic doses of pentobarbital induce cortical and subcortical spindles, and these can obscure the EEG signs of REM sleep in the cat; but REM sleep still occurs, as is especially made clear by the presence of PGO spikes (Jouvet and Delorme, 1965). In the rat, thiopental can inhibit REM sleep, but only at anesthetic doses (Radil-Weiss and Styblova, 1967).

Despite the failure of barbiturates to inhibit REM sleep in animals, they without doubt do so in man (Oswald *et al.*, 1963; Tissot, 1965; Hartmann, 1968b; Kales *et al.*, 1970a). Lester *et al.* (1968) found that secobarbital in man inhibited REM sleep and enhanced slow-wave sleep. Often, the inhibition occurred only in the first part of the night; REM sleep then would tend to return to baseline levels in the second half; even then, however, the occurrence of rapid eye movements was curtailed. There has been much speculation that the rapid eye movements in human REM sleep are connected directly to the dream content (Kleitman, 1963), but proof of this has been lacking. Along these lines, Carroll *et al.* (1969) noted a decline of the profusion of eye movements after amylobarbitone. They wondered if the barbiturate might alter dream content as well as the outward signs of REM sleep. Such was found to be the case; when dreaming did occur after amylobarbitone, it was more conceptual and less perceptual, less vivid, less emotional, or, as the authors stated it, more "thoughtlike" and less "dreamlike."

Oswald and Priest (1965) found that there occurs with chronic use of amylobarbitone a series of changes similar to those seen with amphetamine abuse. Rapid eye movement sleep was initially inhibited, but it then returned to normal within 2 to 3 weeks. When the return to normal was complete, the drug was withdrawn, and the large rebound increase of REM sleep lasted for 5 weeks. During the rebound, which can occur after as few as three nights of barbiturate usage (Kales *et al.*, 1968), there are more rapid eye movements than is typical of placebo REM sleep, and dreams become more vivid than usual, with nightmares common.

Most of the nonbarbiturate hypnotics cause effects similar to those seen with the barbiturates. Glutethimide, 500 and 1000 mg, taken orally, in particular, causes a very profound inhibition of REM sleep, with a postdrug rebound; methyprylon, 300 mg orally, also inhibits REM sleep in man (Kales *et al.*, 1968, 1970a). An important point is discussed by Kales *et al.* (1970a)— the Oswald effect occurs with many drugs which inhibit REM sleep, but not all. In a careful study, Kales *et al.* (1970a) found that with chronic use of glutethimide, REM sleep returned to baseline neither in normal volunteers given the drug for three nights nor in insominac subjects given the drug for fourteen nights (Kales *et al.*, 1970c). Glutethimide, then, unlike most hypnotics, causes a long-lasting inhibition of REM sleep. Further, though REM sleep returns to control levels after a few nights of treatment with methyprylon and pentobarbital, this state of sleep can still be inhibited in the first hours of sleep; a rebound then occurs in the latter half of the night, thus bringing the whole night's amount of REM sleep back to predrug values. All three drugs inhibited REM sleep by shortening the duration of the REM episodes. In addition to their effects upon REM sleep, glutethimide and pentobarbital inhibited stage 4 sleep (Kales *et al.*, 1970a). All three agents (glutethimide, methyprylon, pentobarbital) lead, as stated, to a postdrug rebound of REM sleep. As pointed out by Kales *et al.* (1970c), our knowledge still is not firm enough to say REM inhibition per se is harmful. We can say, however, that a large REM rebound can lead to undesirable clinical effects, such as excessive dreaming, "intense" REM episodes, nightmares, and insomnia. Kales *et al.* (1970b), while stressing that more work is needed, suggest that physicians should avoid REM rebound in patients suffering from conditions known to be exacerbated during REM sleep (for example, coronary artery and duodenal ulcer diseases). Indeed, Kales and Kales (1970) recommend that the labeling and advertisements for hypnotic drugs that suppress REM sleep include a warning and discussion of possible ill effects which may ensue during a postdrug REM rebound.

In marked contrast to the just-mentioned drugs, chloral hydrate (500 and 1000 mg, taken orally) and methaqaulone (150 mg orally) do not suppress REM sleep in humans and do not lead to a postdrug REM rebound; further, flurazepam (30 mg orally) causes only a slight inhibition of REM sleep, and does not cause a postdrug rebound (Kales *et al.*, 1970b, c). Larger doses of methaqualone and flurazepam (300 and 60 mg, respectively) do suppress REM sleep, however, and cause rebounds. In rats, large doses of methaqualone (50–100 mg/kg, given orally) abolish the cortical activation of REM sleep, but fail to inhibit (or augment) the other signs of this sleep stage (Soulairac and Gottesmann, 1967). Does this mean that chloral hydrate, methaqualone, and flurazepam are to be preferred to hypnotics such as glutethimide? Perhaps, especially if REM rebound is to be avoided. However the answer, I must stress, is only "perhaps." A great deal of work still remains to be done. Thus any drug advertisement that claims that for all patients a given hypnotic is better than another because it does not inhibit REM sleep can only be regarded as suspect and misleading.

Alcohol in humans suppresses REM sleep (Gresham *et al.*, 1963). With chronic use, it produces the pattern already mentioned several times—a gradual return of REM sleep to baseline, or even to levels above baseline, and then, on withdrawal, a large, protracted rebound (Yules *et al.*, 1966). Addicts tend to develop very bizarre sleep patterns. Greenberg and Pearlman (1967) noted that as early as 1881, it was claimed that alcoholic delirium was not a delirium but, instead, was a waking dream. The subjects studied by Greenberg and Pearlman showed, during their postalcohol rebound, an increased vividness of dreams with frequent nightmares. Gross *et al.* (1966) claimed even more spectacular effects. They studied a series of patients in acute alcoholic psychosis. The patients were often unable to sleep well, but when they did, almost 100% of their sleep was REM sleep, accompanied by very intense eye movements, mouth movements, and tongue movements. Gross *et al.* called the condition a "REM storm." In some cases the dream content of these patients continued, upon arousal, into the waking hallucinations of the psychosis. Clearly, the authors felt, there was a connection—the brain processes manufacturing the REM storm are probably the same as those creating the waking hallucinations. Is, then, the alcoholic psychosis a waking dream? More study is needed, but the idea is intriguing.

G. Hallucinogens

Marihuana can cause a state of somnolence in dogs; in man it induces first anxiety, then euphoria, and, finally, sleep (Grinspoon, 1969). Marihuana sleep in man is, according to Bromberg (1934), dreamless. Further work is obviously needed, though, because Bromberg's studies did not utilize the EEG and relied instead upon anecdotal data. In the rat, Δ-

9-tetrahydrocannabinol (10 mg/kg, intraperitoneally) causes a pronounced acute inhibition of REM sleep and blocks the rebound of REM sleep after a period of REM-deprivation (Moreton and Davis, 1970).

The only hallucinogen studied in depth by sleep investigators is D-lysergic acid diethylamide (LSD). This drug was first reported to inhibit REM sleep in the cat (Hobson, 1964); the doses tested were 2 and 20 μg/kg, and the cats were kept awake on a treadmill for 15 hours prior to drug treatment. It also seemed to inhibit REM sleep in rabbits (Khazan and Sawyer, 1964), but this and other data concerning REM sleep in rabbits must be taken with a grain of salt—it is only with the most careful management that any REM sleep can be observed in this species, and when one has finally acclimated the apprehensive little animals to the experimental situation, even aspirin will appear to inhibit REM sleep (Goldstein *et al.*, 1967). Later reports suggest that LSD in small doses can enhance REM sleep in rats and in humans (Hartmann, 1967b; Green, 1965). Muzio *et al.* (1966) studied 12 subjects. The initial doses of LSD were 0.41 to 0.57 μg/kg, and these caused awakenings. Smaller doses (0.13–0.31 μg/kg) caused an appreciable prolongation of either the first or second REM episode in 21 of 31 instances of LSD treatment. No changes were ever seen in the third REM episode or thereafter. The usual pattern in the human is for the longer REM episodes to occur in the second half of the night (Kleitman, 1963); the night's first episode tends usually to be brief. After LSD, with the first or second episode unusually long in duration, the normal trend was reversed, and the episodes in the latter half of the night were abnormally short. Thus LSD seems to cause (if the dose is small enough so as not to lead to arousal) a redistribution of REM sleep; with REM sleep so redistributed, the whole night's content of REM sleep may not be higher than baseline; neither is it lower.

It is difficult to reconcile such data—and all other data which point to an acute elevation of REM sleep after a certain drug—with Oswald's hypothesis concerning REM sleep as a repair phenomenon. After LSD, in fact, there appears to be a tiny "negative rebound." Though Oswald's theory may prove to be one with genuine predictive value, it nevertheless, is clear that some drugs can increase REM sleep directly and acutely. Such drugs do not require chronic use and withdrawal before the enhanced REM sleep is evident. One such agent is LSD.

H. Opiates

One might expect from Coleridge's account of how "Kubla Khan" was "dreamt up" that opium, like LSD, can acutely and directly elevate REM sleep. Such an inference might also be drawn from Thomas de Quincey, who wrote of his addiction to opium:

> I now pass to what is the main subject of these...confessions, to the history and journal of what took place in my dreams; for these were the immediate and proximate cause of my acutest suffering.
>
> The first notice I had of any important change going on in this part of my physical economy was from the reawakening of a state of eye generally incident to childhood... . I know not whether my reader is aware that many children, perhaps most, have a power of painting, as it were, upon the darkness, all sorts of phantoms: in some that power is simply a mechanic affection of the eye; others have a voluntary or a semi-voluntary power to dismiss or to summon them... . In the middle of 1817, I think it was, this faculty became positively distressing to me... . A change took place in my dreams; a theater seemed suddenly opened and lighted up within my brain, which presented, nightly, spectacles of more than earthly splendor... . We hear it reported of Dryden, and of Fuseli in modern times, that they thought proper to eat raw meat for the sake of obtaining splendid dreams: how much better, for such a purpose, to have eaten opium... .

These and similar observations helped set off a dream-craze among nineteenth century poets and would-be poets (Hayter, 1969); a number took to opium (and still others to raw meat and onions) in search of inspiration. Most failed.

If opium lights up the dreaming theater, then REM sleep might be expected to increase. Such was found to be the case in one heroin addict (Kaufman *et al.*, 1964), but the examination of the sleep of opiate addicts still awaits a complete, controlled study, and every report except that of Kaufman *et al.* indicates that opiates acutely suppress REM sleep. (The chronic effects of course, may be different.) Kay *et al.* (1969) gave morphine (7.5–30 mg/70 kg intramuscularly) to a small group of postaddicts (at least 4 weeks postdrug) and found a decrease both of the number and of the duration of REM periods; there was also a prolonged REM latency. In fact, morphine—the drug named by its isolator (Serturner) for Morpheus, the Roman diety who was thought to produce the human figures (*morphai*) seen in dreams—tended to diminish the deeper stages of slow-wave sleep and lead to a net increase of wakefulness. It also produced a variety of unusual EEG patterns. Heroin has been studied in humans by Lewis *et al.* (1970); 7.5 mg of this drug was given for seven successive nights. A depression of REM sleep was an early effect, but REM sleep drifted back toward control values as the drug nights came to a close; then in some of the subjects there followed the familiar rebound increase, lasting for as long as 2 months; in others, the rebound was slight or absent.

In rabbits, morphine seems to cause inhibition of REM sleep altogether for varying periods of time (Khazan and Sawyer, 1964). In rats, it greatly suppresses REM sleep during the first few days of administration and simultaneously leads to increased wakefulness. After 3 days of regular administration, and with steadily increasing doses (up to 40 mg/kg/hour), slow-wave sleep and REM sleep returned to normal levels (Khazan *et al.*, 1967a). In cats (Takle and Jewett, unpublished observations), morphine, in small doses (0.2 mg/kg, administered subcutaneously), caused an abrupt inhibition of all the stages of sleep. Echols and Jewett (in preparation) extended these preliminary observations. In cats, a dose of 0.3 mg/kg of morphine caused a period of insomnia which lasted for about 12 hours. This effect could be blocked by naloxone for several hours. The authors wondered whether the arousal reaction might be mediated by central catecholamines; to test this they pretreated their cats with α-methylytrosine. The pretreatment did not modify in any way the arousal caused by morphine. Nor was morphine's effect modified by pretreatment with 5-hydroxytryptophan.

In summary, then, opiates seem to inhibit REM sleep and total sleep, and seem to promote arousal, not only in species which are excited by these agents, such as the cat, but even in species which are depressed by these drugs, such as man and the rat. We still do not know why the theater lit up inside Thomas de Quincey's brain.

I. Miscellaneous Drugs

Here, I would like to mention several agents that defy classification with the other drugs which modify REM sleep.

As has already been mentioned, streptomycin can inhibit REM sleep (Dement, 1968). Penicillin, according to Dement (1968), can cause some "very unexpected effects" on sleep, but just what these effects might be has not been described in any detail at all.

The suppression by acetazolamide of REM sleep has also already been mentioned; the mechanism of this drug effect is obscure.

Jewett (unpublished observations) has noted that piperazine can provoke a very large increase of REM sleep in the cat; the observation needs to be followed up, though, and the meaning of the effect is, again, obscure.

Lithium carbonate is now being used to treat mania; it may also diminish the recurring episodes of depression in manic-depressive psychoses. Kupfer *et al.* (1970) studied seven patients being treated with lithium; one of the patients was depressed, the rest were either manic or hypomanic. In all, the drug produced a sustained inhibition of REM sleep.

Several antihistaminic drugs can inhibit REM sleep: chlorpheniramine, tripelennamine, and phenindamine are notably potent. Meclizine has no effect (Prinz, 1968). Does this mean that REM sleep is mediated by central histamine? Certainly not. The anti-REM effect of the antihistaminics is correlated neither with their ability to block histamine peripherally nor with their sedative potency. And, in addition, most of these agents have some anticholinergic actions, which could be partly responsible for their anti-REM effects.

Cohen *et al.* (1968) have noted that diphenylhydantoin inhibits REM sleep sharply in the cat and in man. In the cat, the REM periods become less frequent. Total sleep is also diminished, and wakefulness increased. Tolerance to the REM-suppressive effect of the drug never develops, even after 24 days of continuous treatment. On withdrawal, there is no rebound. This lack of rebound came as a surprise to this group of workers (as might be expected, since one of their number, Dement, had discovered the rebound phenomenon). The workers extended their postdrug observations for a number of days, waiting for the rebound which never came. This was, they said, the first demonstration of a drug which markedly inhibits REM sleep and which does not then lead to a rebound. The mechanism of the effect is vague. Cohen *et al.* speculated that diphenylhydantoin may interfere with catecholamine metabolism, but they finally concluded that the drug has a "pronounced and rather puzzling effect on REM sleep."

Finally, melatonin has been claimed to inhibit REM sleep (Hishikawa *et al.*, 1969). These data were from chicks. In the cat, melatonin applied topically to the preoptic area can cause cortical EEG synchronization and behavioral sleep (Marczynski *et al.*, 1964).

J. Cholinergics and Anticholinergics

Evidence, both indirect and direct, suggests the participation of a cholinergic system in sleep and dreaming. Diisopropyl fluorophosphate (DFP), for example, tends to cause excessive dreaming in humans (as judged by subjective reports); atropine can prevent this effect to a degree (Grob *et al.*, 1947). In cats, DFP increases REM sleep (Belenky *et al.*, 1968). Eserine can augment the PGO spikes of REM sleep (Jouvet *et al.*, 1965a) and can lead to longer periods of REM sleep (Jouvet and Michel, 1960; Velluti and Hernandez-Peon, 1963). Eserine also increases the frequency of the rapid eye movements in cats (Delorme, 1966). Nicotine can significantly increase REM sleep, without disturbing the amount of slow-wave sleep (Jewett and Norton, 1966); the effect is blocked by mecamylamine (Domino and Yamamoto, 1965). Acetylcholine (ACh) itself, injected into the lateral ventricle or directly into the hypothalamus of cats can cause sleep (Dikshit, 1934). This drug, applied topically to certain sites in the brain, can elicit in cats slow-wave sleep followed by REM sleep

(Hernandez-Peon, 1964). Carbachol, say some investigators (Hernandez-Peon, 1965a; Mandell and Mandell, 1965), can induce REM sleep. Baxter (1969) has made a similar claim; he applied 10 μg of carbachol to various midbrain sites in a group of cats and obtained first "emotional behavior" (i.e., hissing, growling, attack or escape, piloerection) and then an extended term of "REM sleep." The last two words are in quotation marks because if this was really REM sleep it was a different kind of REM sleep than that ever seen by anyone else: Baxter's animals could not be aroused, not by the usual sensory stimuli, not even by surgical incision of the skin. Natural REM sleep is deep, but not that deep. This was, then, really a new form of anesthesia, "REM anesthesia," it might as well be called. Carbachol induces the effect directly from the waking state, without any prior period of slow-wave sleep. The duration of the REM anesthesia was 38–52 minutes. Baxter's data clearly show, as he himelf points out, that the effect is not one mediated by the midbrain; instead it depends upon migration of the carbachol from the midbrain to some other site. The effect is decidely odd, even unique. Khazan *et al.* (1967b) found that in rats neostigmine and eserine are both able to block the REM-inhibitory effects of chlorpromazine and imipramine. The data were intrepreted to implicate anticholinergic effects for chlorpromazine and imipramine, and a cholinergic role in the production of REM sleep.

Itil (1969) has noted what others have noted before, i.e., that atropine can induce sleepiness in man, associated with slow waves and spindles in the cortical EEG—an EEG pattern, it might be added, which persists when the subject "wakes up" and shows every sign of consciousness behaviorally. This is the well-known behavioral dissociation between the EEG and behavior which atropine can induce. Signs of REM sleep were absent from the atropine sleep. Domino and co-workers (Sagales *et al.*, 1969) found that scopolamine, in doses of 0.006 mg/kg, can clearly delay the onset of REM sleep in man and inhibit REM sleep over the course of the full night's sleep. The results were taken to imply the participation of cholinergic mechanisms in sleep. As noted in the last section, electroshock in cats seems to decrease the "need" for REM sleep, even after periods of REM sleep deprivation (Cohen *et al.*, 1967), and electroshock can alter brain ACh levels. Electroshock, however, also may alter the permeability of the blood–brain barrier to catecholamines (Rosenblatt, *et al.*, 1960), and, in the rat, does increase the turnover of central norepinephrine (Kety *et al.*, 1967). Atropine, as might be expected, can inhibit REM sleep or suppress its appearance altogether in cats (Jouvet and Jouvet, 1963; Khazan and Sawyer, 1964; Weiss *et al.*, 1964; Delorme, 1966). Atropine also can prevent the appearance of sleep caused by application of ACh to the brain (Velluti and Hernandez-Peon, 1963) or by electrical stimulation of the preoptic area (Hernandez-Peon, 1964). A more careful analysis suggests that atropine does not inhibit all of the signs of REM sleep; the PGO spiking activity is not entirely blocked by doses of atropine that do inhibit the other signs of REM sleep (Jouvet *et al.*, 1965a). If this is true—if, that is, there is at least some facet of REM sleep which is not cholinergically mediated—then the unitary theory of sleep of Hernandez-Peon cannot be entirely correct.

This hypothesis (Hernandez-Peon, 1962; 1965a,b; Hernandez-Peon and Sterman, 1966) was developed largely through an extensive series of experiments in which a great many areas of the cat's brain were stimulated electrically and chemically. The product of all this work has been the mapping of a system which Hernandez-Peon believed to be (1) responsible for all the stages of sleep, including REM sleep, and (2) exclusively cholinergic. Acetylcholine, which, when applied topically to some areas of the brain, could evoke alertness or even rage (Hernandez-Peon *et al.*, 1963), evoked in the proposed hypnogenic circuit only sleep—first slow-wave sleep and then REM sleep. Atropine, applied topically to one part of the circuit, could block the sleep normally caused by electrical or ACh stimulation of another part (Velluti and Hernandez-Peon, 1963). Norepinephrine, applied to the sites where ACh called forth sleep, produced only alertness and arousal; nialamide caused no discernible effects at the same sites (Hernandez-Peon and Chavez-Ibarra, 1963).

The proposed hypnogenic pathway has two converging parts; these unite to form a final common pathway. The two converging parts are (*1*) an ascending segment, arising in the spinal gray at the thoracic level and climbing through the medulla to the pons and (*2*) a descending segment, leading from the limbic cortex through the midbrain to the medulla, and represented by the structures of Nauta's limbic-midbrain circuit, plus corticofugal projections to this pathway, arising from the prepyriform, pyriform, and periamygdaloid cortex of the temporal lobe, from the orbital surface of the frontal lobe, and from the perisylvian cortex. In addition, there are contributions from midline and intralaminary thalamic nuclei, from the caudate, from the globus pallidus, and from several other areas (Hernandez-Peon, 1965a). Cholinergic stimulation of any portion of this extensive system leads to sleep. The ascending and descending limbs of the system are thought to converge in the brainstem to form the final, common hypnogenic path. From the site of confluence, in the posterior pontine and/or rostral bulbar tegmentum, the final pathway ascends into the pons, the midbrain, and the hypothalamus, and all along the way sends inhibitory connections to the arousal systems of those areas. Electrolytic lesions of the final, common pathway prevent the sleep which otherwise would have occurred after ACh application to some peripheral part of the system.

The operation of the complex is envisaged as follows: the primary hypnogenic stimuli arise in the peripheral neurons of the ascending and decending segments, as, for example, somatic sensory stimuli in the ascending limb and postcoital stimuli (arising in the limbic lobe) and conditioned stimuli, associated with habits (arising in the neocortex), in the descending limb. These influences converge, then arise in the final pathway to cause a progressively spreading inhibition. As the inhibition begins to ascend, mesencephalic arousal neurons become quiescent. These neurons when active supposedly send a tonic inhibition to the thalamus; once they are inhibited, the inhibition of the thalamus is removed. Thalamic recruiting neurons, now disinhibited, organize the thalamic–cortical activity which is recorded as spindles and slow waves. The animal is said to be in slow-wave sleep. The wave of inhibition continues to ascend, and eventually reaches the midline thalamic recruiting nuclei; inhibition of these structures releases the cortex; the cortex now shows fast, low-voltage activity. Simultaneously, somehow, recruitment of bulbopontine inhibitory neurons occurs; the result is an abrupt fall of the tone in neck muscles, inhibition of vasopressor and respiratory neurons, and inhibition of spinal reflexes. All the signs of REM sleep now are observed. Some of these, the inhibition of muscle tone, for example, are a direct effect of the activity in the hypnogenic circuit. Others, the rapid eye movements, for example, or the myoclonic twitches, or the fluctuations of the blood pressure, are due to momentary wanings of that activity. (According to this view, that is, a burst of rapid eye movements is due not to an active influence, but to a momentary *lack* of an active influence.)

Sleep, then, said Hernandez-Peon, not only is cholinergic but is unitary. Slow-wave sleep and REM sleep are not separate states, but are only different manifestations of the same basic process. A wave of inhibition rises, then falls, then rises again within a single circuit, and produces along the way the different stages of sleep.

Hernandez-Peon's arguments are forceful and his conception brings unity to an extensive diversity. But unity can also mean oversimplification. There is too much evidence to the contrary to say that sleep is exclusively cholinergic (though cholinergic mechanisms are undoubtedly involved). There is too much anatomical evidence to the contrary to say that sleep is the function exclusively of the circuit pictured by Hernandez-Peon (though part or all of that circuit is undoubtedly involved). And there is too much evidence, both anatomical and pharmacological, to the contrary to say the sleep is unitary. Thus, the two basic kinds of sleep can be selectively abolished by lesions at different sites in the brainstem (Jouvet and Jouvet, 1963), and the two types of sleep can be altered independently of one another by different drugs or groups of drugs. Although it is true that REM sleep normally occurs only after a preliminary period of slow-wave sleep, one would not expect that one phase could be altered independently of the other were sleep truly unitary. As pointed out by Jouvet (1967), REM sleep in infants often is not preceded by slow wave sleep: the newborn of several species pass directly from wakefulness into REM sleep. The implication is that a REM sleep center is mature at birth, whereas a slow-wave sleep system is not yet fully developed.

Further criticisms of the unitary theory involve Hernandez-Peon's techniques. Nowhere does this worker state the dose of the drugs being applied topically to the brain. Everywhere, dose is stated as "a few minute crystals." A crystal, no matter how minute, when iserted into a small area will most likely deliver a huge dose to the immediate locale. The effects so obtained may have more to do with toxic overdosage than with normal physiology. Also, as pointed out by Mandell and Mandell (1965), large amounts of a polar compound like ACh may have physiochemical effects that are entirely different from the drug's usual effects. One must interpret data obtained with the microinjection technique with caution; the supposedly very specific technique really offers no trustworthy advantage over other techniques in reference to specifiicity. Routtenberg *et al.* (1968) clearly showed how nonspecific the implantation technique can be. They studied the movement of carbachol, norepinephrine, and dopamine in the rat's brain. The agents were allowed to diffuse away from the site of implantation for 1 or 10 minutes; the brain was then removed and frozen. The results with dopamine showed not only a localized, spherical diffusion, but also a diffusion along nerve tracts for relatively long distances, through and to areas which normally contain no dopamine. Diffusion extended even to the contralateral side and into the ventricles and the choroid plexus of either side. The diffusion was for distances considerably greater than had been shown before. The authors conclude that attempts to ascribe anatomical localization to behavioral changes resulting from chemical stimulation of the brain should take into account the widespread movement of the chemical from its original site of application. This, of course, is something that Hernandez-Peon never did. A final drawback to his data is coincidence. The cat is a sleepy species; it is hazardous to say that a topical drug treatment which, after 5 minutes or so, induces sleep in a cat has really induced anything—the animal may simply have gone to sleep of its own accord.

In conclusion, the unitary theory cannot stand as presently presented; there is little doubt, however, the cholinergic mechanisms are involved in sleep.

K. Drugs That Can Interact with the Brain's Monoamines

Reserpine, inhibitors of monoamine oxidase (MAO), and certain other agents can change the brain's levels of monoamines; these drugs also can change sleep patterns.

1. *Distribution of Amines*

The monoamines of brain include norepinephrine (NE), dopamine (DA), and serotonin (5-hydroxytryptamine, 5-HT).

In a series of beautiful papers, the biosynthetic steps in the formation of these amines have been elucidated, largely by the work of Udenfriend, Sjoerdsma, and their associates (see Udenfriend *et al.*, 1966; Schildkraut and Kety, 1967). Tyrosine is taken up by the cell and hydroxylated to dihydroxyphenalanine (dopa); Dopa is decarboxylated by L-aromatic amino acid decarboxylase to form DA; DA is then beta-hydroxylated to form NE. Tryptophan is taken into the cell and hydroxylated by tryptophan hydroxylase to 5-hydroxytryptophan (5-HTP); 5-HTP is then decarboxylated by L-aromatic amino acid decarboxylase to 5-HT. In each pathway, the initial hydroxylation is the rate-limiting step. Epinephrine is not normally present in brain (Schildkraut and Kety, 1967). Despite this, the enzyme, phenylethanolamine *N*-methyl transferase, which converts NE to epinephrine—and which was for a long time regarded to reside only in the mammalian adrenal medulla—has now also been detected in the mammalian brain. Ciaranello *et al.* (1969) report that the enzyme is located, in rat and dog brain, chiefly in the rostral brainstem and in the hypothalamus and diencephalon; smaller amounts were found in midbrain and pons. Pohorecky *et al.* (1969) also find the enzyme in the hypothalamus but report much higher amounts in the olfactory tubercle and the olfactory bulb. Significant amounts appear also in the pons and medulla, and small quantities in the cortex, the hippocampus, and the cerebellum. Thus, although endogenous epinephrine itself has not yet been demonstrated in mammalian brain, the enzyme required for its synthesis has been. It is possible, then, that epinephrine will soon join the other monoamines as possible central neurohumors.

The distribution of phenylethanolamine *N*-methyl transferase follows in a rough fashion the distributions of NE, DA, and 5-HT. Vogt (1954), using bioassay techniques to detect NE, produced a mapping that localized NE chiefly to the area postrema, the hypothalamus, and the gray stratum around the aqueduct; lesser amounts were found in the medulla, pons, medial thalamus, and the limbic cortex. A fluorescence technique, developed by Hillarp and associates (Falck *et al.*, 1962) has confirmed and amplified Vogt's findings. The technique involves a condensation of NE, DA, and 5-HT with formaldehyde; tetrahydroisoquinoline derivates are formed; these then react with protein to form insoluble complexes. The NE and DA form a green fluorescing complex, 5-HT a yellow one; special techniques now allow the separation of NE and DA (Hillarp *et al.*, 1966). No amine appears in glia and little in the neuron's cell body. The fluorescence appears almost exlcusively in the ends of the axons, in minute varicosities. The axons of NE and DA neurons end upon cell bodies of other NE and DA neurons, and upon 5-HT neurons; the axons of 5-HT neurons, however, end only on cells that do not contain monoamines.

All three amines are present in the hypothalamus (Falck, 1964). In the pons and medulla, NE and DA cells are most rich in lateral structures, whereas 5-HT cells congregate in the midline, especially in the nucleus raphe dorsalis and the nucleus raphe medianus (Hillarp *et al.*, 1966). The median eminence and the caudate are peculiarly rich in DA (Falck, 1964). Some NE and 5-HT appears in various neocortical areas (Hillarp *et al.*, 1966).

In some areas of the cat's brain, the levels of NE and 5-HT are stable throughout the day, but in others the amines display a complex series of diurnal rhythms. These rhythms are not synchronous in the various areas; instead, the different areas seem to behave independently of one another. These observations were first made by Reis and Wurtman (1968) and have been extended by Reis *et al.* (1968, 1969). The biochemical mechanisms that control these rhythms remain, for now, obscure, as do the functional consequences (if any) for the animal. It is possible, though, that the rhythms of body temperature and hormonal secretions secretions may be linked to these amine rhythms.

Of the three amines, NE appears to be especially labile to various forms of stress. As noted, electroconvulsive shock in the rat can lead to a prolonged increase in the turnover of central NE (Kety *et al.*, 1967). So, too, can lesser forms of stress, such as mild electric shocks applied to the animal's footpads (Thierry *et al.*, 1968), the deprivation of REM sleep (Pujol *et al.*, 1968), immobilization (Corrodi *et al.*, 1968), and crowding (Bliss and Ailion, 1969). Similar stressful situations can also increase DA and 5-HT turnover at times (Bliss *et al.*, 1968), and 5-HT turnover is increased after deprivation of REM sleep (Glowinski *et al.*, 1969). It is difficult at this time to say just what all these findings might mean.

2. Role of Brain Amines

The amines no doubt have an important role in the brain. As pointed out by Kirshner (1966) the enzymes of their formation and destruction are present in high content; if the amines had no role, all this elaborate machinery would be meaningless. Further, the turnover rate of the amines is high (Udenfriend and Zaltman-Nirenberg, 1963). Just what the role might be, however, is still unknown. Neurohumoral mediation and neurohumoral modulation are much discussed, and the possible connection between NE and mood appears intriguing (Schildkraut and Kety, 1967). Perhaps the area which is becoming most clear is the function of DA in the substantia nigra and the caudate nucleus. These functions and their relationship to Parkinsonism have been reviewed by Hornykiewicz (1966).

Beyond this, however, there is little that can be said with certainty. Speculation in the field is abundant, whereas proven facts are rare.

3. Reserpine

This drug can lower brain amine levels (Brodie *et al.*, 1960); its effects on sleep may or may not be connected with these changes.

One of the subjective side effects of reserpine in man is excessive dreaming, "bizarre" dreaming, frequent nightmares (Muller *et al.*, 1955; Hartmann, 1966). Tissot (1965) found a fairly large increase of REM sleep in humans after reserpine (3–4 mg); the amount of REM sleep rose from a control level of 22% of total sleep time to 41%; the average number of REM sleep episodes rose from 3.0 to 4.6 per night. Hartmann (1966) also found an increase of REM sleep in humans after reserpine. Slow-wave sleep was not changed. The effect reached its peak 1–2 days after a single dose (1–2 mg) and then slowly disappeared; the predrug baseline was reached in about a week. Hoffman and Domino (1969), in a careful study, observed the effects in man of large doses of reserpine (0.01, 0.04, and 0.14 mg/kg, administered intramuscularly). There was a clear, dose-dependent reduction of non-REM sleep; the effect lasted for 96 hours. By contrast there was a large, dose-related increase after reserpine of stage 1 and REM sleep. On the night of the drug's administration, most of this increase was due to elevated stage 1 sleep; REM sleep was slightly inhibited, perhaps because of drug-induced discomfort. There then followed a prolonged period of increased REM sleep. This REM sleep was somewhat different from placebo REM sleep—the rapid eye movements were spaced further apart. The authors commented that it was almost as if, with the reduction of slow-wave sleep, REM could "pursue a more leisurely, indolent course." Rapid eye movement latency was greatly shortened. In rabbits, reserpine may also increase the frequency and length of REM sleep periods (Khazan and Sawyer, 1964). In monkeys, reserpine clearly increases REM sleep. This was shown by Reite *et al.* (1969) who worked with *Macaca mulatta;* their dose of reserpine was 0.25 mg/kg. The drug was given at noon. The polygraph studies were begun at 10:00 P.M. and continued until 7:00 A.M. The animals, who served as their own controls, were not allowed to sleep during the day. The drug increased minutes of REM sleep, REM sleep as a percent of total sleep, and the mean number of REM episodes. However, REM latency was greatly reduced, and total sleep time was not significantly changed. Reite *et al.* declined to speculate about any biochemical basis of the changes. Oswald (1969), however, thinks that increased REM sleep after reserpine may reflect not so much changes in amine levels as changes in the synthesis of new protein, i.e., the new storage granules. He relies here on some observations of Iverson that recovery after reserpine depends not upon the restocking of old "cupboards" (the old, depleted amine granules) with new amines, but upon the synthesis of new cupboards themselves. Obviously, though, the situation is too complex and ill-understood to make any such arbitrary deductions at this time.

One might think that reserpine has clearly now been shown to increase REM sleep. But such is not the case. For it is usually held (Jouvet, 1967, 1968, 1969) that reserpine inhibits REM sleep in a very special way. This is largely because Jouvet and his co-workers (Matsamoto and Jouvet, 1964; Delorme *et al.*, 1965; Delorme, 1966) found quite a different response to the drug in cats. The dose used was 0.5 mg/kg (0.25 mg/kg caused no changes in the cat's sleep cycle). Soon after the drug was given, both slow-wave sleep and REM sleep were abolished altogether; but the PGO spikes were greatly stimulated by reserpine. They appeared about 45 minutes after an intravenous dose and persisted, with a greater than normal voltage and frequency, for 30 to 50 hours. During that period, slow-wave sleep and REM sleep gradually began to reappear. Slow-wave sleep came back first; the PGO spiking continued on into this slow-wave sleep. The REM sleep was abolished for 20 hours or more. If, however, during the initial period, the cat were given dopa, the agitation would subside, and there would appear first a period of slow-wave sleep and then periods of typical REM sleep. The dopa effect persisted for about 6 hours, and then the reserpine syndrome reasserted itself. Jouvet interpreted these results to indicate that the dopa temporarily replenished the stores of central NE, and this NE then led to the restoration of REM sleep. Such an interpretation is unwarranted. As Oswald (1968) points out, it is difficult to make any interpretation at all, due to uncertainties in current knowledge concerning the distortion of brain chemistry by the large initial dose of reserpine.

Further, it has been shown (Glowinski and Iverson, 1966) that exogenous dopa leads chiefly to an increase of brain DA but to little or no increase in brain NE, and that this may occur prominantly in 5-HT neurons and in glial cells, both of which possess L-aromatic amino acid decarboxylase and both of which lack dopamine–β-hydroxylase. The situation is even more altered in the reserpinized animal (Corrodi and Fuxe, 1967)—after reserpine, dopa not only fails to elevate brain NE stores, but can even fail to change brain DA levels. Thus we do not really have any idea of how dopa might confer a restoration of REM sleep upon the reserpinized cat. The mechanism could just as likely be peripheral (an improvement of some function depressed by reserpine, thus easing some reserpine-induced discomfort) as central.

Hoffman and Domino (1969) have repeated in the cat some of the findings of Jouvet; they used intramuscular doses of reserpine comparable to the doses which they found to increase REM sleep in man. Their highest dose (0.16 mg/kg) induced the onset of PGO spiking. The cortical EEG showed a low-voltage, desynchronized pattern for several hours after the administration of the drug. Despite this, the cats seemed lightly somnolent. In any case, non-REM sleep was suppressed. In addition, REM sleep was suppressed promptly and for a long time. It never tended to increase, as it had in humans. Thus, the cat and man respond quite differently to equivalent doses of reserpine.

Gottesmann (1966) set out to duplicate in the rat what Jouvet had found in the cat. The doses of reserpine used in trying to inhibit the rat's REM sleep were the following (all given intraperitoneally): 0.5, 0.75, 1.0, 1.25, 1.5, 1.75, 2.0, 2.25, 2.5, 2.75, 3.0, 3.25, 4.0, 5.0, and 7.0 mg/kg. The "lower" doses (0.5–2.5 mg/kg) produced a reserpine syndrome, with initial agitation, then sedation, irregular respiration, and diarrhea—and no change in REM sleep. That is to say, no suppression. In some animals, though, there was a slight "rebound effect." (The author does not explain in any way what he means by that.) The doses between 2.75 and 5 mg/kg only made things worse—severe agitation followed by prostration, but still no or little inhibition of REM sleep. (One can only admire the animals' hardiness.) Finally, with the 7-mg/kg dose, the desired end was achieved—a "systematic elimination" of REM sleep. The rats, it might be added, were also comatose. In other words, this was not sleep at all; it was a systematic elimination not of REM sleep but of consciousness and arousability. Despite the quality of these data, Jouvet (1968) cites them as evidence pointing toward the involvement of central amines, especially NE, in the production of REM sleep.

Tabushi and Himwich (1969), in a careful study, found that reserpine in the rabbit caused a biphasic response—initial arousal and then a period of slow-wave sleep with a dose-dependent inhibition of REM sleep. The drug (0.05–1.0 mg/kg) was given intravenously. These results, of course, differ sharply with those of Khazan and Sawyer (1964), cited previously. The reason for the discrepancy is not clear.

In summary, it is clear that reserpine increases REM sleep in primates. The same may or may not be true of rabbits. The cat, however, responds to the alkaloid in a bizarre manner: REM sleep per se is suppressed, but one of its phasic signs, the PGO spikes, is markedly increased. The study of the drug in the rat awaits an unbiased trial.

4. Monoamine Oxidase Inhibitors

The short-acting MAO inhibitors, such as harmaline, cause in the cat a suppression of REM sleep for 12 to 18 hours. The longer-acting, irreversible inhibitors of the enzyme, such as iproniazid and nialamide, lead to a total suppression of REM sleep for about 4 days; slow-wave sleep, at the same time, is augmented (Jouvet *et al.*, 1965b). The signs of REM sleep slowly reappear, led by the PGO spiking activity, which returns first. In man, MAO inhibitors also can abolish REM sleep; this deprivation is followed by a large rebound effect—a tranylcypromine addict spent 75.7% of his first withdrawal night in REM sleep (Legassicke *et al.*, 1965). The rebound effect has not been noted in cats (Delorme, 1966).

Delorme *et al.* (1966) noted that hydroxybutyrate will quickly induce REM sleep in the cat after atropine pretreatment but will not do so after nialamide. The authors feel that this, as well as the results mentioned above, support the idea that MAO has an important, central role in the initiation of REM sleep. The shift from slow-wave sleep to REM sleep might be MAO-mediated. How? Perhaps, say Delorme *et al.*, some metabolite of 5-HT triggers the REM sleep center into action.

The effects of MAO inhibitors in the cat have been reproduced in the rat by Jouvet's group (Mouret *et al.*, 1968a); nialamide was the agent used, at 400 mg/kg. The initial effect was intense agitation, which persisted for up to 2 days; some of the animals had nasal hemorrhages during this period. Slow-wave sleep returned between the twelfth and forty-eighth hours; REM sleep was suppressed for 48 to 72 hours. It then gradually returned and was back to baseline at 84 to 144 hours after drug administration. There was no rebound. Again, the interpretation given these data is that some metabolite of 5-HT is needed to trigger REM sleep. Another interpretation is that toxic doses of any drug can inhibit REM sleep.

Small doses of MAO inhibitors tend to elevate REM sleep in man, whereas large doses do the opposite. Wyatt *et al.* (1969) studied a series of depressed patients treated with low doses (5–10 mg/day) of phenelzine. In each of 5 patients, there was an increase of REM sleep, which was sustained throughout the drug's administration. Higher doses (60–75 mg/day) inhibited REM sleep; after varying periods of therapy (7–30 days), REM sleep was abolished. This abolishment, it might be added, was accompanied by sustained clinical improvement. Abrupt cessation of the high dose led to a REM rebound. Akindele *et al.* (1970) found a similar effect with phenelzine (60–90 mg/day) in depressed patients. Doses which elevated mood also tended to abolish REM sleep completely. Further, the enhancement of mood tended to coincide with the onset of REM abolishment. One patient went through a period of fifty-two successive nights without any sign of REM sleep; she suffered no obvious ill consequences. In normal volunteers, too, phenelzine tended to produce a simultaneous elevation of mood and inhibition of REM sleep. Rebound followed inhibition.

Reite *et al.* (1969) found inhibition of REM sleep by iproniazid in monkeys; tranylcypromine had a similar but weaker effect.

What can we conclude from all this? Not very much. At least one thing seems clear, however, i.e., in humans, REM sleep is not a sine qua non for mental well-being—at least not if the patient is being given an MAO inhibitor. This kind of REM inhibition, indeed, enhances mood and combats depressive illnesses. Beyond that, little is clear. The role of MAO as the triggerer of REM sleep is far from being proven. The MAO inhibitors, especially the long-lasting, irreversible ones, have an array of actions other than inhibition of MAO; there is no proof that the effect of these drugs is due to inhibition of MAO or to changes in amine levels. I can only conclude that MAO inhibitors have variable effects on REM sleep. I also would plead for the use in animals of nontoxic doses in the study of so delicate an entity as REM sleep. The activities of the MAO inhibitors are not fully understood, even after 20 years of study, and theories of sleep based on MAO inhibitor data are bound to be shaky.

5. *Other Amine Mobilizers*

Studies with certain other drugs can lead to even more shaky conclusions. If MAO inhibitors are not yet well understood, these newer, more complicated drugs, such as the arylalkylamine, RO 4–6861, are even less so. Delorme (1966) found that RO 4–6861 (which supposedly liberates 5–HT but also inhibits MAO) caused a two-part syndrome in cats: agitation for 16 hours, followed by a period of reserpine-like signs, including numerous PGO spikes. Other amine mobilizers, such as the benzoquinolizines, RO 4–9288 and RO 4–9571, caused reserpine-like syndromes in cats without a period of agitation.

6. *Disulfiram*

Dusan-Peyrethon and Froment (1968) studied several doses of disulfiram in cats. This drug, like reserpine and the MAO inhibitors, has a variety of actions. One of these is inhibition of dopamine–β-hydroxylase—this can lead to a lowering of NE and an increase of DA in the brain. A "low" dose of disulfiram (200 mg/kg) caused no changes in sleep patterns (did it alter amine metabolism? the question is not answered, and the low dose is not discussed further). A "high" dose (500 mg/kg) provoked a distinct inhibition of REM sleep, and also killed the cats. A working dose of 400 mg/kg was chosen. It produced these effects: hypotonia, trembling, difficulty in walking, ataxia, athetoid movements, mydriasis, an increase of slow-wave sleep, and an inhibition of REM sleep. The inhibition was maximal between the twenty-fourth and thirtieth hours after drug administration. The amplitude and frequency of the PGO spikes were both diminished. Interpretation—NE mediates REM sleep and has an important role in the genesis of the PGO spikes. Possible alternative interpretation—sick cats have sick sleep.

7. *Amine-Depleting Drugs*

In addition to drugs that alter monoamine metabolism in complicated, ill-understood ways, there are now several agents which have a more specific kind of effect.

a. Parachlorophenylalanine (PCPA); a "Drive-Serotonin" Hypothesis of REM Sleep. Pletscher *et al.* (1964) noted that some chlorinated aryalkylamines deplete the brain of 5-HT. No behavioral effects were noted. Fuller *et al.* (1965) found that several chloramphetamine derivatives could deplete the brain of 5-HT. The mode of action was unknown; the drugs did not inhibit tryptophan hydroxylase or the uptake of 5-HTP into the brain. Further, there were behavioral effects (central stimulation) not correlated with the decline of 5-HT. Koe and Weissman (1966) developed PCPA, which is a close structural analog of parachloromethamphetamine. In mice, rats, and dogs, PCPA depleted the brain of 5-HT. The effect was quite slow in onset—maximal depletion occurred only 3 days after a single dose. No great change of the NE or tryptamine levels occurred. No behavioral effects were seen. In humans treated with 1000 mg/day, however, there were noticeable subjective effects: tiredness, dizziness, light-headedness, nausea, uneasiness, paresthesias, and headache (Cremata and Koe, 1966). *In vitro,* the drug inhibited tryptophan hydroxylase. Tyrosine hydroxylase was weakly inhibited. Treatment of a PCPA-treated animal with a MAO inhibitor led to an increase of the brain's

NE level, but no change occurred in the 5-HT content. There were no effects on the brain's uptake of 5-HTP. The conclusion was that PCPA depleted tissues of 5-HT by a specific inhibition of tryptophan hydroxylase. Unanswered was why the effect took so long to appear—perhaps some metabolite of the drug was the active agent.

Delorme (1966), working with Jouvet, treated four cats with PCPA (100–350 mg/kg). He found marked behavioral changes, perhaps the most remarkable changes in the pattern of sleep yet produced by any drug. No effects were seen during the first 16 hours. Then there was a fairly abrupt increase of wakefulness. There was no agitation; the animals were calm, with mydriasis and a retracted nictitating membrane. Slow-wave sleep and REM sleep both declined, without, however, totally disappearing. Sixty hours after PCPA, slow-wave sleep was at a minimum, with only short periods of spindling. At this time there was an inversion of the usual slow-wave/REM sleep ratio—REM sleep was now more abundant than slow-wave sleep. Also, the REM episodes now were double the control value in length. And a phenomenon which is never observed normally occurred—the direct transition from wakefulness into REM sleep. Delorme called the syndrome "experimental narcolepsy." The return to the baseline values took a week. The syndrome was attributed to a depletion of the brain's 5-HT. No actual measurements of amine levels were made, nor was an attempt made to reverse the syndrome with 5-HTP.

Delorme *et al.* (1967) also found a suppression of total sleep by parachloromethamphetamine, but this agent, unlike PCPA, also led to signs of agitation.

Koella *et al.* (1968) confirmed Delorme's findings and extended them. Four doses of PCPA were used in cats, and brain 5-HT levels were studied; in addition, 5-HTP was given during the period of PCPA's actions. Again, PCPA was found to have a long latency of action, as long as 24 hours. After this initial period, all stages of sleep began to fall. The maximal effect occurred at 48 to 72 hours after the drug. The effect was dose-related. At the time of the maximal production of insomnia, occasional REM periods intruded directly into wakefulness. Except for the insomnia, there were no behavioral abnormalities. The 5-HTP quickly (within 10 minutes) reversed the insomnia, conferring 8 hours of sleep (mainly slow-wave sleep) upon the animals: the PCPA effect then reasserted itself. The levels of 5-HT were markedly depressed in various brain areas, but the changes in amine levels followed the course of the insomnia rather poorly—sleep returned to normal well before 5-HT did. The latter was not back to baseline until 16 to 20 days after the single dose of PCPA.

Mouret *et al.* (1968b) found a similar insomnia in rats treated with

PCPA. What follows is the time table of the effects after a single intraperitoneal injection of PCPA (500 mg/kg).

Hours 1–4: acute abdominal distress

Hours 4–16: nothing unusual, except for a mild inhibition of REM sleep

Hours 16–40: total abolition of REM sleep; the EEG showed an almost continuous tracing of low-voltage, fast activity (yet, on occasion, the animals seemed to be asleep)

Hours 40–76: here the peak effects were seen; very little sleep of any variety, and distinct behavioral changes—hyperactivity, hyperhagia, hyperdipsia, agitation, fighting

Hours 76–88: REM sleep returned, though only tentatively; slow-wave sleep continued to be suppressed

Hours 88-280: a gradual return of all the stages of sleep

Hours 280–292: the predrug baseline was finally reattained.

The levels of brain 5-HT fell quickly. They were clearly down at the twelfth hour; maximal depletion was at about the hundredth hour; there then began a gradual return to normal.

Weitzman *et al.* (1968) found a similar picture in monkeys treated with 330–1000 mg/kg of PCPA. Slow-wave sleep was inhibited more profoundly than was REM sleep. Thus, REM sleep as a percent of total sleep rose. Serotonin levels were reduced in seven of eight brain areas; an odd finding was a rise of 5-HT in the cerebellum.

Such results have prompted many to conclude that 5-HT is essential for the occurrence of sleep. Koella (1968) has even suggested changing the name of 5-HT from serotonin to "somnotonin."

Engelman *et al.* (1967) have studied the action of PCPA in patients suffering from the carcinoid syndrome. A hallmark of this condition is, of course, an overproduction of 5-HT. The PCPA induced a clear reduction of urinary indoles, but failed to alter blood 5-HT levels. Nevertheless, the gastrointestinal symptoms of the disorder were greatly alleviated. The characteristic flush of the syndrome, however, was only faintly reduced, if at all, perhaps indicating the nonparticipation of 5-HT in the genesis of this sign. Only 1 patient (of 5) developed insomnia. The others, however, did develop certain other CNS symptoms: delusions, hallucinations, ataxia, and mental agitation. These symptoms sometimes required the cessation of drug therapy.

What can we gather from all these data? They strongly indicate that central 5-HT is important for the occurrence of sleep. However, there are some suggestions of a dissociation between the EEG and the animal's behavior. This all-important point has not been kept in mind in these studies. Further, the correlation between brain 5-HT levels and the EEG changes is quite poor, indeed. In addition, the consequences of phenylaline hydroxylase inhibition are not considered and have been insufficiently studied. Yet to be explained, too, is the very prolonged onset of the drug's actions; this is all the more mysterious when one considers the fast turnover rate of central 5-HT. It is of interest that 5-HTP confers upon the PCPA-treated animal a restoration of sleeplike behavior. But might not other drugs behave similarly? Drugs that have no effects upon central 5-HT levels? The question remains unanswered.

The importance, if any, of brain 5-HT for the generation of sleep remains unsettled. The evidence is so imperfect that Hobson (1969b) has questioned whether 5-HT is involved at all. Despite this, one probably can tentatively accept the idea that brain 5-HT, along with brain ACh, are somehow involved in the production of sleep. More certainly, it does appear to be shown now that 5-HT is, after all, important for normal brain functioning. It is definitely too early, however, to rename 5-HT "somnotonin."

I now must mention a curious series of experiments conducted by Dement and his associates with PCPA (Ferguson *et al.*, 1969a, b; Cohen *et al.*, 1969; Barchas *et al.*, 1970). This group of workers had previously shown that when cats are deprived of REM sleep for very long periods of time, there occurs a change in the animals' behavior. After several months of continuous REM deprivation, certain drive-related patterns of behavior become common: hypersexuality, hyperphagia, fighting, and so on (Dement, 1969). Similar changes were induced by PCPA. The drug (75–300 mg/kg) was given to a group of cats every day for periods of up to 37 days. (Why? Is not the effect of one dose marked enough?) Some cats were allowed to sleep *ad lib.*, but others were kept awake for 12 or 16 hours a day by placing them on a treadmill (Why? Is the drug itself not stress enough?)

The chronic drug treatment reduced 5-HT levels in the brain and kept them reduced throughout the study. As expected, insomnia developed. In addition, PGO spikes began to intrude into the waking EEG. As the drug was continued, sleep, both slow-wave and REM, returned somewhat, but kept below the predrug baseline. At this time, PGO spiking was about as frequent in wakefulness and slow-wave sleep as it was in REM sleep. When animals in this state were then subjected to REM deprivation, they failed to show a postdeprivation rebound. This is taken to prove that it is the loss of the phasic events of REM sleep (especially the PGO spikes) which lead to increased REM "pressure" and the rebound. The PCPA animals were having abundant phasic activity in slow-wave sleep and wakefulness, and so did not need to rebound.

The behavioral effects of the chronic PCPA treatment were bizarre.

These abnormal forms of behavior were first seen as the PGO spikes began to appear in wakefulness. Hallucinatory activity was common. For example, a cat would watch the movements of an animal that was not really there; a marked burst of PGO spikes would usually accompany the hallucination. Most of the cats also showed increased drive behavior—hypersexuality and hyperphagia were common. So, too, were rage reactions and agitation. Some of the cats continued to act oddly throughout the study. Others collapsed and died.

Monkeys treated similarly developed insomnia and, after 8 to 12 days of chronic PCPA treatment, began to hallucinate.

Chlorpromazine, given to cats showing the chronic PCPA syndrome, reduced the waking PGO spikes, corrected the odd behavior, and induced sleep. The same occurred when 5-HTP was given instead of chlorpromazine. Both agents temporarily brought the "psychosis" under control. Therefore, the authors suggest that chlorpromazine can "substitute" for brain 5-HT.

Dement (1969), commenting on these findings, wrote that there is probably a "special neuronal system" in the brain which acts as a "drive system" to energize "motivational behaviors." He considers REM sleep as a "safety valve" for this drive system—a valve that allows it to discharge harmlessly and, along the way, cause dreaming. Serotonergic neurons supposedly inhibit and modulate this discharge of the drive system. With serotonin depleted, REM activities and drive behaviors appear in the waking state in an uncontrolled fashion. This could account for many of the symptoms of human psychotic illnesses.

Such, then, is a recent version of Dement's theories of REM sleep. Thus, REM sleep is still connected with psychosis; it is the function that dispels drives which otherwise would render us insane. Serotonin has been added to the picture as the central neurohumor which keeps us sane. Without REM sleep and 5-HT, we would all land in Bedlam.

The basic idea is not new. The Elizabethan-Jacobean writer Thomas Dekker saw a connection between sleep and sanity:

> Do but consider what an excellent thing sleep is: it is so inestimable a jewel that, if a tyrant would give his crown for an hour's slumber, it cannot be bought: of so beautiful a shape is it, that though a man lie with an Empress, his heart cannot beat quiet till he leaves her embracements to be at rest with the other: yea, so greatly indebted are we to this kinsman of death, that we owe the better tributary, half of our life, to him: and there is good cause why we should do so: for sleep is that golden chain that ties health and our bodies together. Who complains of want? or wounds? of cares? of great men's oppressions? of captivity? whilst he sleepeth? Beggars in their beds take as much pleasure as kings: can we therefore surfeit on this delicate Ambrosia? Can we drink too much of that whereof to taste too little tumbles us into a churchyard,

> and to use it but indifferently throws us into Bedlam? No, no, look upon Endymion, the moon's minion, who slept three score and fifteen years, and was not a hair the worse for it.

As Kleitman (1963) notes, Kant stated that the lunatic is a wakeful dreamer, and Schopenhauer declared that a dream is a short-lasting psychosis, and a psychosis is a long-lasting dream. The study of dreams and sanity crested with Freud. Now another crest may be rolling in.

Has Dement really shown a connection between dreams and insanity? A connection between insanity and 5-HT? Pharmacologists in the 1950s thought they had shown the latter; the ideas today are shopworn. Has Dement resurrected this earlier work and brought Freud up to date?

The results found by Mouret *et al.* (1968b), in which PCPA induced behavioral changes in rats may support Dement's notions. The data of Brodie and his co-workers (Tagliamonte *et al.*, 1969) may also offer support—these investigators found that large doses of PCPA (100 mg/kg intraperitoneally, daily for 4 days) caused a profound sexual excitation in male rats. Finally, the data of Engelman *et al.* (1967) may add further support—PCPA in humans caused striking psychotic-like symptoms in some of the patients. Is an altered metabolism of central 5-HT, then, the cause of schizophrenia?

I am unconvinced, though willing to wait and watch the future developments with interest. But I am disturbed at the heavy-handed approach of Dement's experiments. Why continue to jolt the animals day after day with PCPA, when one dose alone has such pronounced and long-lasting effects? Why, also disregard so completely the other known biochemical effects of PCPA? Udenfriend and his co-workers (Lipton *et al.*, 1967) showed that PCPA inhibits phenylalanine hydroxylase just as readily as it inhibits tryptophan hydroxylase; they suggested, therefore, that PCPA might be a useful tool for the production in animals of experimental phenylketonuria. The drug does, in fact, cause some of the signs of phenylketonuria—increased levels of phenylpyruvic acid in the blood and urine, for example. Hence Dement's cats and monkeys probably had experimental phenylketonuria. Beyond that there remains the fact that toxic psychoses can be produced with various drugs. Further, if 5-HT keeps us out of Bedlam, they why did it take 8–12 days of chronic PCPA treatment before the monkeys began to behave oddly? Might this not simply be the result of a severe toxic state, due to prolonged and heavy overuse of the drug? My answer will be yes until more careful, less stressful, and less extreme experiments are at hand to convince me otherwise.

b. α-Methyldopa (α-MDOPA). This drug, studied first as an inhibitor of L-aromatic amino acid decarboxylase, inhibits both the decarboxylation of 5-HTP and of dopa; but it induces a depletion of catecholamines which is so rapid that some other mechanism must be at work, perhaps the formation of false transmitters (Sourkes *et al.*, 1961; Carlsson, 1964). No depletion of 5-HT occurs. Delorme (1966) found that in cats, α-MDOPA caused first a fleeting episode of agitation, then a state of calm, with miosis and hypotension. A total lack of PGO spikes occurred rather quickly; somewhat later, REM sleep disappeared altogether. Sleep was characterized mainly by spindles; slow-wave activity had disappeared too. After 10 hours, slow waves and a few PGO spikes reappeared; REM sleep returned several hours later. Recovery was complete after 24 hours. There was no rebound increase of REM sleep.

Dusan-Peyrethon *et al.* (1968) found similar effects in cats which had been deprived of REM sleep for 3 days. In these animals, α-MDOPA, given at the end of the deprivation period, caused a suppression of REM sleep for about 12 hours (where, of course, one normally would have seen a postdeprivation rebound.) After the 12 hours, a rebound did finally occur, but it was small. Completely lacking here, however, is any proof of specificity. The assumption is that the α-MDOPA delayed the REM rebound because it depleted the brain of NE, the would-be mediator of the REM rebound. But is it not possible that other drugs might also delay the rebound—drugs that suppress REM sleep without simultaneously altering NE metabolism? Perhaps an antihistamine, or atropine, or diphenylhydantoin could act as effectively as α-MDOPA.

c. *α-Methyl-m-tyrosine* (*α-MMT*). This drug inhibits the same enzyme inhibited by α-MDOPA (Sourkes *et al.*, 1961) but probably also depletes tissues of catecholamines by the formation of a false transmitter (Carlsson, 1964). Delorme (1966) studied α-MMT in 4 cats. The first 2 hours after injection were marked by an awake, mydriatic animal, but there was no agitation. The polygraph showed intense electromyographic activity, rapid cortical activity, numerous rapid eye movements, and spikes similar to PGO spikes, but of a lesser amplitude. Then, after 2 hours, slow waves invaded the tracing to occupy more than 80% of the total time. The REM sleep was suppressed, but only for about 3 hours; thereafter it rapidly returned. The PGO activity never disappeared at all. As REM sleep returned, slow-wave sleep declined back to the baseline. The effects were attributed to NE depletion, but no amine levels were measured. Also not considered is the possibility that REM sleep may actually be inhibited by brain NE and by false transmitters formed from drugs such as α-MDOPA and α-MMT. As will be seen, Jouvet feels that brain NE has an important role in the production of REM sleep. The data obtained with α-MDOPA and α-MMT could be easily taken to indicate just the opposite.

d. α-Methyltyrosine (α-MT). This agent has been used by several groups in studies of sleep; the results have been conflicting. Part of the conflict is probably due to the drug's toxicity. With this as with other drugs, toxicity can lead to wayward conclusions.

After tyrosine is taken up into the cell, as has been mentioned, it can be converted to DA and NE. The first enzyme in the sequence of steps leading to the amines is tyrosine hydroxylase. The conversion of tyrosine to dopa is the rate-limiting step (Levitt *et al.*, 1965; Udenfriend *et al.*, 1966).

A number of agents can inhibit tyrosine hydroxylase. Among these are certain L-aromatic amino acids. This inhibition is due to competition with the substrate. Of these amino acids, α-MT is among the most potent (Nagatsu *et al.*, 1964).

Spector *et al.* (1965) found that α-MT causes a fairly rapid depletion of NE stores. A single dose (80 mg/kg) caused in guinea pigs a maximal depletion in 8 hours; the NE of brain fell to about 50% of the control level; thereafter repletion began, complete within 24 to 36 hours. No change occurred in the 5-HT levels. Repeated doses (80 mg/kg at 3-hour intervals for 24 hours) caused the brain NE and DA levels to fall into an undetectable range; adrenal catecholamines, owing to their lower turnover rate, fell only slightly. The drug was shown not to deplete NE by a release mechanism. More importantly, no false transmitters were formed. Nor did α-MT inhibit the ability of tissues to take up and bind exogenous NE—an action which is seen with both reserpine and α-MMT. The evidence, then, pointed toward the inhibition of tyrosine hydroxylase *in vivo* as well as *in vitro.* Thus the drug greatly inhibited the incorporation of tyrosine-^{14}C into DA, NE, and epinephrine but did not inhibit the incorporation of dopa-^{3}H. The dose of α-MT that inhibits whole-brain tyrosine hydroxylase by 50% in rats is about 29 mg/kg (intraperitoneally) (Weissman *et al.*, 1966).

Inhibition of the enzyme and reduced levels of tissue catecholamines go pretty much hand-in-hand. This was shown by Udenfriend *et al.* (1966). They gave guinea pigs *l*-α-MT (100 mg/kg) and, then, at different time intervals, tyrosine-^{14}C—the conversion of which to labeled DA and NE was taken as a measure of enzyme inhibition. The activity of the enzyme in brain fell quickly; the drop of brain catecholamines was somewhat more slow, but the curves were in general parallel, with maximal effects between the sixth and tenth hours. At this time enzyme activity was almost completely absent, and catecholamine levels were down by 60 to 70%. Recovery was well under way after 16 hours and was complete in 36 hours. Tissue levels of the drug itself followed a parallel curve.

α-Methyltyrosine may, of course, also alter the activities of many other enzymes, but, thus far, beside tyrosine hydroxylase, only tyrosine transaminase has been found to be affected. Black and Axelrod (1968) noted that α-MT induced hepatic tyrosine transaminase in the rat. This effect coincided with the lowering of the brain's catecholamine levels. Reserpine has the same effect. Thus it might be that the daily rhythm of hepatic tyrosine transaminase—a rhythm which reaches its nadir at 6:00 A.M., just when the rhythm of brainstem NE is reaching its highpoint—is under nervous control. When α-MT induction of liver tyrosine transaminase is at a peak level, treatment of the animal with dopa will bring the enzyme activity back to normal. Further, MAO inhibitors abolish the rhythm of liver tyrosine transaminase, coincidentally with their elevation of brain NE (Axelrod and Black, 1968).

Gibb and Webb (1969) have found, for the first time, that there is tyrosine transaminase in rat brain. Its activity there is so great that the conversion of tyrosine to *p*-hydroxyphenylpyruvate is about 100 times greater than the conversion of tyrosine to dopa. Tyrosine transaminase might obviously be involved, then, in the regulation of brain catecholamine stores. Reserpine and α-MT strongly inhibit brain tyrosine transaminase (just the opposite of what they do to the liver enzyme). Dopa reverses the inhibition. These changes are, thus, probably mediated by the catecholamines themselves, with low levels of DA and NE "turning off" transamination in brain and, perhaps, shunting more tyrosine through the hydroxylation step. So this effect of α-MT is probably an indirect one, and the only direct action now known is the inhibition of tyrosine hydroxylase.

Maitre in 1965 wrote that α-MT, especially on chronic use, may lead to the formation of false transmitters, but this is probably not so, at least not to any great extent. If studies in man are applicable to other species, it can be held that false-transmitter formation is a very minor aspect of α-MT's actions. Engelman *et al.* (1968a) studied the metabolism of α-MT in humans, both after a single dose and after chronic treatment. After a single dose, all of the drug was recovered from the urine in unaltered form. It is only upon chronic treatment that some biotransformation occurs. This leads to the formation of α-MDOPA, α-methyldopamine and α-methylnorepinephirine. No decarboxylation of α-MT to α-methyltyramine could be detected. And even when metabolites were discovered, they altogether accounted for only 1% of the total dose excreted, the other 99% being the unaltered parent compound.

The *d*-isomer of α-MT has no effects either on tyrosine hydroxylase or on tissue catecholamine levels (Porter *et al.*, 1966). Curiously, though, the *d*-form potentiates not only α-MT, but certain other catecholamine depletors as well, for example, α-MDOPA and α-MMT. The mechanism of the effect is not known. In addition to potentiating *l*-α-MT, the *d*-isomer extends the time course of catecholamine depletion. Whereas with *l*-α-MT the peak depletion occurs 8 hours following the drug, with *dl*-α-MT, the peak effect does not occur until 16 hours after the drug, and recovery requires about 64 hours.

The reduction of catecholamines after α-MT is greater in brain than in other tissues; this probably is so because the turnover of catecholamines is higher in brain than elsewhere (Brodie *et al.*, 1966). Anden *et al.* (1966) gave a group of rats a huge dose of *dl*-α-MT (500 mg/kg) and followed the effects of the drug on brain amines by use of fluorescence microscopy. Some of the animals had previously received a transection of the spinal cord, and this led to an important finding. Two hours after the drug, there was no discernible change in catecholamine fluorescence at any site. After 4 hours, a small reduction was seen. After 8 hours, the catecholamine nerve terminals in almost all areas of the brain showed clear and sharp reductions of their typical green fluorescence. A few areas, however, showed little if any change; these included several hypothalamic nuclei. Twelve hours after the drug, the picture was about the same as that seen at 8 hours. Recovery was clearly detectable 24 hours after the drug. At no time after α-MT were 5-HT neurons affected. The depletion of fluorescence occurred, of course, in the spinal cord as well as in the brain. But in those animals whose cords had been transected, there was a clear-cut difference above and below the section—8 hours after the drug, there was marked depletion of catecholamine fluorescence above the cut, but no discernible depletion below. All of these NE terminals in the cord derive from cells that are located in the medulla. These results indicate the importance of neuronal activity for the disappearance of NE and DA after synthesis has been blocked. Depletion of catecholamines after α-MT, unlike the depletion caused by reserpine, α-MMT, and α-MDOPA, requires ongoing activity of the neuron. Thus electrical stimulation in the amygdala or medulla will significantly enhance the effects of α-MT, leading to an accelerated loss of catecholamines, both in the brain and in the spinal cord.

The toxicity of α-MT is a major problem attending its use. It is such a toxic drug that it probably will never be a useful therapeutic agent in man (though its use in humans is justified in certain very special cases). The toxicity apparently stems from the drug's insolubility. When the amino acid is given, it must be taken by mouth, or injected intraperitoneally as a suspension; the amino acid is soluble only at extreme pH ranges. The methyl and ethyl esters of the drug have been synthesized, and these are readily soluble at neutral pH; once inside the body, however, the ester link is hydrolyzed, and the ester forms of the drug become as toxic as the amino acid form. The toxicity is chiefly renal; the drug precipitates in the convoluted tubules, and can lead to renal failure (Moore, 1966a, K. E. Moore *et al.*, 1967; Hook and Moore, 1969). In the rat, this leads to polyuria, emaciation, lethargy, and death within 28–48 hours, with an LD_{50} of about 160 mg/kg. Proteinuria and glycosuria are prominent; the blood urea nitrogen rises, and areas of the kidney become necrotic; the adrenals become markedly hemorrhagic.

The toxicity must always be kept in mind in order not to mistake a toxic reaction for a pharmacological one. Both reactions, it should be remembered, are in the same general direction—toxicity leads to lethargy and coma; the pharmacological action leads to sedation. Thus the two can be easily confused (and have been in several publications). Unless it can be shown that a given species (for example, a monkey) differs from the rat in its LD_{50}, then doses exceeding 150 mg/kg cannot lead to clear-cut results. A way around this problem—and one which has been used frequently—is to give the drug in multiple injections, administered at intervals of 3–4 hours; this procedure markedly reduces the toxicity (K. E. Moore *et al.*, 1967) and can allow the use of fairly large doses.

The effects of α-MT include acute sedation; this is seen in humans (Sjoerdsma *et al.*, 1965; Engelman *et al.*, 1968b) and in animals (Spector *et al.*, 1965). In man, withdrawal of the drug can cause anxiety and insomnia (Sjoerdsma *et al.*, 1965). The drug has no antipsychotic effects, but leads to improved nighttime sleep both in schizophrenics and in normals (Gershon *et al.*, 1967; Charalampous and Brown, 1967). This effect on sleep, I must emphasize, was deduced from subjective experience; no objective EEG studies have been carried out in man.

In animals, α-MT inhibits the conditioned avoidance response (Moore, 1966b; Rech *et al.*, 1966), and other behavioral parameters (Schoenfeld and Seiden, 1969). The body of the evidence suggests that these effects are not agonistic effects of α-MT itself, but are correlated with a lowering of brain DA and NE levels (Dominic and Moore, 1969).

If central NE is the key that unlocks REM sleep, then α-MT should clearly jam the lock.

Crowley *et al.* (1968) claimed that, in monkeys, α-MT dramatically inhibits REM sleep. Their dose, however, was in excess of 400 mg/kg. This high dose would kill a rat, a guinea pig, a cat. The LD_{50} of α-MT in monkeys is unknown. The best we can say, then, is that the dose used by Crowley *et al.* was too high to indicate anything, one way or the other, unless the monkey handles the drug in a way different from the way it is handled by other species.

Torda (1968) used 80 mg/kg of α-MT, repeated 3 times at 6-hour intervals, in rats. The REM sleep went down and slow-wave sleep went up; NE went down. The study was blemished by the way the drug was administered—it was "surgically implanted," i.e., the dry powdered form of the drug was inserted into the animal's peritoneal cavity by way of an incision through the skin and peritoneum. Animals were also given α-MT as a suspension, injected intraperitoneally, but the author does not state which animals were used for the sleep studies and which were used for brain amine studies. Nor were there any surgically implanted placebo studies. In view of all this surgery, anesthesia, trauma, and discomfort, the results of the study are of doubtful value.

Iskander and Kaelbling (1969) gave α-MT to a group of cats. The dose was 80 mg/kg, repeated 4 times at 6-hour intervals. The form of the drug used was the insoluble *l*-amino acid. The animal's EEG was recorded continuously for 4 days prior to the drug treatment, during the drug treatment, and then for 7 more days. Control cats were handled similarly, except that they were given vehicle injections. The drug caused a 50% inhibition of REM sleep during the period of its administration. During this time, brain NE levels were presumed to have gone to zero or near zero (though actual amine determinations were not made). The discrepancy between the presumed 100% reduction of central NE and the 50% reduction of REM sleep is not commented upon. After the last injection of α-MT, REM sleep quickly rose to 300% above the predrug baseline. The authors reason that this huge quantity of REM sleep was being mediated by new NE, being synthesized by a disinhibited tyrosine hydroxylase. Such an interpretation ignores everything that is currently known concerning the time course of the effects of α-MT. A more plausible interpretation is that the 50% reduction was due to discomfort and perhaps nausea caused by the drug, and that the 300% increase of REM sleep coincided with very low central catecholamine levels.

King and Jewett (1968), in contrast to the above findings, had reported that several doses of *l*-α-MT increase REM sleep in cats. We gave the animals a single dose of the drug (50, 100, and 150 mg/kg, intraperitoneally) and then recorded continuously for 23 hours. The animals served as their own controls. There was no effect in the first 4-hour period after the drug's administration. Then there was a clear enhancement of REM sleep which lasted for up to 16 hours.

We have since extended these studies to include two further doses (25 and 3.125 mg/kg) and an analysis of several brain areas for NE after 100 mg/kg of α-MT, intraperitoneally. There was an enhancement of REM sleep, even after the smallest dose. The effect was dose-related—the smallest dose caused fleeting changes, the higher ones being larger and more long-lasting changes. Further, as the dose was raised, the drug began to increase non-REM sleep as well as REM sleep, but REM sleep was the stage most consistently elevated. This came at a time when NE levels were decreased in several areas of the brain, including the medulla, pons, and midbrain. We concluded that the clearest interpretation of our data was that in the cat central catecholamines inhibit REM sleep, or, more precisely, inhibit those signs of REM sleep that we measured—cortical EEG activation, hippocampal theta rhythm, PGO spikes, skeletal muscle atony, and rapid eye movements. We felt that perhaps some other aspect of REM sleep may be a function of central catecholamines but concluded that the function has yet to be discovered.

Our studies are incomplete and should be extended. The augmentation of REM sleep was always over by the sixteenth to twentieth hours after drug administration. Unanswered is whether or not, after the augmentation of REM sleep, there might not be a "negative rebound" in the second 24-hour period following the drug. If REM- deprivation leads to a REM rebound, then might not a period of REM overabundance lead to a period showing a poverty of REM sleep? Our studies have left this and similar questions unexplored.

Weitzman *et al.* (1969) gave monkeys 125 mg/kg of *l*-α-MT. A distinct, heavy inhibition of REM sleep was the result. This came about chiefly as a result of a greatly increased cycle length, i.e., the periods of REM sleep were separated from one another by very long episodes of non-REM sleep. Total sleep was augmented. The drug was given both as an intraperitoneal injection and by way of a nasogastric tube. In the case of the intraperitoneal injections, there were some signs of possible toxicity—lethargy and decreased appetite for food and water. Such signs did not follow the oral administration of the drug. Both methods of dosage suppressed REM sleep equally well. Weitzman (personal communication) thinks there may be some species difference between monkey and cat in their response to α-MT.

α-Methyltyrosine has been studied in the rat by Marantz and Rechtschaffen (1967) and by Marantz *et al.* (1968). The experimental design of both studies was excellent. In the first, polygraph recordings were continued for 19 consecutive days, in a room lighted half the day, and in darkness for the rest. At 4-day intervals, the rats received a series of three intraperitoneal injections either of *l*-α-MT (as the amino acid) or of vehicle. The animals served as their own controls, and the drug and placebo injections were given in one sequence to one group of rats, and in the opposite sequence to another group. Determinations of brain NE and 5-HT levels were carried out on a separate group of rats, some given vehicle, the others drug. The results of the amine determinations were the expected ones: reduction of NE and no change of 5-HT. The results of the sleep studies were entirely negative. The drug changed nothing—no decrease and no increase of any sleep parameter. In the second study (Marantz *et al.*, 1968), rats were deprived of REM sleep for 90 hours by the flower pot method. At the eighty-sixth hour of deprivation, there began a series of four intraperitoneal injections of *l*-α-MT, 75 mg/kg of the amino acid suspended in water and given at 2-hour intervals; control animals were given four injections of saline. Recovery sleep was then allowed. A separate group of rats was handled in the same way, i.e., deprived, injected, allowed to experience some recovery sleep (12 hours of it), and then were sacrificed for amine determinations. As in the first study, α-MT had no effects. Both groups of animals, drug and placebo, rebounded from the period of REM deprivation, and both rebounds were equally large. Two rats (out of 18) developed toxic signs, and died 36–48 hours after α-MT; their EEGs became bizarre, and they were not included in the data presented. The other rats showed no signs of toxicity. Clearly, the authors concluded, the synthesis of brain NE is not essential for REM sleep in the rat.

In summary, it is clear that, in cats, α-MT augments REM sleep and that, in rats, it has no effect one way or the other. These results fail to support the monoamine hypothesis of REM sleep, but do not disprove it either. Clearer evidence would come from a drug regimen that selectively lowers brain NE levels without at the same time altering DA concentrations. In monkeys, α-MT appears to inhibit REM sleep. The striking species differences between cat, rat, and monkey await an explanation.

8. Alpha-Adrenergic Blockage

In 1967, Matsumoto and Watanabe (cited in Jouvet, 1968) treated cats with phenoxybenzamine and Dibenamine (15 mg/kg). There followed an "elective" suppression of REM sleep and an increased amount of slow-wave sleep. Nethalide, a beta-adrenergic blocking agent, caused no changes. The doses of these drugs were very high; interpretation of the results as indicating an elective blockage of REM sleep by an action on central alpha-adrenergic receptors is not justified. High doses of these drugs can cause marked peripheral effects, and these could cause the sleep patterns to be abnormal.

9. Precursors of the Amines; the Amines

Work with precursors of the amines, as well as with the amines themselves, may indicate further a role for 5-HT in sleep. A note of caution is necessary, however. Experiments in which the animal is flooded with a particular amino acid can lead to many nonspecific effects. As pointed out by Mandell and Mandell (1965), loads of one precursor inhibit the transport of other similar substances, bind cofactors, create amino acid imbalances which inhibit many enzymes, activate others, and alter pH. Further, there is the striking finding of McGeer *et al.* (1963) that after treating an animal with 5-HTP or dopa, there is an inverse relationship between 5-HT or NE content before treatment and the amine content after treatment—areas which normally contain little or no monoamine end up with the greatest percentage increase, and vice versa. Carlsson (1964) discounts these effects; he admits that dopa administration, for example, will lead to a buildup of NE in areas normally lacking NE, but he feels that since NE normally is not present in the area neither will NE's receptor be there; only those areas where NE has some physiological role will contain NE's receptor. Thus the effects of dopa treatment will be similar to the effects of endogenous NE. This, of course, may not be so. It is highly possible that loading with precursor can lead to physiologically spurious results. Thus it has been shown, for example, that cells in the CNS which normally contain catecholamines can take up 5-HTP and 5-HT (Lichtensteiger *et al.*, 1967). Therefore it is impossible to say how much of the following is valid.

a. Tryptophan. Tryptophan was administered by Pollin *et al.* (1961) to a group of schizophrenic patients treated with iproniazid. A transient phase of somnolence was an early effect; this was followed by mood elevation and increased extroversion, with cases of euphoria and marked amorous feelings. In a group of normal volunteers, tryptophan (30–90 mg/kg, taken orally) caused drowsiness, diminished interest, listlessness, frequent yawning, and sleep. All subjects could easily be aroused. On awakening, the volunteers became euphoric, talkative, and overactive; 3 (out of 7) became so uninhibited in their conversation that the nurses in attendance complained. One volunteer became hilarious, laughing inappropriately. All 7 sustained nystagmus (Smith and Prockop, 1962). Oswald *et al.* (1966) administered tryptophan to a group of 16 normal volunteers. Marked effects included euphoria and lewd conversation. In 5 of the subjects, REM latency was reduced. Two of the people showed this effect consistently; 1 showed a latency of less than 1 minute. After ingestion of tryptophan, 6 narcoleptics who typically fell directly into REM sleep showed an increased REM sleep duration (more than double the control duration) and seemed to have more "intense" REM sleep—more rapid eye movements and nightmares (Evans and Oswald, 1966). Hartmann (1967b) found in 8 volunteers a slight but significant increase in REM time after tryptophan (6–9 gm, at bedtime); total sleep time also rose, and there was a slight decrease of the length of the sleep-dream cycle. Hartman *et al.* (1966) found that though a tryptophan-free diet in rats decreased brain 5-HT only by 20–40%, nevertheless there followed a significant increase in the mean length of time between one REM episode and the next.

b. 5-Hydroxytryptophan. This immediate precursor of 5-HT characteristically causes arousal, tremor, even convulsions in animals (Carlsson, 1964); 5-HT can cause the same effects (Koella and Czicman, 1966). But 5-HTP also can lead to CNS depression. It can diminish the conditioned avoidance response in rats (Joyace and Hurwitz, 1964). In dogs treated with tranylcypromine, it induced transient drowsiness; this was followed by a phase of agitation, with hyperthermia, ataxia, increased hostility, and motor hyperactivity with spontaneously occurring orgasms (Himwich and Costa, 1960). Injected directly into the pons of rabbits, 5-HTP can induce slow-wave sleep and REM sleep (Ledbur and Tissot, 1966). Oral 5-HTP can also lead to sleep in monkeys (Macchitelli *et al.*, 1966). Delorme (1966) studied the effects of 5-HTP (30–50 mg/kg) in 10 cats. The animals showed no phase of excitement, instead were calm, with miosis, and a retracted nictitating membrane. Slow waves dominated the EEG tracing, with fewer spindles than normal; PGO spikes disappeared, as did REM sleep. As the animal recovered, PGO activity reappeared first, then the other signs of REM sleep. A large REM rebound dominated the recovery period. The 5-HTP suppressed REM sleep even in animals deprived of REM sleep for 3 days. In humans, by contrast, 5-HTP (3 mg/kg, taken orally) can increase REM-sleep (Zarcone and Dement, 1970).

c. 5-Hydroxytryptamine. At most sites, 5-HT itself does not pass the blood–brain barrier (Udenfriend *et al.*, 1957). Koella and Czicman (1966), however, find in the brainstem a discrete area of high permeability to to 5-HT—the area postrema. The actions of 5-HT at the site lead to EEG synchronization, miosis, and behavioral sleep. Intracarotid 5-HT causes a dual response—initial arousal and then sleep. The arousal comes from a receptor area other than the area postrema, some more rostral site. Parenteral 5-HT in the mouse can cause sedation, central depression of motor activity, and a potentiation of the hypnotic effects of alcohol and barbiturates (Shore *et al.*, 1957). In cats, application of 5-HT to the preoptic area or the nucleus centralis medialis of the thalamus leads to drowsiness and high-voltage, slow-wave activity in the EEG (Yamaguchi *et al.*, 1963). The raphe area of the brainstem is the center proposed by Jouvet

(1967) and others as the anatomical locus of the serotonergic sleep-inducing neurons. Destruction of the area yields a persistently wakeful animal. Electrical stimulation of the site brings about a neurally mediated release of 5-HT in the rat's forebrain (Aghajanian *et al.*, 1967). Methysergide, a lysergic acid derivative and a potent 5-HT blocker (Karja *et al.*, 1961), causes insomnia as a frequent adverse reaction (Graham, 1964). In rabbits, methysergide inhibits sleep, both REM and non-REM, and augments wakefulness (Tabushi and Himwich, 1970).

There is thus a mass of evidence pointing toward a role of 5-HT in sleep. The evidence that NE is involved in sleep, especially in REM sleep, is as yet less convincing.

d. Dopa. The usual effect of dopa administration is arousal; this extends even to the reversal of the reserpine syndrome (Carlsson, 1964). Delorme (1966) found that dopa (30–75 mg/kg) in 7 cats produced a calm state of wakefulness with mydriasis. The electromyographic activity was intense; cortical EEG activity was fast and low in voltage. There were many rapid eye movements; PGO spikes were abolished, as were REM and slow wave sleep. When DOPA and 5-HTP were administered together, the picture was similar to that seen after 5-HTP alone. Dopa, applied topically to the pons and medulla, can induce neocortical desychronization, hippocampal theta rhythms, and some abatement of neck muscle tone (Ledbur and Tissot, 1966). These results, however, are subject to several limitations: The species used (rabbit) and the usual objections to topical applications of drugs to the brain. The controversy about whether or not dopa replenishes central NE stores should also be kept in mind. The effects of parenteral dopa may reflect mainly an increased central DA level.

Matsumoto *et al.* (1968) investigated the influence of fatigue on sleep. In a control experiment, rats were placed upon a nonoperating treadmill for 4 hours; the animals were kept awake manually, but not exercised. Then they were allowed to sleep; the first REM sleep period came after 123 minutes. Then the animals were exercised on the now operative treadmill for 4 hours; this exercise retarded the appearance of REM sleep (it now came after 367 minutes). If such animals, however, were given dopa (50 mg/kg) after the period of exercise, the first REM episode came after only 106 minutes. The authors suggest that the exercise stress lowered the brain's NE and, thus, retarded the appearance of REM sleep. The combination of exercise plus dopa supposedly refilled the NE stores and abolished the inhibition by exercise of REM sleep. Actual amine determinations were not done, however; and it is not stated whether the same animals were used in the three experimental situations; nor were any statements concerning statistical significance given.

e. Dihydroxyphenylserine (DOPS). This amino acid was once considered to be a possible natural precursor of NE; it is not, but it is converted by tissus directly to NE (Blaschko *et al.*, 1950), presumably by L-aromatic amino acid decarboxylase. Unlike DOPA, DOPS leads to tissue accumulations of NE alone; no DA is built up. Havlicek (1967) studied the effects of DOPS in rats. The agent (500 mg/kg) was given by way of an indwelling catheter in the jugular vein. Saline was the placebo. The drug caused no changes in the first hour after its administration but led to an increased "sleep" in the second hour. It was an unusual kind of sleep, however. Whereas in the control experiments the animals slept in a normal huddled-up posture, after the drug they were found in unusual postures, lying on their sides with their backs and legs extended. There was a very slight increase in REM sleep, but no statements were made concerning statistical significance. Dihydroxyphenylserine was also given after pretreatment of the animals with an MAO inhibitor, a catechol-*O*-methyl transferase inhibitor, and an alpha-adrenergic blocking agent (phentolamine—this was to inhibit peripheral alpha-adrenergic effects of the NE being formed from the DOPS). In such animals, 500 mg/kg of DOPS caused stupor and death; 200 mg/kg caused CNS depression. It is difficult to say what all this means; toxicity and an abnormal state of CNS depression seem to be the clearest interpretations.

f. Norepinepherine—A Dualistic Theory of Sleep. The NE itself, as noted by Spooner and Winters (1965) and by Jouvet (1967), can induce in young birds and kittens, whose blood–brain barrier is permeable, behavioral sleep. When applied to certain brain sites, it can lead to sleep in adult cats (Yamaguchi *et al.*, 1963). Peripheral adrenergic discharges often occur during REM sleep (Gottschalk *et al.*, 1966).

In rats, according to Pujol *et al.* (1968), there is an increased turnover of central NE during the rebound which follows REM sleep deprivation. As Oswald (1968) has pointed out, however, the experiments were poorly controlled. Furthermore, as Thierry *et al.* (1968) mention, the increased NE turnover can be interpreted as a nonspecific response to the chronic stress of REM sleep deprivation.

Jouvet (1967) feels that REM sleep is generated by structures within the rostral pons, notably the locus coeruleus. This nucleus in rats and mice is rich in its NE content. In fact, according to Dahlstrom and Fuxe (1964) it is unique—all of its neurons contain NE. Pin *et al.* (1968) have shown that this is also true in the cat. Roussel *et al.* (1967) studied the effects of bilateral destruction of the locus coeruleus in the cat. The REM sleep was abolished altogether; slow-wave sleep and waking continued unchanged. The lesion at the same time caused a notable decline of NE concentrations in all areas of the brain rostral to the area coagulated. Destruction of areas immediately caudal or lateral to the locus coeruleus caused changes neither in the stages of sleep nor in CNS monoamines. There, thus, seems to exist in the cat as ascending noradrenergic system with its hub at the locus coeruleus. And the function of the system seems to have nothing to do either with wakefulness or slow-wave sleep; it is, according to Jouvet, the REM system.

Similar lesions of the midbrain raphe system cause insomnia and a generalized decline of 5-HT levels (Jouvet *et al.*, 1967).

There are, of course, nuclei that contain NE and DA in the midbrain as well as in the pons. Jones *et al.* (1968, 1969) report that lesions of the substantia nigra led to a dimunition of DA rostral to the lesion, and caused a comatose state marked by a general motor stiffness. The EEG of such cats is, despite the coma, generally unaffected—there are alternating periods of sleep and of EEG waking. Destruction of NE nuclei in the dorsolateral pontine tegmentum (rostral to the locus coeruleus) and in the midbrain cause a decline in NE levels rostral to the lesions and a decline of the waking pattern of the EEG.

What do these data indicate? Three things, says Jouvet: (*1*) a system arises in the locus coeruleus which is noradrenergic and which generates all the signs of REM sleep; (*2*) a system arises in the midbrain which is dopaminergic and which is responsible for behavioral waking; and (*3*) a system arises mainly in the midbrain which is noradrenergic and which is responsible for the EEG activation of wakefulness.

Parts of the data are already being challenged. Henley and Morrison (1969) studied the effects of large electrolytic lesions in the rostral pons, lesions which destroyed the locus coeruleus and surrounding tissue. Only one sign of REM sleep was abolished—the loss of skeletal muscle tone. The other signs of REM sleep persisted. This meant that the animals, upon entering REM sleep, would move and twitch violently; sometimes they would get up and run, or even leap in a convulsive manner. On occasion, the strong jerks of the body ended in arousal. Henley and Morrison suggested that Jouvet may have misinterpreted the effects of his pontine lesions. If the cat is awakened by the spasmodic movements that occur in REM sleep, then this, and not the lesion, could account for the 100% abolition of REM sleep seem by Jouvet's group.

I think that at present no conclusions are possible. A great deal of further work is needed. As of now, however, I can find in the literature not one single, firm, convincing bit of data to indicate that central NE is in any way essential for the production of REM sleep.

Both 5-HT and NE play a part, however, in Jouvet's dualistic theory of sleep. The evidence upon which the theory is based has already been mentioned.

Structurally, it is claimed, REM sleep and slow-wave sleep can be separated. Slow-wave sleep is triggered by the midbrain. The pons alone is sufficient to initiate all the signs of REM sleep. The 5-HT-containing neurons of the raphe complex appear to be the slow-wave sleep cells. The NE-containing neurons of the pons trigger all the signs of REM sleep. A duality of sleep is a consequence of the duality of structure. The overwhelming mass of data shows that the two states are separable. In Jouvet's formulation, 5-HT initiates slow-wave sleep, and NE is necessary for REM sleep; in addition, a cholinergic system is also somehow required for the shift from slow-wave to REM sleep (Jouvet, 1967, 1969).

Delorme (1966) was more specific. The typical sequence, resulting from interactions between the two sleep centers, is

$$\text{wakefulness} \longrightarrow \text{slow-wave sleep} \longrightarrow \underset{\text{with PGO spikes}}{\text{slow-wave sleep}} \longrightarrow \text{REM sleep}$$

The 5-HT initiates slow-wave sleep; MAO catabolizes 5-HT to 5-hydroxyindoleacetic acid (5-HIAA); 5-HIAA rises in concentration, and at a critical level both (*1*) initiates the PGO activity and (*2*) triggers a group of cholinergic neurons that interconnect the raphe system and the rostral pons. The cholinergic neurons stimulate the noradrenergic neurons of the locus coeruleus, which, in turn, trigger the signs of REM sleep. I stress that this formulation is Delorme's; Jouvet's is similar, only less explicit.

What does the evidence say? Sleep is dualistic; perhaps. As Ursin (1968) has noted, it is even more complicated; but at least it seems clear that there are at least two separate states of sleep, and they can be modified in various directions, both together and separately. Serotonin and ACh both may be important in the active generation of the two stages of sleep. There the evidence stops. The monoamine basis of the dualistic theory of sleep has not at this time been established. Some evidence suggests, in a ragged, circumstantial way, that NE has a role to play in the genesis of sleep, but firmer evidence argues against such a role. Brain NE may well be involved in the production of some of the signs of sleep. What those signs might be, however, remains unclear.

IV. Conclusion

We shall not cease from exploration
And the end of all our exploring
Will be to arrive where we started
And know the place for the first time.

T. S. Eliot

Is wakefulness cholinergic? Certainly, and more. Is wakefulness noradrenergic? Certainly, and more. Is wakefulness dopaminergic? Certainly, and more.

Is it an oversimplification to say that a state so complicated as wakefulness is mediated by some single would-be neurohumor? Certainly. Is it an oversimplification to say the same of sleep? Again, the answer is certainly.

I do not mean by this to declare that a kind of nihilism exists upon the investigation of the central neurohumoral bases of the various states of consciousness. Such investigations can only add to our total store of knowledge. But I do say that it is a gross oversimplification to say that so exquisitely complicated a state as REM sleep is mediated by any single neurohumor, or by two or three neurohumors. As Mandell and Spooner (1968) have pointed out, the 5-HT–NE theory of sleep was almost an inevitability. 5-Hydroxytryptamine and NE have been of central importance in recent neurochemical studies, and, hence, it was "only too predictable" that they should enter into concepts concerning the central neurohumoral basis of the states of sleep.

Thus, wakefulness is not a cholinergic function, though cholinergic mechanisms are without doubt involved. Nor is it exclusively a noradrenergic function, nor a dopaminergic function.

Sleep may be no less complicated than wakefulness. It is different but, perhaps, just as intricate. Sleep is not "negative"; it is "positive" and enormously complex. I have no doubt that cholinergic mechanisms are involved in sleep, and noradrenergic, dopaminergic, serotonergic mechanisms also. Nor would I be surprised to find that Pappenheimer's peptide is involved, as well as prostaglandins, melatonin, and progesterone.

Schizophrenia cannot, I predict, be attributed to the action of one neurohormone; it is not caused merely by altered 5-HT metabolism and disturbed sleep mechanisms. As Hobson (1969a) has noted, sleep research has thus far had little if any practical consequence in psychiatry.

The current theories of sleep remind us of how ignorant we are. We shall not cease, however; and, in the end, we shall finally begin to understand.

Acknowledgments

The author would like to thank Dr. Neil C. Moran and Dr. Harry L. Williams for their help and encouragement and would like to acknowledge the generous support and help of Dr. Robert E. Jewett.

References

Adey, W. R., Kado, R., and Rhodes, J. (1963). *Science* **141,** 932.
Aghajanian, G. K., Richards, J. A., and Sheard, M. H. (1967). *Science* **156,** 402.

Agnew, H. W., Webb, W. B., and Williams, R. L. (1967). *Perceptual and Motor Skills* **24,** 851.

Akindele, M. O., Evans, J. I., and Oswald, I. (1970). *Electroencephalogr. Clin. Neurophysiol.* **29,** 47.

Allison, T., and Goff, W. R. (1968). Report to the Association for the Psychophysiological Study of Sleep. *Psychophysiology* **5,** 200. (Abstr.)

Allison, T., and vanTwyver, H. (1970). *Exp. Neurol.* **27,** 564.

Amin, A. H., Crawford, T. B. B., and Gaddum, J. H. (1954). *J. Physiol.* (*London*) **126,** 596.

Anden, N. E., Corrodi, H., Dahlstrom, A., Fuxe, K., and Hokfelt, T. (1966). *Life Sci.* **5,** 561.

Anton-Tay, F., Chou, C., Anton, S., and Wurtman, R. J. (1968). *Science* **162,** 277.

Aserinsky, E., and Kleitman, N. (1953). *Science* **118,** 273.

Axelrod, J., and Black, I. B. (1968). *Nature* (*London*) **220,** 161.

Baekland, F. (1967). *Psychopharmacologia* **11,** 388.

Barchas, J. D., Dement, W. C., Ferguson, J., Cohen, H. B., and Henriksen, S. (1970). *Fed. Proc. Fed. Amer. Soc. Exp. Biol.* **29,** 747.

Baust, W. (1967). *Electroencephalogr. Clin. Neurophysiol.* **22,** 365.

Baust, W., and Bohnert, B. (1969). *Exp. Brain Res.* **7,** 169.

Baxter, B. L. (1969). *Exp. Brain Res.* **23,** 220.

Belenky, G., Henriksen, S., McGarr, C., Ferguson, J., Cohen, H. B., and Dement, W. C. (1968). Report to the Association for the Psychophysiological Study of Sleep. *Psychophysiology* **5,** 243. (Abstr.)

Bizzi, E., and Brooks D. C. (1963). *Arch. Ital. Biol.* **101,** 666.

Black, I. B., and Axelrod, J. (1968). *Proc. Nat. Acad. Sci. U.S.* **58,** 1231.

Blaschko, H., Burn, J. H., and Longemann, H. (1950). *Brit. J. Pharmacol.* **5,** 431.

Bliss, E. L., and Ailion, J. (1969). *J. Pharmacol. Exp. Ther.* **168,** 258.

Bliss, E. L., Ailion, J., and Zwanziger, J. (1968). *J. Pharmacol. Exp. Ther.* **164,** 122.

Bowers, M. B., Hartmann, E. L., and Freedman, D. X. (1966). *Science* **153,** 1416.

Brannen, J. O., and Jewett, R. E. (1969). *Arch. Gen. Psychiat.* **21,** 284.

Brebbia, D. R., and Paul, R. C. (1969). Report to the Association for the Psychophysiological Study of Sleep. *Psychophysiology* **6,** 229. (Abstr.)

Bremer, F. (1935). *C. R. Soc. Biol.* **118,** 1235.

Bremer, F. (1936). *C. R. Soc. Biol.* **122,** 464.

Brodie, B. B., Finger, K. F., Orlans, F. B., Quinn, G. P., and Sulser, F. (1960). *J. Pharmacol. Exp. Ther.* **129,** 250.

Brodie, B. B., Costa, E., Dlabac, A., Neff, N. H., and Smookler, H. H. (1966). *J. Pharmacol. Exp. Ther.* **154,** 493.

Bromberg, W. (1934). *Amer. J. Psychiat.* **91,** 303.

Brooks, D. C. (1968). *Exp. Neurol.* **22,** 603.

Candia, O., Favale, E., Giussani, A., and Rossi, G. F. (1962). *Arch. Ital. Biol.* **100,** 216.

Carlsson, A. (1964). *Progr. Brain Res.* **8,** 9.

Carroll, D., Lewis, S. A., and Oswald, I. (1969). *Nature* (*London*) **223,** 865.

Charalampous, K. D., and Brown, S. (1967). *Psychopharmacologia* **11,** 422.

Ciaranello, R. D., Barchas, R. E., Byers, G. S., Stemmle, D. W., and Barchas, J. D. (1969). *Nature* (*London*) **221,** 368.

Clemes, S. R., and Dement, W. C. (1967). *J. Nerv. Ment. Dis.* **144,** 485.

Cohen, H. B., and Dement, W. C. (1966). *Science* **154,** 396.

Cohen, H. B., Duncan, R. F., and Dement, W. C. (1967). *Science* **156,** 1646.

Cohen, H. B., Duncan, R. F., and Dement, W. C. (1968). *Electroencephalogr. Clin. Neurophysiol.* **24,** 401.

Cohen, H. B., Henriksen, S., Ferguson, J., Barchas, J. D., and Dement, W. C. (1969). Report to the Association for the Psychophysiological Study of Sleep. *Psychophysiology* **6,** 221. (Abstr.)

Corrodi, H., and Fuxe, K. (1967). *Life Sci.* **6,** 1345.

Corrodi, H., Fuxe, K., and Hokfelt, T. (1968). *Life Sci.* **7,** 107.

Cremata, V. Y., and Koe, B. K. (1966). *Clin. Pharmacol. Ther.* **7,** 768.

Crowley, T. J., Smith, E., and Lewis, O. L. (1968). Report to the Association for the Psychophysiological Study of Sleep. (Unpublished.)

Dahlstrom, A., and Fuxe, K. (1964). *Acta Physiol. Scand. Suppl.* **232.**

Delorme, F. (1966). "Monoamines et Sommeils." Imprimerie L.M.D., Lyon.

Delorme, F., Jeannerod, M., and Jouvet, M. (1965). *C. R. Soc. Biol.* **159,** 900.

Delorme, F., Riotte, M., and Jouvet, M. (1966). *C. R. Soc. Biol.* **160,** 1457.

Delorme, F., Froment, J. L., and Jouvet, M. (1967). *C. R. Soc. Biol.* **160,** 2347.

Dement, W. C. (1958). *Electroencephalogr. Clin. Neurophysiol.* **10,** 291.

Dement, W. C. (1960). *Science* **131,** 1705.

Dement, W. C. (1968). *In* "Mind as a Tissue" (C. Rupp, ed.), pp. 214–236, 260–262. Harper & Row, New York.

Dement, W. C. (1969). *Stanford M.D.* **8,** 2.

Dement, W. C., and Kleitman, N. (1957). *Electroencephalogr. Clin. Neurophysiol.* **9,** 673.

Dement, W. C., Rechtschaffen, A., and Gulevich, G. (1964). *Electroencephalogr. Clin. Neurophysiol.* **17,** 608.

Derbyshire, A. J., Rempel, B., Forbes, A., and Lambert, E. F. (1936). *Amer. J. Physiol.* **116,** 577.

Dewson, J. H., Dement, W. C., Wagener, T. E., and Nobel, K. (1967). *Science* **156,** 403.

Dikshit, B. B. (1934). *J. Physiol.* (*London*) **83,** 42P.

Dominic, J. A., and Moore, K. E. (1969). *Arch. Int. Pharmacodyn. Ther.* **178,** 166.

Domino, E. F., and Yamamoto, K. (1965). *Science* **150,** 637.

Doust, L. J. W., and Schneider, R. A. (1952). *Brit. Med. J.* **1,** 449.

Dusan-Peyrethon, D. and Froment, J. L. (1968). *C. R. Soc. Biol.* **162,** 2141.

Dusan-Peyrethon, D., Peyrethon, J., and Jouvet, M. (1967). *C. R. Soc. Biol.* **161,** 2530.

Dusan-Peyrethon, D., Peyrethon, J., and Jouvet, M. (1968). *C. R. Soc. Biol.* **162,** 116.

Duval, M. M. (1895). *C. R. Soc. Biol.* **47,** 74.

Echols, S. D., and Jewett, R. E. In preparation.

Engelman, K., Lovenberg, W., and Sjoerdsma, A. (1967). *New Engl. J. Med.* **277,** 1103.

Engelman, K., Jequier, E., Udenfriend, S., and Sjoerdsma, A. (1968a). *J. Clin. Invest.* **47,** 568.

Engelman, K., Horwitz, D., Jequier, E., and Sjoerdsma, A. (1968b). *J. Clin. Invest.* **47,** 577.

Evans, J. I., and Oswald, I. (1966). *Brit. J. Psychiat.* **112,** 401.

Evarts, E. V., Bental, E., Bihari, B., and Huttenlocher, P. R. (1962). *Science* **135,** 726.

Falck, B. (1964). *Progr. Brain Res.* **8,** 28.

Falck, B., Hillarp, N. A., Thieme, G., and Torp, A. (1962). *J. Histochem. Cytochem.* **10,** 348.

Faure, J. (1964). *Electroencephalogr. Clin. Neurophysiol.* **17,** 444.

Ferguson, J., and Dement, W. C. (1968). Report to the Association for the Psychophysiological Study of Sleep. *Psychophysiology* **5,** 238. (Abstr.)

Ferguson, J., Cohen, H., Henriksen, S., McGarr, K., Mitchell, G., Hoyt, G., Barchas, J. D., and Dement, W. C. (1969a). Report to the Association for the Psychophysiological Study of Sleep. *Psychophysiology* **6,** 220. (Abstr.)

Ferguson, J., Henriksen, S., Cohen, H. B., Hoyt, G., Mitchell, G., McGarr, K., Rubenson, D., Ryan, L., and Dement, W. C. (1969b). Report to the Association for the Psychophysiological Study of Sleep. *Psychophysiology* **6,** 221. (Abstr.)
Foulkes, W. D. (1962). *J. Abnorm. Soc. Psychol.* **65,** 14.
Freeman, F. R., Agnew, H. W., and Williams, R. L. (1965). *Clin. Pharmacol. Ther.* **6,** 172.
Freeman, F. R., McNew, J. J., and Adey, W. R. (1969). *Exp. Neurol.* **25,** 129.
Fuller, R. W., Hines, C. W., and Mills, J. (1965). *Biochem. Pharmacol.* **14,** 483.
Gershon, S., Hekimian, L. J., Floyd, A., and Hollister, L. E. (1967). *Psychopharmacologia* **11,** 189.
Gibb, J. W., and Webb, J. G. (1969). *Proc. Nat. Acad. Sci. U.S.* **63,** 364.
Gibbs, E. L., and Gibbs, F. A. (1947). *Res. Publ. Ass. Res. Nerv. Ment. Dis.* **26,** 366.
Gloor, P. (1969). *Electroencephalogr. Clin. Neurophysiol.* **27,** 649.
Glowinski, J., and Axelrod, J. (1964). *Nature (London)* **204,** 1318.
Glowinski, J., and Iverson, L. L. (1966). *J. Neurochem.* **13,** 655.
Glowinski, J., Durand, M., Hery, F., and Pujol, J. F. (1969). *Proc. Int. Pharmacol. Meet. 4th, Basel, Switzerland,* p. 38.
Goldstein, L., Gardocki, J. F., Mundsschenk, D. L., and O'Brien, G. (1967). *Fed. Proc. Fed. Amer. Soc. Exp. Biol.* **26,** 506.
Gottesmann, C. (1966). *C. R. Soc. Biol.* **160,** 2056.
Gottschalk, L. A., Stone, W. N., Gleser, G. C., and Iacono, J. M. (1966). *Science* **153,** 654.
Graham, J. R. (1964). *New Engl. J. Med.* **270,** 67.
Green, W. J. (1965). *J. Nerv. Ment. Dis.* **140,** 417.
Greenberg, R., and Dewan, E. M. (1969). *Nature (London)* **223,** 183.
Greenberg, R., and Pearlman, C. (1967). *Amer. J. Psychiat.* **124,** 133.
Greenberg, R., Kelty, M., and Dewan, E. M. (1969). Report to the Association for the Psychophysiological Study of Sleep. *Psychophysiology* **6,** 226. (Abstr.)
Gresham, S. C., Webb, W. B., and Williams, R. L. (1963). *Science* **140,** 1226.
Gresham, S. C., Agnew, H. W., and Williams, R. L. (1965). *Arch. Gen. Psychiat.* **13,** 503.
Grinspoon, L. (1969). *Sci. Amer.* **221,** 17.
Grob, D., Lilienthal, J. L., Harvey, A. M., and Jones, B. F. (1947). *Bull. Johns Hopkins Hosp.* **81,** 217.
Gross, M. M., Goodenough, D., Tobin, M., Halpert, E., Lepore, D., Perlstein, A., Sirota, M., Dibianco, J., Fuller, R. W., and Kishner, I. (1966). *J. Nerv. Ment. Dis.* **142,** 493.
Gyermek, L. (1967). *Proc. Soc. Exp. Biol. Med.* **125,** 1058.
Hartmann, E. L. (1965). *New Engl. J. Med.* **273,** 30, 87.
Hartmann, E. L. (1966). *Psychopharmacologia* **9,** 242.
Hartmann, E. L. (1967a). "The Biology of Dreaming." Thomas, Springfield, Illinois.
Hartmann, E. L. (1967b). Report to the Association for the Psychophysiological Study of Sleep. See also, Hartmann, E. L. (1967a).
Hartmann, E. L. (1968a). *J. Nerv. Ment. Dis.* **146,** 165.
Hartmann, E. L. (1968b). *Psychopharmacologia* **12,** 346.
Hartmann, E. L., and Freedman, D. X. (1966). Report to the Association for the Psychophysiological Study of Sleep. See also, Hartmann, E. L. (1967a).
Hartmann, E. L., Freedman, D. X., Zack, M., and Kluft, R. (1966). Report to the Association for the Psychopysiological Study of Sleep. See also, Hartmann, E. L. (1967a).
Harvey, E. N., Loomis, A. L., and Hobart, G. A. (1937). *Science* **85,** 443.

Havlicek, V. (1967). *Int. J. Neurophamacol.* **6,** 83.
Hawkins, D. R., and Mendels, J. (1966). *Amer. J. Psychiat.* **123,** 682.
Hayter, A. (1969). "Opium and the Romantic Imagination." Univ. of California Press, Berkeley, California.
Hediger, H. (1969). *Proc. Roy. Soc. Med.* **62,** 153.
Heiner, L., Godin, Y., Mark, J., and Mandel, P. (1968). *J. Neurochem.* **15,** 150.
Henley, K., and Morrison, A. R. (1969). Report to the Association for the Psycho-physiological Study of Sleep. *Psychophysiology* **6,** 245. (Abstr.)
Hernandez-Peon, R. (1962). *Electroencephalogr. Clin. Neurophysiol.* **14,** 423.
Hernandez-Peon, R. (1964). *Electroencephalogr. Clin. Neurophysiol.* **17,** 444.
Hernandez-Peon, R. (1965a). *J. Nerv. Ment. Dis.* **141,** 623.
Hernandez-Peon, R. (1965b). *In* "Aspects Anatomo-Fonctionnels de la Physiologie du Sommeil" (M. Jouvet, ed.), pp. 63–88.C.N.R.S., Paris.
Hernandez-Peon, R., and Chavez-Ibarra, G. (1963). *Electroencephalogr. Clin. Neurophysiol. Suppl.* **24,** 188.
Hernandez-Peon, R., and Sterman, M. B. (1966). *Annu. Rev. Psychol.* **17,** 363.
Hernandez-Peon, R., Chavez-Ibarra, G., Morgane, P. J., and Timo-Iaria, C. (1963). *Exp. Neurol.* **8,** 93.
Hess, R., Jr. Koella, W. P., and Akert, K. (1953). *Electroencephalogr. Clin. Neurophysiol.* **5,** 75.
Hess, W. R. (1929). *Amer. J. Physiol.* **90,** 386.
Hess, W. R. (1932a). *Lancet* **ii,** 1199.
Hess, W. R. (1932b). *Lancet* **ii,** 1259.
Hess, W. R. (1949). *J. Physiol. (Paris)* **41,** 61A.
Hess, W. R. (1965). *Progr. Brain Res.* **18,** 3.
Heuser, G., Ling, G. M., and Kluver, M. (1967). *Electroencephalogr. Clin. Neurophysiol.* **22,** 122.
Hillarp, N. A., Fuxe, K., and Dahlstrom, A. (1966). *Pharmacol. Rev.* **18,** 727.
Himwich, W. A., and Costa, E. (1960). *Fed. Proc. Fed. Amer. Soc. Exp. Biol.* **19,** 838.
Hishikawa, Y., Nakai, K., Ida, H., and Kaneko, Z. (1965). *Electroencephalogr. Clin. Neurophysiol.* **19,** 518.
Hishikawa, Y., Cramer, H., and Kuhlo, W. (1969). *Exp. Brain Res.* **7,** 84.
Hobson, J. A. (1964). *Electroencephalogr. Clin. Neurophysiol.* **17,** 52.
Hobson, J. A. (1967). *Electroencephalogr. Clin. Neurophysiol.* **22,** 113.
Hobson, J. A. (1969a). *New Engl. J. Med.* **281,** 1343.
Hobson, J. A. (1969b). *New Engl. J. Med.* **281,** 1468.
Hoffer, B. J., Siggins, G. R., and Bloom, F. E. (1969). *Science* **166,** 1418.
Hoffman, J. S., and Domino, E. F. (1969). *J. Pharmacol. Exp. Ther.* **170,** 190.
Honda, Y., Takahashi, K., Takahashi, S., Azumi, K., Irie, M., Sakuma, M., Tsushima, T., and Shizume, K. (1969). *J. Clin. Endocrinol. Metab.* **29,** 20.
Hook, J. B., and Moore, K. E. (1969). *J. Pharmacol. Exp. Ther.* **168,** 310.
Hornykiewicz, O. (1966). *Pharmacol. Rev.* **18,** 925.
Horton, E. W. (1964). *Brit. J. Pharmacol.* **22,** 189.
Iskander, T. and Kaelbling, R. (1969). Report to the Association for the Psychophysiological Study of Sleep. *Psychophysiology* **6,** 219. (Abstr.)
Itil, T. M. (1969). *Psychopharmacologia* **14,** 383.
Jewett, R. E. (1968). *Exp. Neurol.* **21,** 368.
Jewett, R. E. (1971). In preparation.
Jewett, R. E., and Norton, S. (1966). *Exp. Neurol.* **15,** 463.
Johnson, F. H., and Russell, G. V. (1952). *Anat. Rec.* **112,** 348.

Jones, B. E., Bobillier, P., and Jouvet, M. (1968). *C. R. Soc. Biol.* **163,** 176.
Jones, B. E., Bobillier, P., and Jouvet, M. (1969). Report to the Association for the Psychophysiological Study of Sleep. *Psychophysiology* **6,** 245. (Abstr.)
Jouvet, D., and Delorme, F. (1965). *C. R. Soc. Biol.* **159,** 387.
Jouvet, M. (1967). *Physiol. Rev.* **47,** 117.
Jouvet, M. (1968). *In* "Psychopharmacology, a Review of Progress, 1957–1967" (D. H. Efron, ed.), Publ. No. 1836, pp. 523–540. U.S. Pub. Health Serv., Washington, D.C.
Jouvet, M. (1969). *Science* **163,** 32.
Jouvet, M., and Jouvet, D. (1963). *Electroencephalogr. Clin. Neurophysiol. Suppl.* **24,** 133.
Jouvet, M., and Michel, F. (1960). *J. Physiol. (Paris)* **52,** 130.
Jouvet, M., Michel, F., and Courjon, J. (1959a). *C. R. Soc. Biol.* **153,** 101.
Jouvet, M., Michel, F., and Courjon, J. (1959b). *C. R. Soc. Biol.* **153,** 1024.
Jouvet, M., Michel, F., and Mounier, D. (1960). *Rev. Neurol.* **103,** 189.
Jouvet, M., Jeannerod, M., and Delorme, F. (1965a). *C. R. Soc. Biol.* **159,** 1599.
Jouvet, M., Vimont, P., and Delorme, F. (1965b). *C. R. Soc. Biol.* **159,** 1595.
Jouvet, M., Bobillier, P., Pujol, J. F., and Renault, J. (1967). *C. R. Soc. Biol.* **160,** 2343.
Joyace, D., and Hurwitz, H. M. B. (1964). *Psychopharmacologia* **5,** 424.
Kahn, E., and Fisher, C. (1969). *J. Nerv. Ment. Dis.* **148,** 477.
Kales, A., and Kales, J. D. (1970). *Pharmacology for Physicians* **4** (Sept.), 1.
Kales, A., Hoedemaker, F. S., Jacobson, A., and Lichtenstein, E. L. (1964). *Nature (London)* **204,** 1337.
Kales, A., Jacobson, A., Kales, J. D., Marusak, C., and Hanley, J. (1968). *Psychophysiology* **4,** 391.
Kales, A., Preston, T. A., Tan, T.-L., and Allen, C. (1970a). *Arch. Gen. Psychiat.* **23,** 211.
Kales, A., Kales, J. D., Scharf, M. B., and Tan, T.-L. (1970b). *Arch. Gen. Psychia.* **23,** 219.
Kales, A., Allen, C., Scharf, M. B., and Kales, J. D. (1970c). *Arch. Gen. Psychiat.* **23,** 226.
Karadzic, V., and Mrsulja, B. B. (1968). *J. Neurochem.* **16,** 29.
Karja, J., Karki, N. T., and Tala, E. (1961). *Acta Pharmacol. Toxicol.* **18,** 255.
Kaufman, E., Roffwarg, H. P., and Muzio, J.N., (1964). Report to the Association for the Psychophysiological Study of Sleep. (Unpublished.)
Kay, D. C., Eisenstein, R. B., and Jasinski, D. R. (1969). *Psychopharmacologia* **14,** 404.
Kety, S. S., Javoy, F., Thierry, A.-M., Julou, L., and Glowinski, J. (1967). *Proc. Nat. Acad. Sci. U.S.* **58,** 1249.
Khatri, I. M., and Freis, E. D. (1967). *J. Appl. Physiol.* **22,** 867.
Khazan, N., and Sawyer, C. H. (1964). *Psychopharmacologia* **5,** 457.
Khazan, N., Weeks, J. R., and Schroeder, L. A. (1967a). *J. Pharmacol. Exp. Ther.* **155,** 521.
Khazan, N., Bar, R., and Sulman, F. G. (1967b). *Int. J. Neuropharmacol.* **6,** 279.
Killam, E. K. (1962). *Pharmacol. Rev.* **14,** 175.
King, C. D., and Jewett, R. E. (1968). *Pharmacologist* **10,** 160.
Kirshner, N. (1966). *J. Neurosurg.* **24,** 165.
Klein, M., Michel, F., and Jouvet, M. (1964). *C. R. Soc. Biol.* **158,** 99.
Kleitman, N. (1963). "Sleep and Wakefulness," Univ. of Chicago Press, Chicago, Illinois.
Koe, B. K., and Weissman, A. (1966). *J. Pharmacol. Exp. Ther.* **154,** 499.
Koella, W. P. (1968). *In* "Psychopharmacology, a Review of Progress, 1957–1967" (D. H. Efron, ed.), Publ. No. 1836, pp. 541–543. U.S. Pub. Health Serv., Washington, D.C.

Koella, W. P., and Czicman, J. (1966). *Amer. J. Physiol.* **211,** 926.
Koella, W. P., Feldstein, A., and Czicman, J. S. (1968). *Electroencephalogr. Clin. Neurophysiol.* **25,** 481.
Kupfer, D. J., Wyatt, R. J., Greenspan, K., Scott, J., and Snyder, F. (1970). *Arch. Gen. Psychiat.* **23,** 35.
Lanoir, J., and Killam, E. K. (1968). *Electroencephalogr. Clin. Neurophysiol.* **25,** 530.
Ledbur, X., and Tissot, R. (1966). *Electroencephalogr. Clin. Neurophysiol.* **20,** 370.
Legassicke, J., Ashcroft, G. W., Eccleston, D., Evans, J. I., Oswald, I., and Ritson, E. B. (1965). *Brit. J. Psychiat.* **111,** 357.
Legendre, R., and Pieron, H. (1910). *C. R. Soc. Biol.* **68,** 1077.
Legendre, R., and Pieron, H. (1911). *C. R. Soc. Biol.* **70,** 190.
Legendre, R., and Pieron, H. (1912a). *C. R. Soc. Biol.* **72,** 210.
Legendre, R., and Pieron, H. (1912b). *C. R. Soc. Biol.* **72,** 274.
Lester, B. K., Coulter, J. D., Cowden, L. C., and Williams, H. L. (1968). *Psychopharmacologia* **13,** 275.
Levitt, M., Spector, S., Sjoerdsma, A., and Udenfriend, S. (1965). *J. Pharmacol. Exp. Ther.* **148,** 1.
Lewis, S. A., and Evans, J. I. (1969). *Psychopharmacologia* **14,** 342.
Lewis, S. A., and Oswald, I. (1969). *Brit. J. Psychiat.* **115,** 1403.
Lewis, S. A., Oswald, I., Evans, J. I., and Akindele, M. O. (1970). *Electroencephalogr. Clin. Neurophysiol.* **28,** 374.
Lichtensteiger, W., Mutzner, U., and Langemann, H. (1967). *J. Neurochem.* **14,** 489.
Lindsley, D. B., Schreiner, L. H., Knowles, W. B., and Magoun, H. W. (1950). *Electroencephalogr. Clin. Neurophysiol.* **2,** 483.
Lipton, M. A., Gordon, R., Guroff, G., and Udenfriend, S. (1967). *Science* **156,** 248.
Loomis, A. L., Harvey, E. N., and Hobart, G. A. (1935a). *Science* **81,** 597.
Loomis, A. L., Harvey, E. N., and Hobart, G. A. (1935b). *Science* **82,** 198.
Macchitelli, F. J., Fischetti, D., and Montanarelli, N. (1966). *Psychopharmacologia* **9,** 447.
McGeer, P. L., McGeer, E. G., and Wada, J. A. (1963). *Arch. Neurol.* (*Chicago*) **9,** 81.
McGinty, D. J., and Sterman, M. B. (1968). *Science* **160,** 1253.
Magni, F., Moruzzi, G., Rossi, G. F., and Zanchetti, A. (1959). *Arch. Ital. Biol.* **97,** 33.
Maitre, L. (1965). *Life Sci.* **4,** 2249.
Mandell, A. J., and Mandell, M. P. (1965). *Amer. J. Psychiat.* **122,** 391.
Mandell, A. J., and Spooner, C. E. (1968). *Science* **162,** 1442.
Mandell, A. J., Chaffey, F., Brill, P., Mandell, M. P., Rodnick, J., Rubin, R. T., and Sheff, R. (1966). *Science* **151,** 1559.
Marantz, R., and Rechtschaffen, A. (1967). *Perceptual and Motor Skills* **25,** 805.
Marantz, R., Rechtschaffen, A., Lovell, R. A., and Whitehead, P. K. (1968). *Communications in Behavioral Biology, Part A* **2,** 161.
Marczynski, T. J., Yamaguchi, N., Ling, G. M., and Grodzinska, L. (1964). *Experientia* **20,** 435.
Matsumoto, J., and Jouvet, M. (1964). *C. R. Soc. Biol.* **158,** 2137.
Matsumoto, J., Nishisho, T., Suto, T., Sadahiro, T., and Miyoshi, M. (1968). *Nature* (*London*) **218,** 177.
Matsuzaki, M., Takagi, H., and Tokizano, T. (1964). *Science* **146,** 1328.
Michel, F., Klein, M., Jouvet, D., and Valatx, J. (1961). *C. R. Soc. Biol.* **155,** 2389.
Micic, D., Karadzic, V., and Rakic, L. M. (1967). *Nature* (*London*) **215,** 169.
Mink, W. D., Best, P. J., and Olds, J. (1967). *Science* **158,** 1335.

Mongold, R., Sokoloff, L., Conner, E., Kleinerman, J., Therman, P.-O. G., and Kety, S. S. (1955). *J. Clin. Invest.* **34,** 1092.

Monroe, L. J. (1969). *Psychophysiology* **6,** 330.

Monti, J. M. (1968). *Experientia* **24,** 1143.

Moore, K. E. (1966a). *Fed. Proc. Fed. Amer. Soc. Exp. Biol.* **25,** 688.

Moore, K. E. (1966b). *Life Sci.* **5,** 55.

Moore, K. E., Wright, P. F., and Bert, J. K. (1967). *J. Pharmacol. Exp. Ther.* **155,** 506.

Moore, R. Y., Heller, A., Wurtman, R. J., and Axelrod, J. (1967). *Science* **155,** 220.

Moreton, J. E., and Davis, W. M. (1970). *Pharmacologist* **12,** 258.

Moruzzi, G., and Magoun, H. W. (1949). *Electroencephalogr. Clin. Neurophysiol.* **1,** 455.

Mott, F. (1924). *Lancet* **ii,** 1161.

Mouret, J., Jeannerod, M., and Jouvet, M. (1963). *J. Physiol. (Paris)* **55,** 305.

Mouret, J., Vilppula, A., Franchon, N., and Jouvet, M. (1968a). *C. R. Soc. Biol.* **162,** 914.

Mouret, J., Bobillier, P., and Jouvet, M. (1968b). *Eur. J. Pharmacol.* **5,** 17.

Muller, J. C., Pryor, W. W., Gibbons, J. E. G., and Orgain, E. S. (1955). *J. Amer. Med. Ass.* **159,** 836.

Muzio, J. N., Roffwarg, H. P., and Kaufman, E. (1966). *Electroencephalogr. Clin. Neurophysiol.* **21,** 313.

Nagatsu, T., Levitt, M., and Udenfriend, S. (1964). *J. Biol. Chem.* **239,** 2910.

Norton, S., and Jewett, R. E. (1965). *J. Pharmacol. Exp. Ther.* **149,** 301.

Nowlin, J. B., Troyer, W. G., Collins, W. S., Silverman, G., Nichols, C. R., McIntosh, H. D., Estes, E. H., and Bogdonoff, M. D. (1965). *Ann. Intern. Med.* **63,** 1040.

Oswald, I. (1968). *Pharmacol. Rev.* **20,** 273.

Oswald, I. (1969). *Nature (London)* **223,** 893.

Oswald, I., and Priest, R. G. (1965). *Brit. Med. J.* **ii,** 1093.

Oswald, I., and Thacore, V. R. (1963). *Brit. Med. J.* **ii,** 427.

Oswald, I., Berger, R. J., Jaramillo, R. A., Keddie, K. M. G., Olley, P. C., and Plunkett, G. B. (1963). *Brit. J. Psychiat.* **109,** 66.

Oswald, I., Ashcroft, G. W., Berger, R. J., Eccleston, D., Evans, J. I., and Thacore, V. R. (1966). *Brit. J. Psychiat.* **112,** 391.

Pappenheimer, J. R., Miller, T. B., and Goodrich, C. A. (1967). *Proc. Nat. Acad. Sci. U.S.* **58,** 513.

Parker, D. C., Sassin, J. F., Mace, J. W., Gotlin, R. W., and Rossman, L. G. (1969). *J. Clin. Endocrinol. Metab.* **29,** 871.

Pasnau, R. O., Naitoh, P., Stier, S., and Kollar, E. J. (1968). *Arch. Gen. Psychiat.* **18,** 496.

Peyrethon, J., and Dusan-Peyrethon, D. (1968). *C. R. Soc. Biol.* **163,** 181.

Pin, C., Jones, B. E., and Jouvet, M. (1968). *C. R. Soc. Biol.* **162,** 2136.

Pletscher, A., Bartholini, G., Bruderer, H., Burkard, W. P., and Grey, K. F. (1964). *J. Pharmacol. Exp. Ther.* **145,** 344.

Pohorecky, L. A., Zigmond, M., Karten, H., and Wurtman, R. J. (1969). *J. Pharmacol. Exp. Ther.* **165,** 190.

Pollin, W., Cardon, P. V., and Kety, S. S. (1961). *Science* **133,** 104.

Porter, C. C., Totaro, J. A., Burcin, A., and Wynosky, E. R. (1966). *Biochem. Pharmacol.* **15,** 583.

Prinz, P. N. (1968). Report to the Association for the Psychophysiological Study of Sleep. *Psychophysiology* **5,** 205. (Abstr.)

Pujol, J. F., Mouret, J., Jouvet, M., and Glowinski, J. (1968). *Science* **159,** 112.

Radil-Weiss, T., and Styblova, V. (1967). *Psychopharmacologia* **11,** 52.

Ramwell, P. W., and Shaw, J. E. (1966). *Amer. J. Physiol.* **211,** 125.

Ravenscroft, K., and Hartmann, E. L. (1968). *Psychophysiology* **4,** 396.

Rech, R. H., Borys, H. K., and Moore, K. E. (1966). *J. Pharmacol. Exp. Ther.* **153,** 412.

Rechtschaffen, A., and Maron, L. (1964). *Electroencephalogr. Clin. Neurophysiol.* **16,** 438.

Rechtschaffen, A., and Verdone, P. (1964). *Perceptual and Motor Skills* **19,** 947.

Reich, P., Driver, J. K., and Karnovsky, M. L. (1967). *Science* **157,** 336.

Reis, D. J., and Wurtman, R. J. (1968). *Life Sci.* **7,** 91.

Reis, D. J., Weinbren, M., and Corvelli, A. (1968). *J. Pharmacol. Exp. Ther.* **164,** 135.

Reis, D. J., Corvelli, A., and Conners, J. (1959). *J. Pharmacol. Exp. Ther.* **167,** 328.

Reite, M. L., and Pegram, G. V. (1968). *Electroencephalogr. Clin. Neurophysiol.* **25,** 36.

Reite, M. L., Pegram, G. V., Stephens, L. M., Bixler, E. C., and Lewis, O. L. (1969). *Psychopharmacologia* **14,** 12.

Reivich, M., Isaacs, G., Evarts, E. V., and Kety, S. S. (1967). *Trans. Amer. Neurol. Ass.* **92,** 70.

Reivich, M., Isaacs, G., Evarts, E. V., and Kety, S. S. (1968). *J. Neurochem.* **15,** 301.

Rhodes, J., Reite, M. L., Brown, D., and Adey, W. R. (1965). *In* "Aspects Anatomo-Fonctionnels de la Physiologie du Sommeil" (M. Jouvet, ed.), pp. 451–472. C.N.R.S., Paris.

Ritvo, E. R., Orn tz, E. M., Lafranchi, S., and Walter, R. D. (1967). *Electroencephalogr. Clin. Neurophysiol.* **22,** 465.

Roldan, E., Weiss, T., and Fifkova, E. (1963). *Electroencephalogr. Clin. Neurophysiol.* **15,** 775.

Rosenblatt, S., Chanley, J. D., Sobotka, H., and Kaufmann, M. R. (1960). *J. Neurochem.* **5,** 172.

Roussel, B., Buguet, A., Bobillier, P., and Jouvet, M. (1967). *C. R. Soc. Biol.* **161,** 2537.

Routtenberg, A., Sladek, J., and Bondareff, W. (1968). *Science* **161,** 272.

Ruckenbusch, Y. (1963a). *Arch. Ital. Biol.* **101,** 111.

Ruckenbusch, Y. (1963b). *C. R. Soc. Biol.* **157,** 840.

Ruckenbusch, Y., and Morel, M. T. (1968). *C. R. Soc. Biol.* **162,** 1346.

Sagales, T., Erill, S., and Domino, E. F. (1969). Report to the Association for the Psychophysiological Study of Sleep. *Psychophsiology* **6,** 258. (Abstr.)

Sassin, J. F., Parker, D. C., Mace, J. W., Gotlin, R. W., Johnson, L. C., and Rossman, L. G. (1969. Report to the Association for the Psychophysiological Study of Sleep. *Psychophysiology* **6,** 218. (Abstr.)

Sawyer, C. H., and Kawakmi, M. (1959). *Endocrinology* **65,** 622.

Schildkraut, J. J., and Kety, S. S. (1967). *Science* **156,** 21.

Schoenfeld, R. I., and Seiden, L. S. (1969). *J. Pharmacol. Exp. Ther.* **167,** 319.

Selye, H. (1942). *Endocrinology* **30,** 437.

Shimizu, A., and Himwich, H. E. (1968). *Psychopharmacologia* **13,** 161.

Shore, P. A., Pletscher, A., Tomich, E. G., Carlsson, A., Kuntzman, R., and Brodie, B. B. (1957). *Ann. N.Y. Acad. Sci.* **66,** 609.

Shurley, J. T., Serafetinides, E. A., and Brooks, R. E. (1969). Report to the Association for the Psychophysiological Study of Sleep. *Psychophysiology* **6,** 230. (Abstr.)

Siegel, J., and Langley, T. D. (1965). *Experientia* **21,** 740.

Sjoerdsma, A., Engelman, K., Spector, S., and Udenfriend, S. (1965). *Lancet* **ii,** 1092.

Smith, B., and Prockop, D. J. (1962). *New Engl. J. Med.* **267,** 1338.

Soulairac, A., and Gottesmann, C. (1967). *Life Sci.* **6,** 1229.

Sourkes, T. L., Murphey, G. F., Chavez, B., and Zielinska, M. (1961). *J. Neurochem.* **8,** 109.

Spector, S., Sjoerdsma, A., and Udenfriend, S. (1965). *J. Pharmacol. Exp. Ther.* **147,** 86.
Spooner, C. E., and Winters, W. D. (1965). *Experientia* **21,** 256.
Spreng, L. F., Johnson, L. C., and Lubin, A. (1968). *Psychophysiology* **4,** 311.
Sterman, M. B., Krauss, T., Lehmann, D., and Clemente, C. D. (1965). *Electroencephalogr. Clin. Neurophysiol.* **19,** 509.
Stern, M., Roffwarg, H. P., and Duvoisin, R. (1968). *J. Nerv. Ment. Dis.* **147,** 202.
Tabushi, K., and Himwich, H. E. (1969). *Psychopharmacologia* **16,** 240.
Tabushi, K., and Himwich, H. E. (1970). *Fed. Proc. Fed. Amer. Soc. Exp. Biol.* **29,** 384.
Tagliamonte, A., Tagliamonte, P., Gessa, G. L., and Brodie, B. B. (1969). *Science* **166,** 1433.
Takahashi, Y., Kipnis, D. M., and Daughaday, W. H. (1968). *J. Clin. Invest.* **47,** 2079.
Tauber, E. S., and Weitzman, E. D. (1969). Report to the Association for the Psychophysiological Study of Sleep. *Psychophysiology* **6,** 230. (Abstr.)
Thierry, A.-M., Javoy, F., Glowinski, J., and Kety, S. S. (1968). *J. Pharmacol. Exp. Ther.* **163,** 163.
Tissot, R. (1965). *Progr. Brain Res.* **18,** 175.
Torda, C. (1968). *Brain Res.* **10,** 200.
Trask, C. H., and Cree, E. M. (1962). *New Engl. J. Med.* **266,** 639.
Udenfriend, S., and Zaltman-Nirenberg, P. (1963). *Science* **142,** 394.
Udenfriend, S., Weissbach, H., and Bogdanski, D. F. (1957). *J. Biol. Chem.* **224,** 803.
Udenfriend, S., Zaltman-Nirenberg, P., Gordon, R., and Spector, S. (1966). *Mol. Pharmacol.* **2,** 95.
Ursin, R. (1968). *Brain Res.* **11,** 347.
Van den Noort, S., and Brine, K. (1970). *Amer. J. Physiol.* **218,** 1434.
vanTwyver, H., and Webb, W. B. (1968). Report to the Association for the Psychophysiological Study of Sleep. (Unpublished.)
Velluti, R., and Hernandez-Peon, R. (1963). *Exp. Neurol.* **8,** 20.
Vogel, G. (1960). *Arch. Gen. Psychiat.* **3,** 421.
Vogt, M. (1954). *J. Physiol.* (*London*) **123,** 451.
Wallach, M. B., Winters, W. D., Mandell, A. J., and Spooner, C. E. (1969a). *Electroencephologr. Clin. Neurophysiol.* **27,** 563.
Wallach, M. B , Winters, W. D., Mandell, A. J., and Spooner, C. E. (1969b). *Electroencephalogr. Clin. Neurophysiol.* **27,** 574.
Weiss, T., and Roldan, E. (1964). *Experientia* **20,** 280.
Weiss, T., Bohdanecky, Z., Fifkova, E., and Roldan, E. (1964). *Psychopharmacologia* **5,** 126.
Weissman, A., Koe, B. K., and Tenen, S. S. (1966). *J. Pharmacol. Exp. Ther.* **151,** 339.
Weitzman, E. D. (1961). *Electroencephalogr. Clin. Neurophysiol.* **13,** 790.
Weitzman, E. D., Rapport, M. M., McGregor, P., and Jacoby, J. (1968). *Science* **160,** 1361.
Weitzman, E. D., McGregor, P., Moore, C., and Jacoby, J. (1969). *Life Sci.* **8,** 751.
Whitman, R. M., Kramer, M., and Baldridge, B. (1963). *Arch. Gen. Psychiat.* **8,** 277.
Whitman, R. M., Pierce, C. M., Maas, J. W., and Baldridge, B. (1966). *Comprehensive Psychiatry* **2,** 219.
Williams, H. L., Hammack, J. T., Daly, R. L., Dement, W. C., and Lubin, A. (1964). *Electroencephalogr. Clin. Neurophysiol.* **16,** 26).
Wyatt, R. J., Kupfer, D. J., Fram, D. H., and Snyder, F. (1969). Report to the Association for the Psychophysiological Study of Sleep. *Psychophysiology* **6,** 258. (Abstr.)

Yamada, Y., Yamamoyo, J., Fujiki, A., Hishikawa, Y., and Kaneko, Z. (1967). *Electroencepgalogr. Clin. Neurophysiol.* **22,** 558.

Yamaguchi, N., Marczynski, T. J., and Ling, G. M. (1963). *Electroencephalogr. Clin. Neurophysiol.* **15,** 154.

Yules, R. B., Freedman, D. X., and Chandler, K. A. (1966). *Electroencephalogr. Clin. Neurophysiol.* **20,** 109.

Zarcone, V. P., and Dement, W. C. (1970). *Pharmacologist* **12,** 219.

The Pharmacology of Peripheral Auditory Processes; Cochlear Pharmacology*

PAUL S. GUTH AND RICHARD P. BOBBIN

Department of Pharmacology, Tulane University, New Orleans, Louisiana

I. Introduction

Audition and, indeed, all sensory modalities have for too long been outside the purview of pharmacology. It is a purpose of this article to acquaint pharmacologists with the research potential of the auditory system. Pharmacology has much to gain from and much to give to the study of audition. There is to be gained the enhanced stature from the development of new regions of interest; there is also to be gained the recognition and esteem of a segment of biological scientists whose hitherto unsolved problems may finally yield to pharmacological examination.

* Much of the work reported herein was supported by grants from the Deafness Research Foundation.

Some problems in audition by their nature and from the beginning should have been pharmacology's. Specifically, the problems of ototoxicity and the study of drugs used empirically by the otolaryngologists (e.g., vasodilators and remedies for motion sickness) by definition belong to pharmacology, yet they have received little or no attention from pharmacologists. Little or no progress has been made toward understanding the mechanisms underlying the actions of either ototherapeutic or ototoxic drugs.

Another aspect of audition which may prove fruitful for pharmacologists involves the use of auditory physiological preparations as models by which other sensory or homeostatic processes may be studied. For example, pharmacological studies with the olivocochlear or the cochleoinhibitory tract could illuminate inhibitory processes in other areas such as the spinal cord. Central inhibitory processes share a sensitivity to strychnine. The cochlea, however, has the advantage of being physically isolatable from the rest of the central nervous system. The problems of communication between sensory and nerve cells in general could well yield to pharmacological techniques employed in the cochlea. In fact, the author's interest in the pharmacology of audition was really born with the prospect of perfusion of the cochlea, full of interesting junctions as it is, and relatively isolated from the rest of the body.

The power of pharmacology's special tools, drugs, for the solution of problems appears to be appreciated by physiologists and biochemists as well as by pharmacologists. However, lacking both expertise in drug application and the awareness of the limitations of drugs, biomedical specialists other than pharmacologists may be misled by the results of experiments dependent on interpretation of drug action. On this basis, the application of drugs for the solution of problems in biology ought to be carried out by pharmacologists.

The relatively novel nature of this subject dictates the introduction of a special section on technical references. This section includes references on background information in anatomy, physiology, and biochemistry as well as descriptions of special techniques, which should prove useful to the neophyte auditory pharmacologist.

An extensive review of the literature has been made of the period between 1940 and mid-1970. Occasional key references before and since that time period have been included. In many instances the work seemed to be of such poor quality that judgment dictated its exclusion from this article. This article is, therefore, not all-inclusive. Studies on the effects of drugs on vestibular apparatus could have been included on many of the same bases that were used to justify the writing of this review, but lack of time, space, and expertise likewise dictated their exclusion from this article.

II. Methods in Cochlear Pharmacology

Introductory material on methodology may be found in otolaryngology, physiology, anatomy, or physics texts. Advanced techniques are essentially adaptations from other areas. A monograph of particular interest for its introductory material and completeness in regard to cochlear mechanics and experimentation is Georg von Békésy's "Experiments in Hearing" (1960). This monograph reviews and summarizes all of the author's experiments and includes a review of other work in the area. An excellent publication complementary to von Békésy's is E. A. Wever's "Theory of Hearing" (1949). More advanced monographs include Engström *et al.* (1966), Iurato (1967), Spoendlin (1966) (on structure), and Dittrich (1963) (on biophysics). Many reviews and symposia also include excellent surveys of methodology (Bishop, 1967; Bredberg, 1968; Davis, 1957; Fex, 1962; Hawkins, 1964; Johnstone, 1967, Lawrence, 1968; Rasmussen and Windle, 1960; Schwartzkopf, 1967; Tasaki, 1957).

The gross surgical approaches to the cochlea have been described for the guinea pig (Tasaki, 1954) and the cat (Gulick and Cutt, 1962a). The guinea pig is often favored because its cochlea protrudes from its temporal bone.

The methods of recording cochlear potentials vary. Placement of an active electrode near or on the round window (Fig. 1) with a reference electrode nearby is the simplest method (Amaro *et al.*, 1966; Rosenblith and Rosenzweig, 1951; Wever and Lawrence, 1955; Wever *et al.*, 1949). The electrical activity recorded by this means is of limited value for studying intracochlear phenomena. Therefore, a method of "differential" intracochlear recording developed by Tasaki *et al.* (1952) is used to obtain a greater number and better separation of electrical parameters. Other recording methods include the use of electrodes inserted into the middle scala (Fig. 1) (Tanaka and Katsuki, 1966; von Békésy, 1952) and the use of microelectrodes to measure intracochlear and eighth nerve unit activity (Tasaki *et al.*, 1954); chronically implanted electrodes have been placed on the eighth nerve (Farkashity *et al.*, 1963) or on the round windows of cats (Simmons, 1967; Simmons and Beatty, 1962) or guinea pigs (Bũno *et al.*, 1966).

Many methods for application of chemicals are available. Application onto the round window (Davis *et al.*, 1934) and through the round window (Adrian *et al.*, 1931) are simple and are thought to elicit a localized response. This is in contrast to an intra-arterial application involving cannulation of the axillary artery and advancing the cannula to the level of the vertebral artery (Amaro *et al.*, 1966; Daigneault and Brown, 1966a) or a direct catheterization of the vertebral artery. A method of perfusing

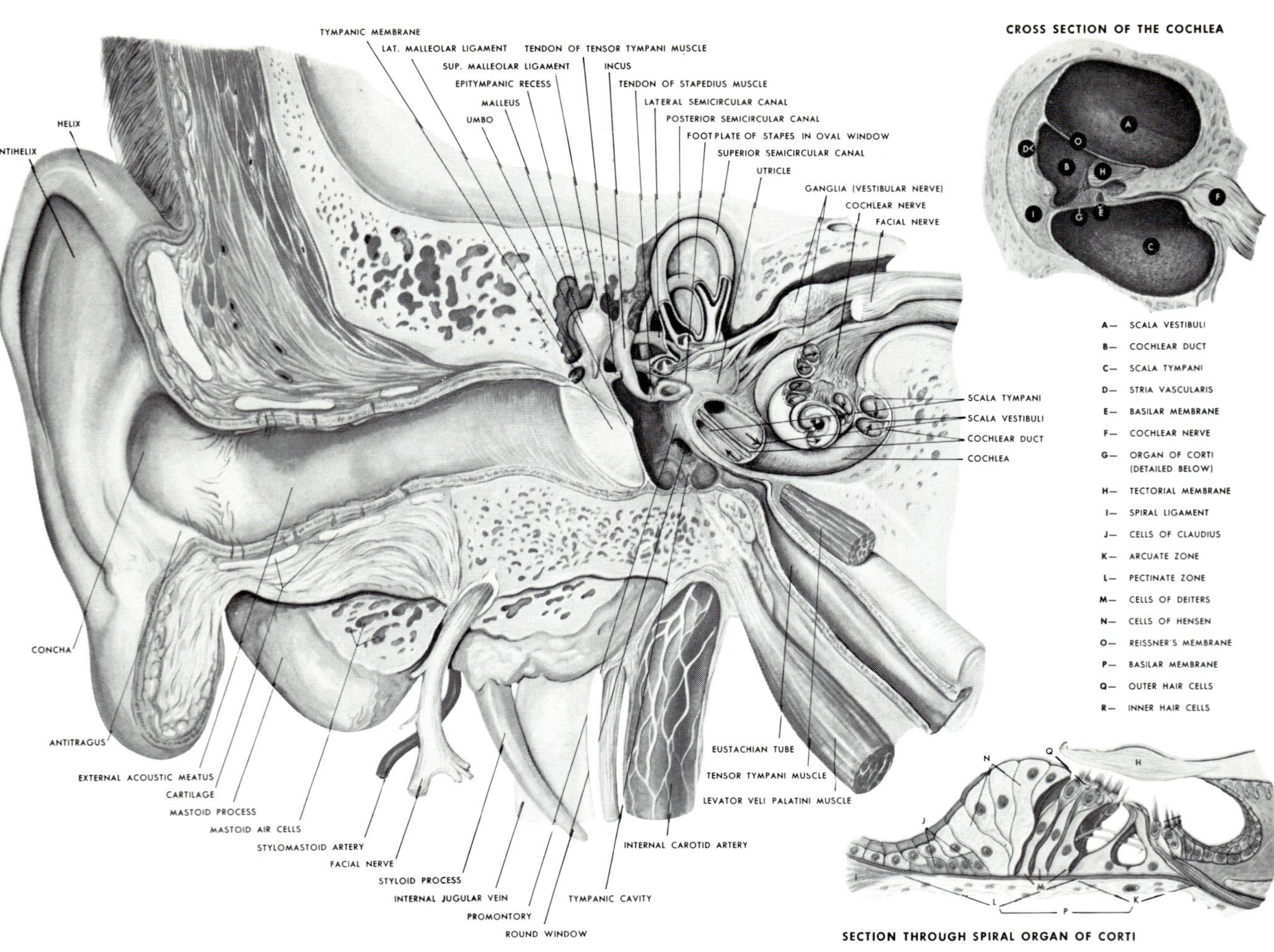
TYMPANIC MEMBRANE
LAT. MALLEOLAR LIGAMENT
TENDON OF TENSOR TYMPANI MUSCLE
SUP. MALLEOLAR LIGAMENT
INCUS
EPITYMPANIC RECESS
TENDON OF STAPEDIUS MUSCLE
MALLEUS
LATERAL SEMICIRCULAR CANAL
UMBO
POSTERIOR SEMICIRCULAR CANAL
FOOTPLATE OF STAPES IN OVAL WINDOW
SUPERIOR SEMICIRCULAR CANAL
UTRICLE
GANGLIA (VESTIBULAR NERVE)
COCHLEAR NERVE
FACIAL NERVE
HELIX
ANTIHELIX
SCALA TYMPANI
SCALA VESTIBULI
COCHLEAR DUCT
COCHLEA
CONCHA
ANTITRAGUS
EXTERNAL ACOUSTIC MEATUS
CARTILAGE
MASTOID PROCESS
MASTOID AIR CELLS
STYLOMASTOID ARTERY
FACIAL NERVE
STYLOID PROCESS
INTERNAL JUGULAR VEIN
PROMONTORY
ROUND WINDOW
TYMPANIC CAVITY
INTERNAL CAROTID ARTERY
EUSTACHIAN TUBE
TENSOR TYMPANI MUSCLE
LEVATOR VELI PALATINI MUSCLE
CROSS SECTION OF THE COCHLEA
A— SCALA VESTIBULI
B— COCHLEAR DUCT
C— SCALA TYMPANI
D— STRIA VASCULARIS
E— BASILAR MEMBRANE
F— COCHLEAR NERVE
G— ORGAN OF CORTI (DETAILED BELOW)
H— TECTORIAL MEMBRANE
I— SPIRAL LIGAMENT
J— CELLS OF CLAUDIUS
K— ARCUATE ZONE
L— PECTINATE ZONE
M— CELLS OF DEITERS
N— CELLS OF HENSEN
O— REISSNER'S MEMBRANE
P— BASILAR MEMBRANE
Q— OUTER HAIR CELLS
R— INNER HAIR CELLS
SECTION THROUGH SPIRAL ORGAN OF CORTI

the cochlea via the vascular bed has been developed (Costa *et al.*, 1966) but not used as a means of applying drugs. The application of agents directly into the scala vestibuli and scala tympani (Fig. 1) circumvents extracochlear influences. This method has been used with excellent results by Konishi and Kelsey (1968a) in the guinea pig. Injections into the scala media, though more difficult, have been accomplished by pressure (Tanaaka, 1963) or iontophoresis (Tanaka and Katsuki, 1966). In cats this is more difficult than in guinea pigs, but a method has been described which may be adapted for chemical injection into the cat scala media (Tonndorf and Tabor, 1962).

Procedures have been described for removing extracochlear influences such as section of the middle ear muscles (Fig. 1) (Amaro *et al.*, 1966), section of eighth nerve (von Békésy, 1960), and section of the olivocochlear bundle (Schuknecht *et al.*, 1959). To examine the effect an agent may have on the cochlear vessels, methods of observing them have been developed (Naumann, 1964; Perlman and Kimura, 1965; Tsunao and Perlman, 1965).

Other approaches to the study of the cochlea include the biochemical examination of cochlear fluids (Makimoto *et al.*, 1967; Miyake, 1960; Palva and Raunio, 1967; Savin *et al.*, 1968) and structures (Iinuma, 1967; Kuijpers *et al.*, 1967; Matschinsky and Thalmann, 1967), the microscopic examination of the components of the cochlea (Beck and Holz, 1968; Goldstein and Mizukoshi, 1967; Vinnikov and Titova, 1964), its histology (Engström *et al.*, 1966), and measurement of cochlear fluid pressure (Harkins and Yanof, 1967). Vinnikov and Titova (1964) have described the methods for rapid isolation of the membranous cochlea of the guinea pig in a functional state.

III. Blood Supply and Autonomic Innervation of the Cochlea

Blood is supplied to the cochlea via the internal auditory artery, a branch of either the basilar artery or, more commonly, the inferior cerebellar artery. The internal auditory artery itself divides into vestibular, vestibulocochlear, and cochlear arteries. The cochlear artery enters the modiolus and divides to form spiral arteries supplying the scala tympani, spiral ligament, osseous spiral lamina, and cochlear ganglion throughout the cochlea.

The cochlear drainage consists of the posterior spiral vein, receiving blood from the basal and middle cochlear turns, and the anterior spiral

FIG. 1. Section through human head showing the external, middle, and inner ear with magnified depictions of the organ of Corti and cross section of the cochlea (by courtesy of the Zenith Radio Corporation).

vein, receiving blood from the apical turn. These veins together form the veins of the cochlear aqueduct and empty into the jugular vein.

According to Lorente de No (1926) and Bovero (1914) the sympathetic innervation of the inner ear consists of postganglionic nerve fibers arising from the stellate ganglion and probably from the superior cervical ganglion.

Lichtensteiger and Spoendlin (1967) demonstrated the sympathetic innervation of the basilar, the inferior anterior cerebellar, and the *labyrinthine* arteries by the method of Falck *et al.* (1962). The perivascular green-fluorescing network disappears at the level of the modiolar branches of the cochlear artery; more peripherally, no adrenergic fibers are found with the blood vessels. The fluorescence of the presumed adrenergic nerve fibers disappears after treatment with reserpine (Terayama *et al.*, 1966). No evidence of adrenergic innervation could be found in association with the vessels of the limbus, spiral ligament, stria vascularis, or spiral vessel of the basilar membrane by the fluorescence method. At a recent meeting, Hilding (Hilding and Sugiura, 1970) reported evidence for the presence of catecholamines or indoleamines in the cochlea, and Spoendlin described an autonomic innervation of the basilar membrane vessels.

A large number of green fluorescent fibers (adrenergic) independent of blood vessels are found in the osseous spiral lamina. These fibers appear to travel with the cochlear nerve, but their origin and termination have not been determined.

Thus, there seem to be two distinct sets of adrenergic fibers within the cochlea. One is the perivascular system limited to the larger cochlear arteries, the second set appears independent of blood vessels. For more detailed information, the reader is directed to the excellent monographs of Iurato (1967) and Spoendlin (1966).

Pharmacologists with their specific interest and expertise in matters autonomic might profitably investigate the significance of dual adrenergic innervation of the cochlea. Section of fibers of the stellate ganglion leads to an increase in amplitude of cochlear potentials (Beickert and Terayama, 1965), whereas stimulation of the cervical sympathetic fibers decreases the amplitude of the cochlear microphonic. In seeking a role for the nonvascular sympathetic innervation, Spoendlin (1966) referred to the work of Loewenstein (1956) who demonstrated that sympathetic stimulation lowers the threshold of touch receptors. Cochlear sympathetic fibers may likewise influence auditory sensitivity.

IV. Autonomic Agents Producing Effects within the Cochlea

A. Adrenomimetic and Adrenolytic Agents

Adrenomimetic agents have been applied to the inner ear by several routes. On intracochlear application of epinephrine, Gulick and Cutt

(1962a,b) and Tanaka and Katsuki (1966) found no effect on cochlear microphonic (CM) amplitude (see Glossary). Gulick and Cutt (1962a,b) also applied epinephrine to the round window of the guinea pig and found no effect on CM amplitude by this route. On the other hand, on injecting ephedrine and cobephrin so that blood pressure was affected, Jankowski *et al.* (1962a) found some correlation in time course between the increase of blood pressure and the decrease in CM amplitude which resulted. In a parallel investigation with Hydergin and guanethidine (Jankowski *et al.*, 1962b), there was some correlation in time between the CM decreases and in this case the fall in systemic blood pressure. The authors attributed these changes in CM to the circulatory disturbance and possible compromise of oxygen supply to the organ of Corti. Gisselson (1950) first remarked on the sensitivity of the cochlear potentials to blood pressure changes in 1950; he considered that 40 mm Hg represented a minimal level below which potentials are not sustained.

The relationship between oxygen supply and cochlear potentials has been studied by many authors. Of the cochlear potentials, VIII nerve action potential (N_1) (see Glossary) is more sensitive to oxygen deprivation than CM in that N_1 decreases more rapidly and requires longer to recover than CM does. For more complete discussion of this subject, see Vosteen (1961). This same article discusses the relationships of cochlear blood supply disturbances and hypothermia to oxygen deprivation and subsequent alterations in cochlear potentials. It seems important to mention here that hypothermia may affect both CM and N_1 with CM being the more sensitive potential (Kahana *et al.*, 1950).

B. Cholinomimetic and Cholinolytic Agents

Evidence for the existence of cholinergic innervation of the cochlea rests on (*1*) the demonstration of cochlear staining for cholinesterase (Schuknecht *et al.*, 1959) which disappears upon section and degeneration of the olivocochlear bundle of Rasmussen, (*2*) the demonstration of cholinesterase in endolymph (Gisselson, 1950; Miyake, 1960) and perilymph (Miyake, 1960); and (*3*) the unconfirmed demonstration of the presence of acetylcholine in the perilymph (Martini, 1941). The cholinesterase-containing nerve fibers clearly belong to the olivocochlear bundle and more will be said about them in the next section (Section V, A).

Gisselson, following his demonstration of cholinesterase in endolymph (Gisselson, 1950) reported that the cholinesterase inhibitors physostigmine, metastigmin, and isoflurophate (DFP) injected intra-arterially prolonged the period between the application of sound stimulus and the appearance of CM (Gisselson, 1952). This finding is difficult to interpret. Contrariwise, using a different route of drug administration and a more sophisticated means of measuring latencies, Gannon *et al.* (1966) found the sound–

CM latency to be exceptionally stable and alterable only by imminent death. Likewise, these authors reported that CM–N_1 latency was not influenced by intravenous physostigmine. The route of drug administration may be critical in these studies. Sohmer and Feinmesser (1963) could find no effect of acetylcholine or physostigmine on CM or N_1 either when these agents were injected into perilymph space or when they were applied to the round window. Amaro *et al.* (1966) and Brown *et al.* (1967), however, found physostigmine to inhibit N_1 when given by close intraarterial injection (the axillary artery was cannulated and the cannula advanced approximately to the level of the vertebral artery). Acetylcholine injected by the same route also depressed N_1. Amaro *et al.* (1966) injected acetylcholine and physostigmine intravenously and found acetylcholine to be inactive and the character of the physostigmine-induced N_1 depression to be changed. Physostigmine-injected intra-arterially produces two phases of action in regard to N_1 depression—an initial transient phase I and a later, prolonged phase II (Amaro *et al.*, 1966). Following intravenous physostigmine only phase II inhibition is produced; phase II is prevented from appearing by previous administration of atropine and in time course has the characteristics of physostigmine's anticholinesterase action. Phase I, in contrast, is not antagonized by atropine and appears to be independent of cholinesterase inhibition, since in cats treated with atropine, or with atropine plus enough DFP to inhibit cerebral cholinesterase completely, physostigmine still produces phase I depression (Amaro *et al.*, 1966). However, cochlear cholinesterase may be resistant or at least inaccessible to DFP according to the research of Kaneko (1965). Further confirmation of the N_1 depressive action of cholinomimetic agents comes from the studies of Daigneault and Brown (1966a) using acetylcholine and methacholine by close intra-arterial injection, of Guth (1967) using acetylcholine and neostigmine and nicotine by close intra-arterial injection; and of Katsuki *et al.* (1965) and Tanaka and Katsuki (1966) using acetylcholine and neostigmine by electrophoretic application in the region of the hair cells. A word of explanation is required. Katsuki *et al.* (1965) and Tanaka and Katsuki (1966) make much more of the depressant effect of the cholinomimetic agents of CM than they do on N_1, saying "change in N_1 response due to acetylcholine was not so clear-cut." However, close inspection of the figures in these papers can only lead to the conclusion that N_1 is clearly depressed. Tanaka and Katsuki (1966) went on to measure firing rates of primary auditory neurons under the influence of electrophoretically applied acetylcholine and found a marked decrease in firing rate. This decrease in firing rate could be associated with the reduction in N_1 seen with intra-arterial acetylcholine.

The depression of CM by acetylcholine as first noted by Katsuki *et al.* (1965) has been seen after close intraarterial injection (Guth, 1967) on occasion, but not regularly.

The N_1-depressive action of acetylcholine and physostigmine takes place whether or not the middle ear muscles are severed (Amaro *et al.*, 1966). Daigneault and Brown (1966b) found acetylcholine still active after VIII nerve section which produces a neuronally isolated cochlea. It is, therefore, reasonable to conclude that these cholinomimetics are acting within the cochlea.

It has been reported that atropine sulfate (Amaro *et al.*, 1966; Daigneault and Brown, 1966a) and atropine methylsulfate (Daigneault and Brown, 1966a) block the N_1 depressant effect of acetylcholine. In a later communication, Pruett *et al.* (1967), reported that streptomycin, dihydrostreptomycin, neomycin, quinine, and kanamycin prevented acetylcholine's effect.

Whereas atropine by general consent has no effect on the amplitude of cochlear potentials, in a very interesting paper Gannon and Laszlo (1968) demonstrated the prolongation of the CM–N_1 interval by atropine. In their discussion, Gannon and Laszlo favored the possibilities that atropine is acting on intracochlear synaptic transmission, perhaps at a cholinergic junction, or that it is inhibiting a postulated adrenergic facilitatory influence. In some of the experiments, atropine was applied topically to the round window, and in their view, "It is unlikely that the effect of atropine is due to other general changes because of the rapid effect noticed following local administration. . . ." These authors were careful to note, and rightly so, that the effects of atropine need not imply the presence of a cholinergic junction in the cochlea. Likewise, the effects of cholinomimetics on cochlear potentials ought to be regarded rather conservatively as evidence not for the existence of cholinergic mechanisms but only for the existence of cholinoceptive structures within the cochlea. The action of cholinomimetics on cochlear potentials has a bearing on the discussion of the pharmacology of the olivocochlear bundle and its putative inhibitory transmitter (see Section V).

Comis and Whitfield (1965, 1968) have adduced evidence for cholinergic synapses in the cochlear nucleus. In this instance, however, the cholinomimetics, acetylcholine and acetyl-β-methylcholine, applied locally by microtap produced excitatory effects such as increased resting activity of the neurons and lowered thresholds to sonic stimulation. Furthermore, atropine and dihyro-β-erythroidine antagonized the effects of sonic stimulation, which is excitatory, on these same neurons.

V. The Olivocochlear Bundle

A. Anatomy

Although the nerve fibers now known to belong to the olivocochlear bundle (OCB) were recognized by early anatomists, even to their efferent nature (Spoendlin, 1966), it was Rasmussen (1946) who demonstrated definitively the origin and course of this tract. It arises from the retro-olivary nucleus, crosses the midline along the floor of the fourth ventricle (where it is accessible for the placement of electrodes or sectioning), and joins the vestibular branch of the contralateral VIII nerve. With this nerve, this bundle reaches the basal turn of the cochlea. In 1960, Rasmussen provided evidence for yet another OCB, this one ipsilateral. In the cat, the crossed or contralateral OCB contains 500 fibers and the uncrossed, 100 (Rasmussen and Windle, 1960). By the application of a histochemical method, Schuknecht *et al.* (1959) demonstrated that the acetylcholinesterase of the cochlea was confined to the OCB which by this means could be traced to the inner and outer hair cells.

Many researchers (in Spoendlin, 1966) have confirmed the association of OCB with large nerve endings containing synaptic vesicles which synapse with the hair cells (mainly outer hair cells) and possibly with VIII nerve afferents. The above description of the OCB contains only the barest outline of the anatomical information available. For further elaboration, see Spoendlin (1966) and Iurato (1967).

B. Physiology

The physiological importance of the OCB remains to be discovered. The inhibitory effect of OCB stimulation on N_1 was first noted and studied by Galambos (1956). His original observations made by means of stimulating electrodes on the floor of the fourth ventricle and recording electrodes on the cochlear round window have been confirmed many times (Desmedt and Monaco, 1961; Fex, 1967; Guth and Amaro, 1968). Fex (1962) first showed that OCB stimulation increased the amplitude of the CM response and the endocochlear resting potential. Maximum inhibition of N_1 and increase of CM requires that the OCB be stimulated by 40 pulses at 400 pps (Desmedt, 1962). The inhibitory influence lasts up to 180 msec.

By recording from single fibers of the crossed OCB, Fex (1962) found some of them to exhibit a resting firing rate of 1 to 20 impulses/second. The frequency of firing of these fibers could be increased by sound stimulation up to a maximum of 50 impulses/second. Fex (1962) considered the OCB a part of a feedback system regulating auditory afferent activity.

In support of this proposal, Dewson (1968) has demonstrated that monkeys require an intact crossed OCB in order to discriminate speech sounds in the presence of noise. No deficit of perception was seen in animals with transections of the crossed OCB when speech sounds are presented without a noise background. The OCB may, therefore, function in a filtering capacity, increasing signal-to-noise ratio.

The suggestion of Desmedt (1962) that the crossed OCB produces its effects by hyperpolarizing the hair cell membrane has been substantiated by Fex (1967). Marshalling the data of Iurato (1967) that the crossed OCB endings innervated only the outer hair cells (in the rat) plus his own electrophysiological data suggesting a hyperpolarization of the hair cell, Fex (1967) has proposed that the crossed OCB acts only presynaptically relative to the primary afferents. Specifically, hyperpolarization of the hair cells would result in an increase in current flow through the hair cell membrane explaining the increase in CM, which is thought to be a hair cell potential, and resulting in decreased transmission to the primary afferents explaining the decrease in N_1. The uncrossed OCB, however, has not been shown to affect CM (Desmedt and LaGrutta, 1963; Fex, 1967) although the inhibitory effect on N_1 is seen. On this basis, Fex proposed that the uncrossed OCB synapses only with afferent endings and not with hair cells.

C. Pharmacology

The most reliable antagonist of OCB effects both on CM and N_1 is strychnine. It antagonizes the effects of both the crossed and uncrossed OCBs. Closely related alkaloids, such as brucine and coniine, produce similar antagonistic effects (LaGrutta and Desmedt, 1964). Inactive in this regard are Metrazol, picrotoxin, ammonium chloride, physostigmine, β-erythroidine (Desmedt and Monaco, 1960), and a strychnine-like substance, compound 1757 I.S. (Desmedt and Monaco, 1962). Unpublished data from the author's laboratory permits the conclusion that the crossed OCB contains the ACh-synthesizing enzyme choline acetyltransferase. The presence of both the synthetic and hydrolytic enzymes of ACh strongly supports the hypothesis that the OCB operates by a cholinergic mechanism.

The possibility that the OCB exerts its effects by a neurohumoral mechanism cholinergic in nature was supported by the following evidence: (*1*) OCB endings synapsing with hair cells contain synaptic vesicles (Engström *et al.*, 1966); (*2*) OCB fibers contain acetylcholinesterase (Churchill *et al.*, 1956); (*3*) a factor in the inner ear with acetylcholine-like activity on smooth muscle assay has been reported (Martini, 1941) but not confirmed; (*4*) physostigmine has been alleged (Gisselson, 1952) to prolong the CM–N_1 latency, but this was denied (Gannon *et al.*, 1966); and (*5*) cholinomimetic agents influence the amplitude of auditory nerve action potentials (Amaro *et al.*, 1966; Daigneault and Brown, 1966a).

Evidence damaging to the hypothesis that OCB effects are achieved by cholinergic means is not difficult to find. Cholinomimetics, although mimicking OCB insofar as reduction of N_1 amplitude, do not usually mimic the enhancement of CM caused by OCB stimulation, In fact, several investigators (Guth, 1967; Tanaka and Katsuki, 1966) have reported a decrease in CM amplitude. Daigneault (1967) has occasionally seen an increase in CM amplitude with intra-arterial cholinomimetics. Furthermore, the classic anticholinergic agents, atropine, dihydro-β-erythroidine (Desmedt and Monaco, 1962; Guth and Amaro, 1968), tubocurarine, and mecamylamine (Guth and Amaro, 1968) do not affect OCB-induced effects on N_1. Cholinesterase inhibitors, such as physostigmine, do not seem to enhance or prolong OCB-induced inhibition. The fact that the action of the OCB antagonists, strychnine and related alkaloids, was not known to involve an interaction with cholinomimetic neurohumors has also weighed against the hypothesis. However, now information has appeared concerning the relationship of strychnine to cholinergically mediated processes. In fact, the antagonism of OCB inhibition by strychnine may be accommodated within a cholinergic hypothesis when viewed in the light of the work of McKinstry and Koelle (1967). These authors found that strychnine sulfate reduced the output of acetylcholine from the preganglionically stimulated superior cervical ganglion. The problem of OCB inhibition and its antagonism by strychnine receive extensive consideration in their paper. Strychnine's effects may, therefore, not be produced by an antagonism of an inhibitory transmitter postsynaptically, but by a presynaptic action inhibiting acetylcholine release.

In an investigation into the possible cholinergic nature of OCB-induced inhibition, Guth and Amaro (1968 employed hemicholinium No. 3 (HC-3). As an agent that interferes with cholinergic processes not by antagonizing acetylcholine primarily but by inhibiting the synthesis of acetylcholine (Schueler, 1960) HC-3 was used as yet another pharmacological stratagem whereby acetylcholine's involvement in OCB-induced inhibition could be tested. The HC-3 gradually decreased the OCB inhibitory effect; like other effects of HC-3, this action was reversed on rest or after injection of choline (Guth and Amaro, 1968). Even more convincing evidence of the cholinergic nature of OCB inhibition comes from the work of Fex (1968). He recorded from electrodes within the scala media the slow potential changes induced by repetitive OCB stimulation. Perfusion of the perilymph space with artificial perilymph containing a rather specific cholinergic antagonist, *d*-tubocurarine, tended to reduce the amplitude and rate of rise of the OCB-induced potential changes.

At least two explanations present themselves for the apparently incongruous findings that most cholinolytics do not antagonize OCB-induced inhibition, whereas HC-3, presumably inhibiting acetylcholine synthesis, does. First, is the possibility raised in other seemingly noncholinergic systems affected by HC-3, that acetylcholine is merely an intermediate agent, a link by which the release of the final transmitter is accomplished. This possibility accommodates the activities of HC-3 and strychnine and the inactivity of the classic cholinolytics. The second possibility is that the OCB–hair cell junction represents a new type of cholinergic junction. Autonomic ganglia, neuromuscular junctions, parasympathetic–effector junctions, and motor nerve–Renshaw cell junctions, all cholinergic, differ somewhat in their susceptibilities to blocking agents. It may be that the junction under consideration is likewise cholinergic but will require yet a different type of blocking agent. After all, the OCB–hair cell synapse may be considered functionally different from the junctions mentioned above because it is nerve–nerve (or nerve–hair cell) and inhibitory and influencing a sensory structure.

A series of experiments designed to determine whether γ-aminobutyric acid (GABA) might be the transmitter of OCB inhibition produced no evidence in favor of this hypothesis (Bobbin and Guth, 1970). Although intra-arterially injected GABA produces a decrease in N_1, other chemically unrelated agents, such as dextrose and sodium chloride, do likewise when injected in doses equimolar to the high doses of GABA necessary to evoke this response. Neither GABA antagonists nor agents influencing GABA metabolism were able to influence OCB-induced inhibition of N_1. In the course of these studies, however, a very interesting effect of the GABA transaminase inhibitor, amino-oxyacetic acid, was noted on N_1 (Bobbin *et al.*, 1969) and on behaviorally determined hearing thresholds. This agent produces a long-lasting reversible decrease in N_1 amplitude and a correlated increase in hearing threshold. The actions appear unrelated to any change in GABA metabolism (Bobbin *et al.*, 1969).

VI. Ototoxic Agents

A. Analgesic Antipyretics

1. Quinine and Chloroquine

The neurotoxicity of quinine has been recognized for some time. Auditory changes include tinnitus and decreased auditory acuity. Vertigo is also seen. The damage inflicted upon the inner ear may be irreversible under certain conditions (Ehmke, 1963), such as disturbances in kidney function, pregnancy, and predisposition, as in familial deafness.

Consistent histological damage in quinine intoxication occurs in the stria vascularis and outer hair cells (Fig. 1) (Hennebert and Fernandez, 1959; Ruedi *et al.*, 1952). Vascular contusion and hemorrhage in the cochlea with clear strial damage have been reported. (Ruedi *et al.*, 1952). The outer hair cells show degeneration and cloudy swelling. There is occasional internal hair cell damage (Lurie, 1955; Ruedi *et al.*, 1952). This damage is reflected in the decrease or loss of CM (Hennebert and Fernandez, 1959; Ruedi *et al.*, 1952) and reduction of N_1. With acute administration of quinine, both potentials recover over time (Lurie, 1955), but with chronic administration it is possible to abolish CM permanently. The high oxygen requirement of the stria vascularis and the outer hair cells may be responsible for their sensitivities to quinine and other ototoxic agents. The stria vascularis has been reported (Chou and Rodgers, 1962) to have the highest oxygen consumption in the body. Several authors have attributed the ototoxicity of quinine to an interference with oxygen supply (Ruedi *et al.*, 1952).

Koide *et al.* (1966) studied the histochemical changes of succinic dehydrogenase and diphosphopyridine nucleotide diaphorase in the cochlea after administrating quinine or ototoxic antibiotics. The enzymes in the outer hair cells and nerve endings were most seriously affected. The patterns of damage with quinine and the antibiotics were identical.

Another commonly seen morphological change in quinine poisoning was compression of the organ of Corti resulting from pressure changes in the chambers of the inner ear. For example, Permin (1957) reported endolymphatic compression (i.e., Reissner's membrane and tectorial membrane (Fig. 1) pressed toward organ of Corti). Increased pressure in the scala media was also reported by Hennebert and Fernandez (1959) and Ruedi *et al.* (1952). Supracochlear damage after quinine intoxication is attributed to hair cell degeneration causing changes in the spiral ganglion cells (Ruedi *et al.*, 1952). Although damage to brainstem nuclei has been reported, this does not seem to be a consistent finding. For an extensive review of the earlier literature, see Ruedi *et al.* (1952).

Chloroquine has been reported to produce ototoxicity characterized by tinnitus and imbalance (Hart and Naunton, 1964). Three cases of congenital deafness after treatment of pregnant women with chloroquine have been reported (Hart and Naunton, 1964). Cochlear potentials show the expected changes with both CM and N_1 being depressed (Ishii *et al.*, 1967) as well as changes in amplitude seen with electrodes on VIII nerve and cochlear nucleus (Gold and Wilpizeskie, 1966). Amplitude changes appear greater at low intensity of stimulation (Gold and Wilpizeskie, 1966).

2. Salicylates

The labyrinthine toxicity of salicylates, like that of quinine, manifests itself in tinnitus, loss of auditory acuity, especially for high frequencies, and vertigo (McCabe and Dey, 1965; Myers and Bernstein, 1965; Myers *et al.*, 1965; Perez de Moura and Hayden, 1968). These changes are regarded by most authorities as being reversible, but Ehmke (1963)stressed that under certain conditions, as with quinine, the damage may be permanent.

The hearing deficit seems to be dose related. That is, the increase in hearing threshold (Myers and Bernstein, 1965) is reported to be related to blood levels of salicylate. The hearing loss appears primarily at high frequencies, but audiometric changes at high and low frequencies have also been reported. Interestingly, in patients suffering hearing losses from other causes, salicylates may influence the normal portions of the audiograms more than the abnormal (Myers *et al.*, 1965).

Histological alterations consisting of hyperchromatosis of nuclei or whole cells (Gotlib, 1957), hemorrhage in the cochlea, changes in the spiral ganglion but no ultrastructural changes (Myers and Bernstein, 1965), and constriction of stria vascularis have been seen with acute salicylate administration (Hawkins, 1964). Within 15 minutes after tritiated salicylate administration, Ishii *et al.* (1967) found radioactivity in the stria vascularis and vessels of the spiral ligament but none in the organ of Corti (Fig. 1) or in the spiral ganglion; 60 minutes after drug administration, the stria vascularis and spiral ligament (Fig. 1) still showed radioactivity, and it had begun to appear in the organ of Corti and spiral ganglion. The radioactivity was essentially gone after 360 minutes.

Silverstein *et al.* (1967) monitored electrical activity as well as selected biochemical parameters under the influence of salicylate. Salicylate intoxication was accompanied by a decrease of both CM and N_1 potentials, commencing within 30 to 60 minutes after intraperitoneal injection of sodium salicylate (350 mg/kg, in cats). The sodium, potassium, and total protein concentrations in the inner ear fluids appeared unaffected during salicylate intoxication, but malic dehydrogenase activities of endolymph and perilymph decreased in proportion to rising serum and perilymph salicylate levels. Elevation of serum, endolymph, and perilymph glucose was also found. The site of salicylate ototoxicity is felt to be intracochlear.

The mechanics of salicylate and quinine ototoxicity are unknown. Damage to the stria vascularis seems implicated with alterations in hair cell function resulting from ischemia or compression of the organ of Corti.

The hair cells appear to depend on the diffusion of primary substrates from the stria vascularis of the scala media as well as from vessels in the basilar membrane for their nutrition. The stria also seems to serve a secretory function. Thus, the hair cells may be operating only on minimal concentrations of nutrients and any abridgement of supply may result in functional and eventually morphological changes. The same mechanism may cause antibiotic ototoxicity.

B. Local Anesthetics

Local anesthetics have been used by otolaryngologists for many years. It is reasonable to assume that the local anesthetics which are known to influence other neural processes would likely also alter auditory function. For the most part, these agents have been applied locally into the middle ear or directly on the round window, but some studies have been performed with parenterally administered drugs. Intramuscular lidocaine or mepivacaine caused no change in cochlear electrical activity (Nowak and Dahl, 1966). Intravenous procaine, on the other hand, was reported to cause considerable increases in auditory thresholds of normal humans (Fruttero and Sartoris, 1966). Increased pressure in the inner ear was considered the probable cause of the change in sensitivity.

Both CM and N_1 amplitudes are depressed by the application of local anesthetics to the round window. As noted in Table I, some anesthetics in some concentrations depress CM and N_1 with no signs of recovery for 6 hours in one study (Rahm *et al.*, 1961) and 20 hours in another (Rahm *et al.*, 1961). Epinephrine has been applied both separately (Cutt, 1963; Rahm *et al.*, 1962) and together with the local anesthetics (Cutt, 1963; Nowak and Dahl, 1966). Cutt (1963) found no change in CM with the application of epinephrine, whereas Rahm *et al.* (1962) reported some enhancement of CM. Not unexpectedly dibucaine applied to the VIII nerve sheath produced potential changes equivalent to VIII nerve section (Daigneault and Brown, 1966b). Intraarterial injections of chlorpromazine (5 mg/kg) are capable of obliterating N_1 and reducing CM, presumably by local anesthetic action of the drug (Guth, 1967).

Strother *et al.* (1964) were able to demonstrate that local anesthetics applied to the round window caused increases in behavioral threshold and a decrement in cochlear potentials.

Perfusion of the perilymphatic space with lidocaine also decreases both CM and N_1, with N_1 being much more sensitive (Honrubia and Ward, 1966). Under lidocaine perfusion, a phenomenon resembling recruitment

TABLE I

Effect of Local Anesthetics Applied to the Round Window on Cochlear Potentials

Anesthetic agent	Concentration applied to round window (%)	Recovery time	Ref.
Cocaine	0.5–10	Min–hr	Cutt (1963); Rahm *et al.* (1959)
	10	Irreversible	Rahm *et al.* (1960, 1961, 1962)
Hexylcaine	0.5–10	Min–hr	Cutt (1963)
	1	Irreversible	Rahm *et al.* (1961)
	5	Complete recovery	Rahm *et al.* (1961)
Procaine	0.5–10	Min–hr	Cutt (1963)
	2	Complete recovery (30 min)	Rahm *et al.* (1960, 1961)
Tetracaine	0.5–10	Min–hr	Cutt (1963)
	2	Irreversible	Rahm *et al.* (1961)
Lidocaine	0.5–10	Min–hr	Cutt (1963)
	1	Irreversible (6 hr)	Rahm *et al.* (1962)
	0.5	Recovery	Rahm *et al.* (1962)

(i.e., an unnatural gain in intensity with increasing stimulus) developed. The N_1 was rapidly depressed when 0.05–0.1% procaine was introduced into the scala tympani (Konishi and Kelsey, 1968a); the CM was depressed when procaine was introduced into scala tympani or scala media. The endocochlear potential increased when procaine was applied to the scala media or scala tympani. Konishi and Kelsey (1968a) proposed that procaine interferes with potassium permeability. Potassium-rich endolymph has been shown to be important for the sensitivity of the hair cells to sound stimulation, production of CM, and the inhibitory effect of procaine (Konishi and Kelsey, 1968a).

C. Metabolic Inhibition

1. Tetraethylammonium and Tetrodotoxin

These two agents have in common the ability to interfere with ion permeability. Tetraethylammonium (TEA), like the local anesthetics, can reduce potassium conductance (Katsuki *et al.*, 1966). Tetrodotoxin, on the other hand, is considered to block the sodium channel in the cell membrane

(Kao, 1966). As mentioned just above, a potassium-rich endolymph seems indispensible for high sensitivity of CM. When TEA was introduced into the scala media or the hair cell region by iontophoresis, there was produced a gradual, irreversible decrease of CM (Katsuki *et al.*, 1966). Tetraethylammonium resembled iontophoretically applied acetylcholine in slightly reducing the neural potential. The endocochlear potential was reduced after introduction of TEA in the scala media, but no change occurred after introduction of the drug into the hair cell region.

By comparison, tetrodotoxin caused no change in CM responses but irreversibly depressed N_1 (Katsuki *et al.*, 1966). This implies that different ionic mechanisms are responsible for the two potentials. Changes in potassium conductance appear essential for CM generation, and sodium conductance changes for N_1. Konishi and Kelsey (1968b) supported this hypothesis by perfusing the perilymphatic space with sodium-free solutions and found that N_1 is reversibly inhibited by lack of sodium, whereas the endocochlear potential and CM were only slightly affected and at a later time. Interestingly, replacement of sodium by choline in the perfusion solution occasionally increased CM.

2. Glucose Metabolism

Insulin-induced hypoglycemia was reported to cause marked diminution in CM (Wing, 1959) in cats. On the basis of these findings it was assumed that the cochlea was extremely sensitive to decreases in blood sugar. However, Fernandez and Brenman (1957) found that rather profound hypoglycemia did not affect CM when vascular changes were prevented. Koide *et al.* (1960) confirmed the influence of insulin on CM, reporting that high doses (80 U/kg) decrease CM after many hours. The injection of substrates (glucose, pyruvate, fumarate) produced recovery of CM. These authors also monitored cochlear oxygen tension and concluded in accord with Fernandez and Brenman (1957) that decrease in oxygen tension, probably secondary to insulin hypoglycemia-induced vascular changes, was responsible for the reduction in CM.

3. Anoxia

Several reports have attested to the sensitivity of the cochlear potentials to oxygen deprivation (Bornschein and Krejci, 1950; Fernandez and Alzate, 1959; Wever, 1949). By pressing a probe against the anterior inferior cerebellar artery the blood supply of the cochlea may be shut off immediately. Konishi *et al.* (1961) found that this maneuver abolished N_1

and the endocochlear potential within 45 seconds; CM declined to a constant level in slightly longer time and the summating potential also fell. In general, the endocochlear and summating potentials are more resistant to anoxia than CM and N_1. Butler *et al.* (1962) found that perfusion of the scala vestibuli with Ringer's solution markedly retarded the decline in cochlear potentials during anoxia. The antianoxia effect of Ringer's solution was seen whether it was bubbled with nitrogen or with oxygen. The authors offer two explanations of these results but do not strongly support one over the other: either washing the perilymph space removes accumulated toxic products or perfusion delivers some oxygen to the cochlea even if Ringer's solution is bubbled with nitrogen (or both).

When cochlear anoxia is produced by interference with blood supply or with respiration, all the structures of the cochlea are subject to its effects. Misrahy (1958) applied a method designed to produce localized hypoxia. This consisted of injecting a mixture of glucose and glucose oxidase into the scala media of the various cochlear turns. The enzymatic oxidation of glucose was expected to consume local supplies of oxygen. By this means it was shown that CM generation is an oxygen-dependent process and that the CM-generating structures (hair cells) derive their oxygen largely from endolymph.

The N_1 potential is also very sensitive to oxygen deprivation (in Vosteen, 1961). In fact, N_1 declines more rapidly than CM in the face of anoxia and CM recovers more rapidly (Fernandez and Alzate, 1959).

4. Cyanide and Iodoacetate

Whether applied intra-arterially or intracochlearly, cyanide depresses cochlear potentials (in Vosteen, 1961). Konishi and Kelsey (1968a) applied sodium cyanide by cochlear perfusion and found a reversible depression of all cochlear potentials and the appearance of a new negative potential in the scala media which they attributed to hair cell depolarization. Perfusion of the scala tympani with cyanide was more effective in depressing potentials than perfusion of scala vestibuli. On this basis, the authors reasoned that the stria vascularis is probably not the site of action since the stria is equally accessible from either scala. However, it may mean that the basilar membrane is more permeabile to cyanide than Reissner's membrane. In either case, it may be concluded that the cochlear partitions are permeable to cyanide.

Iodoacetate when added to perilymph perfusion medium depresses CM and flattens the intensity–function curve (Bornschein and Thalmann, 1962).

5. *Ouabain and Erythrophleine*

Iinuma (1967) studied the Na^+- and K^+-activated adenosine triphosphatase (Na^+–K^+ ATPase) present in stria vascularis and spiral ligament. This enzyme was similar in many respects to the enzyme found in other tissues and thought to be responsible for ion transport. The cochlear activity was about one-half that of kidney cortex and about the same as choroid plexus, ciliary body, and gastric mucosa. These results suggest that stria vascularis and spiral ligament are engaged in ion transport.

Rauch (1964) in fact has demonstrated a transport of both K^+ and Na^+ from perilymph to endolymph through Reissner's membrane. Potassium ions were transported 3 times more rapidly than Na^+ ions and both were reabsorbed in the stria vascularis.

Ouabain inhibits the Na^+–K^+ ATPase of the cochlea (Iinuma, 1967). The perilymph perfusion with ouabain or erythrophleine causes a dose-dependent reduction of CM, which is gradually reversible on removal of the ouabain (Kuijpers *et al.*, 1967). Chou (1970) also demonstrated a dose-dependent reduction of CM upon perfusion of the perilymphatic space with ouabain (10^{-7}–10^{-5} M). Furthermore, Chou confirmed the discovery of Glynn (1957) that an increase in potassium concentration antagonized the inhibitory effect of ouabain *in vitro* when, by increasing the potassium content of Ringer's solution perfusate, he lessened the CM reduction by ouabain.

In regard to cochlear Na^+–K^+ ATPase, Kuijpers (1969) determined the activity of this enzyme in stria vascularis and demonstrated that it diminishes as it is monitored from the basal to the apical end of the cochlea. This arrangement of enzymatic activity is reminiscent of the pattern of cochlear degeneration induced by antibiotics in which the damage to the outer hair cells begins at the basal end of the cochlea and proceeds apicalward. Other relationships between the ototoxic antibiotics and ATPase will be discussed below.

6. *Acetazolamide*

This substance influences the electrolyte composition of endolymph (Watanabe, 1963) and perilymph (Varga *et al.*, 1966) as well as perilymphatic carbonic anhydrase and electrical activity (Gieldanowski and Prastowsk, 1966).

Where blood carbonic anhydrase is inhibited to 0 to 20%, the perilymphatic activity of this enzyme is completely depressed. It was reported also that CM is elevated slightly by acetazolamide (Gieldanowski and Prastowsk, 1966). Perilymphatic sodium and potassium increase up to the third hour after drug administration (Varga *et al.*, 1966). In the endolymph, sodium concentration has decreased within 1 hour of drug administration and the capillaries of the stria vascularis are dilated (Watanabe, 1963). Twelve hours after drug administration a depression of Reissner's membrane is seen (Watanabe, 1963), probably indicating an imbalance between perilymph and endolymph production and drainage.

7. *Ethacrynic Acid*

It is now well established that the diuretic agent, ethacrynic acid, is capable of inducing transient or permanent deafness. This is especially true in the presence of renal failure as evidenced by uremia, in which it is presumed that the drug is retained in ototoxic concentrations for inordinately prolonged periods.

The first report of ototoxicity due to ethacrynic acid was by Maher and Schreiner (1965) shortly after the drug appeared on the market. In this report, 5 cases of acute, transient hearing loss occasioned by the use of ethacrynic acid were listed. A cysteine adduct of ethacrynic acid had been withdrawn from clinical use because of its propensity to produce transient hearing loss.

The first report of permanent deafness appeared in 1969 (Pillay *et al.*, 1969). In this study, 5 uremic patients received ethacrynic acid and 3 demonstrated permanent hearing loss. This hearing loss was irregularly accompanied by vertigo and tinnitus, suggesting that ethacrynic acid ototoxicity might be primarily cochlear rather than vestibular.

Matz *et al.* (1969) were able to examine histologically the cochlea of a patient who had demonstrated a bilateral, high-frequency hearing loss 20 minutes after an infusion of ethacrynic acid. Unfortunately, this patient had previously received neomycin. Nonetheless, histological examination revealed severe destruction of the outer hair cells in the basal turn of the cochlea, which is consonant with a high-frequency loss and which resembles the cochlear lesion seen following the ototoxic antibiotics. No ganglion cell destruction was seen. These same investigators studied ethacrynic acid ototoxicity in cats and found that it produced an early reversible and a later irreversible deafness.

Mathog and Klein (1969) reported on 3 individuals who had received combinations of aminoglycoside antibiotics and ethacrynic acid. All of these patients were uremic and all developed permanent, bilateral hearing loss. The doses of antibiotics and diuretics used were not exceptionally high nor were they used for prolonged periods. In fact, the authors quote an F.D.A. report in which permanent deafness followed single doses of kanamycin and ethacrynic acid. Once again, the primary labyrinthine

TABLE II

OTOTOXIC ANTIBIOTICS

Drug[a]	Cochlear toxicity	Vestibular toxicity	Latency	Permanence	Nephro-toxic	Neuro-muscular block	Ref.
Streptomycin (a)	+	++	Yes	Yes	No	Yes	McGee (1961); Wersäll and Lundquist (1968)
Dihydrostreptomycin (a)	++	+	Yes	Yes	No	Yes	McGee (1961); Wersäll and Lundquist (1968)
Neomycin [also (a) framycetin or neo-mycin B]	++	Little	Yes		Yes(++)	Yes	Kohonen (1965); Wersäll and Lundquist (1968)
Kanamycin (a)	++	+	No	Yes	Yes	Yes	Kohonen (1965); Hawkins (1959); Wersäll and Lundquist (1968)
Viomycin (p)	+	++			Yes	Yes	Jelert (1967); Wersäll and Lundquist (1968)
Vancomycin	+			Not always	Yes		Goodman and Gilman (1970) Wersäll and Lundquist (1968)
Ristocetin[b]	+				No		Wersäll and Lundquist (1968)
Paromomycin (a) (aminosidine)	+	+					Marseillan (1965)

							Warner and Sanders (1971)
Gentamicin (a)	+	+	Possible		Possibly	Yes	Küpper (1969); Wersäll and Lundquist (1968)
Capreomycin (p)	+[c]	+ (Mild), infrequent			Yes		Garfield *et al.* (1966); Miller *et al.* (1966); Wersäll and Flock (1964)
Colistimethate (p)[b]	+				Yes	Yes	Meuwissen and Robinson (1967)
Chloramphenicol	+			Yes			Patterson and Gulick (1963); D'Angelo *et al.* (1967)

[a] (a) Aminoglycoside; (p) polypetide.
[b] Not derived from *Streptomyces*. For contradictory opinion, see Gabrielson (1970).
[c] Rarely seen in humans unless previously exposed to other ototoxic agents.

toxicity was cochlear, no vestibular signs having presented themselves. The implication, therefore, is that uremic patients are extraordinarily sensitive to ethacrynic acid and other diuretics should be used in preference to it.

However, furosemide, heretofore not thought to produce ototoxicity, was recently implicated in transient ototoxic effects seen in 5 patients with diminished renal function (Schwartz *et al.*, 1970).

D. Antibiotics

The literature describing the toxic effects of antibiotics on the labyrinth is enormous. Antibiotic ototoxicity is universally recognized, may be regularly reproduced in animals, and has been widely discussed in several excellent review articles (Hawkins, 1970; Kohonen, 1965; Meuwissen and Robinson, 1967; Wersäll and Lundquist, 1968). Nonetheless and despite the attention devoted to it, precise understanding of ototoxicity, its mechanisms and, more urgently, clinically useful means of avoiding it still elude us. This is not to imply that progress is not being made. For instance, certain contradictory statements in the early literature seem to have been reconciled and certain important generalizations about the ototoxic antibiotics may now be made (see Table II).

Whereas it was considered early on that antibiotics influenced hearing by damaging brainstem nuclei, it is now generally accepted (Hawkins, 1970; Kohonen, 1965; Meuwissen and Robinson, 1967; Wersäll and Lundquist, 1968) that the primary site of damage is cochlear. Further evidence that the brainstem nuclei are not primarily and consistently damaged by ototoxic antibiotics comes from a human study (Wersäll and Lundquist, 1968). In this study in patients with dead labyrinths, treatment with streptomycin did not affect the nystagmus exhibited by them. If the streptomycin were acting on brainstem nuclei an influence on nystagmus could be expected.

The clear-cut and reproducible destruction of the cochlear hair cells has led authorities to conclude that these sensory elements were among the prime targets of the ototoxic antibiotics. The patterns of hair cell destruction indicate that the outer hair cells of the basal turn and the inner hair cells of the apical turn of the cochlea are the sensory elements most sensitive to these drugs. Damage then proceeds apicalward in the case of the outer hair cells and basalward in the case of the inner hair cells. The characteristic behavioral effect of the ototoxic antibiotics is a rise in threshold for the higher-frequency pure tones which are transduced into nervous signals by the sensory elements of the basal portion of the organ of Corti. Thus, there is a good agreement between morphological damage to the basal outer hair cells and functional disruption of the frequencies they serve.

Hawkins (1959) has provided further evidence that the hair cells suffer early damage when he demonstrated that the hair cell potential, CM, is diminished in amplitude soon after treatment with kanamycin, streptomycin, and viomycin while N_1 remains intact.

Kohonen (1965) has uncovered a correlation between the distribution of large, richly granulated nerve endings and the degeneration of outer hair cells saying that "the degree of vulnerability of outer hair cells is directly proportional to the size of the nerve endings." This implies that ototoxic antibiotics are concentrated at such synapses or possibly that they influence some trophic function of the nervous elements or that some activity of these particular hair cells lays them open to drug insult.

Kohonen (1965) studying neomycin, kanamycin, and framycetin ototoxicity in guinea pigs agreed that the most characteristic effect seen was the collapse of the sensory cells. Discussing such damage he described the swelling of hair cell nuclei and their breakdown as well as a disarrangement of the hairs themselves. Normally the sensory hairs are arranged in a "W" configuration, but Kohonen reported that antibiotic intoxication causes the hairs to point in different directions and the W figure to be disrupted. Others (Wersäll and Lundquist, 1968) have presented detailed descriptions of hair cell damage listing degeneration of mitochondria, fusion of the hairs, changes in cell membrane, and bulging of the cell toward the endolymph under the influence of streptomycin. Wersäll and Lundquist (1968) divided kanamycin-induced hair cell damage into stages, listing nuclear and ribosomal changes as early reversible and mitochondrial and cell membrane changes in the late irreversible stage. Supporting cells, ganglion cells, and efferent endings all seem substantially less susceptible than the hair cells to damage by antibiotic ototoxins.

That hair cell destruction is secondary to action elsewhere in the cochlea has been suggested by several authors (Hawkins, 1970). Among the suggested primary sites are the stria vascularis (a favorite of ototoxins)especially the mitochondria of the stria vascularis, the pericapillary elements of the outer sulcus with damage extending throughout the spiral ligament, (Hawkins, 1970), spiral limbus, and Reissner's membrane (Fig. 1). The stria vascularis, elements of the spiral ligament, and Reissner's membrane are all involved in secretion or filtration, and a disruption of this function might easily result in severe changes in the environment of the hair cells. Such a change in hair cell environment could account for the diminution in CM as well as the observed morphological changes.

Hawkins (1970) in a cogent discussion of the biochemical bases of ototoxicity, points out the relationship between the ototoxic effects of the antibiotics and their effects on the biochemical processes of bacteria. Selecting streptomycin as his model, Hawkins suggests that the impairment of cell membrane function and the inhibition of protein synthesis in bacteria have their cochlear counterparts. Inhibition of protein synthesis may be the cause of destruction in the spiral ligament and Reissner's membrane, whereas an effect on membrane permeability may cause the immediate effects or hair cell potentials.

In support of these possibilities, Hawkins first quotes studies (Vrabec *et al.*, 1965; Stupp *et al.*, 1967) demonstrating that streptomycin and kanamycin both are concentrated in endolymph and perilymph. An effect on cochlear protein synthesis is based on a statement by Plester (1963) that he found reduced protein metabolism in spiral ligament, and the function of Reissner's membrane as an effective partition between the endolymphatic and perilymphatic spaces was reported by Misrahy *et al.* (1961) as an increase in permeability following kanamycin. The electrical signs of cochlear function depend on the maintenance of the distinctive differences in composition between endolymph and perilymph. Integrity of Reissner's membrane is obligatory for maintaining endolymph–perilymph composition. Cell membrane permeability was invoked to explain the finding by Wersäll and Flock (1964) that potassium reversed the inhibitory influence of streptomycin on lateral line organ, microphonic potential.

The inhibitory influence of streptomycin on mammalian CM is also reversed by potassium (Wersäll and Lundquist, 1968). This reversal of streptomycin-induced reduction in CM by washing the endolymph compartment with high-potassium Ringer's solution brings to mind the parallel antagonism by potassium of ouabain's influence on CM (Chou, 1970) and suggests the possibility that some of the ototoxic antibiotics may be acting to inhibit cochlear Na^+–K^+ ATPase.

The activity of Na^+–K^+ ATPase was studied in cochlear tissues by Kuijpers (1969). The highest activity of this enzyme was found in the stria vascularis of the basal turn with diminishing activity seen in stria closer to the apical turn. As quoted earlier, the inhibitory effect of cardiac glycosides on Na^+–K^+ ATPase has been shown to be reversed by an increase in potassium concentration (Glynn, 1957). This finding of Glynn's led Chou (1970) to attempt and finally succeed in reversing the effect of ouabain on CM by increasing the potassium content of fluid perfusing the perilymphatic space. Thus, it may be assumed that CM amplitude is dependent on the activity of Na^+–K^+ ATPase. The demonstration by Iinuma (1966) that kanamycin intoxication in guinea pigs produced a reduction in ATPase activity of the stria vascularis and spiral ligament provides more circumstantial evidence linking ototoxicity and membrane ATPase. Another such link is the report that the ototoxic diuretic, ethacrynic acid is an inhibitor of renal membrane ATPase (Duggan and Noll, 1965). Therefore the correlation between the ototoxicity of certain antibiotics and their ability to inhibit membrane ATPase, although not conclusively demonstrated, remains tantalizing.

Another captivating suggestion regarding the mechanism of ototoxicity stems from the observation that many of the ototoxic antibiotics are so-called aminoglycoside antibiotics. That is they contain an aminosugar in their structure. Certain aminosugars are known to reduce the uptake of metabolically important sugars such as glucose (Balazs and Jacobson, 1966). Although a mild reduction in glucose uptake in organs such as liver may not be of importance to the economy of these organs because they operate with large metabolic reserves, a similar reduction in uptake in the cochlea, reducing glucose availability to the hair cells may be critical. The metabolic reserve of the hair cells may be too small to survive reduction in supply of glucose. Such a small metabolic reserve would then "select" the hair cells as the structures most susceptible to the ototoxic antibiotics. Some emphasis of this possibility comes from the finding of Owada (1962) that an aminosugar component of the kanamycin molecule, 3-glucosamine, is more ototoxic than the antibiotic itself.

Table II contains a listing of the antibiotics known to cause ototoxicity. Chemically these agents are either aminoglycoside or polypeptide structures. The structures of gentamicin and vancomycin are not fully known, but gentamicin is an aminoglycoside whereas vancomycin contains both amino acids and sugar moieties. All the ototoxic antibiotics have certain strongly basic groups such as guanido or amino groups. The ability to cause nephrotoxicity is not fully correlated with ototoxicity and is seen more regularly with antibiotics containing amino rather than guanido groups. However, it seems reasonable to assume that the cochlea and kidney share certain drug-vulnerable processes. Witness the dual toxicity, nephro and oto, of neomycin, viomycin, and kanamycin and the potent toxic effect of the diuretic agent, ethacrynic acid. Further, it is now clear that ototoxicity of the antibiotics and ethacrynic acid is potentiated by diminished renal function (Meuwissen and Robinson, 1967), presumably because of the failure to excrete the drug with resultant prolonged exposure of cochlear structures to increased concentrations.

The ototoxins are also potentiated by previous exposure of patients to other ototoxins (Miller *et al.*, 1966) or to acoustic trauma (Darrouzet and de Lima Sobrinho, 1962). Deafness has also been reported in the neonate following transplacental transfer of streptomycin (Meuwissen and Robinson, 1967). Furthermore, in the presence of renal disease, sufficient antibiotic may be absorbed from the denuded skin to cause deafness (Meuwissen and Robinson, 1967).

The neuromuscular blockade induced by streptomycin, neomycin, kanamycin, and viomycin is well known among anesthesiologists and pharmacologists. The mechanism is thought to be curare-like. Mückter (1961) has reported on this and other facets of the pharmacology of the basic antibiotics.

Early recognition of the signs of antibiotic ototoxicity and cessation of drug usage may reduce the occurrence of permanent deafness. This seems especially true with kanamycin. The reported early signs are cochlear—feeling of fullness in the ear, tinnitus, and subtle high-frequency threshold changes, as well as vestibular—ataxia, dizziness, and vomiting.

Attempts have been made to reduce antibiotic ototoxicity by combining them with vitamins of the B-complex group or with certain amino acids (Kohonen, 1965). Kanamycin has also been administered as the monopantothenate with one claim of reduced ototoxicity (Brun and Stupp, 1969) and mixed reviews (Hawkins, 1959). Finally an agent called Ozothin (hydrosoluble oxidation products of turpentine oil) has been tried with mixed results (Holz *et al.*, 1968; Brun and Stupp, 1969).

Thus the challenge of the ototoxicity of the antibiotics remains, perhaps, to be taken up by a pharmacologist.

E. Miscellany

1. *Organic Solvents*

Histological lesions as well as perceptive deafness have been reported in people exposed to solvents such as benzene, gasoline, carbon tetrachloride (Pierangeli, 1959), and certain alcohols. Gieldanowski (1965) injected methanol, ethanol, or propanol intravenously and monitored CM in cats at several frequencies. Propanol proved most and ethanol least depressant to CM. Mazzei and Costa (1954) reviewed occupational and experimental gasoline poisonings and auditory sequelae. Perceptive deafness is produced in people. Rabbits chronically exposed to gasoline vapors show lesions of the inner ear and brainstem. The same authors (Costa and Mazzei, 1955) have discussed benzene poisoning and reported that 20% of people chronically exposed to benzene show perceptive deafness. In rabbits chronically exposed to benzene vapors, severe histological lesions were found. These lesions included degenerative changes of neural and sensory elements of the cochlea, the ganglia of Scarpa and Corti, and nerve trunks. The investigators suggested that the damage resulted from vascular insults since they found hemorrhage and serious effusions in the stria vascularis, spiral ligaments, and organ of Corti. They also found some brainstem degeneration. The inner ear may be worthy of greater attention by the toxicologist.

2. *Hexadimethrine* (*Polybrene*)

Tinnitus, deafness, and slight imbalance was seen in some patients receiving hemodialysis with heparin–hexadimethrine for renal failure (Ransome *et al.*, 1966). Five patients of a total of 14 receiving hexadimethrine became deaf. The authors surmised that hexadimethrine acted primarily to block small vessels. There was produced widespread degeneration of the organ of Corti, and changes were also seen in spiral ganglion upon postmortem examination.

3. *Chenopodium Oil* (*Ascaridole*)

Deafness has been reported to occur in 20% of patients treated with chenopodium oil for worm infestations. The deafness varies in intensity from mild losses to complete bilateral loss lasting from several weeks to years (Oppikofer, 1919; Roth, 1918). Oka attributed these effects to degeneration of the spiral ganglia (Oka, 1929), but degeneration of external hair cells was also demonstrated. Little change in internal hair cells was noted (Lurie, 1955).

4. *Endocrinological Distrubances*

Some patients with hypothroidism show progressive deafness characterized by high-frequency losses. With return to the euthyroid state, hearing is recovered. Dennhardt (1965) suggested that changes in mucopolysaccharide metabolism accompanying hypothyroid states, such as myxedema, may influence the mucopolysaccharide complement of the inner ear, thus producing functional disruption of the transducing mechanism.

Adrenal cortical insufficiency, on the other hand, is associated with a lowered pure-tone threshold, but also a loss of speech discrimination. Other sensory modalities, such as taste, also show increases in sensitivity in the presence of adrenal cortical insufficiency. Lassman and Doyle (1969) reported that deoxycorticosterone acetate does not reverse the changes in hearing but that prednisolone and other glucocorticoids do. Glucocorticoids increased neural conduction time and latency but decreased transmission time in the skeletal neuromuscular junction.

F. Other Agents Influencing Audition

Other drugs affecting hearing include arsenicals—atoxyl, arsacetin (Crema, 1953; Tschirren, 1957), oxophenarsine, acetarsol (Gieldanowski, 1963)—and study of the reversal of arsenical ototoxicity by British anti-Lewisite (BAL) (Moretto, 1958); tetanus antitoxin (von Békésy, 1960); sulfapyridine, Phenergan, Multergan, thiopental (Gieldanowski, 1963); pentobarbital (Henriksen and Merlis, 1950); adenosine triphosphate (Faltynek, 1965); isoniazid (Ancetti, 1956; Kluyskens, 1953; Riser *et al.*, 1959); halothane (D'Anna, 1965); fusidic acid (Goldbaum *et al.*, 1965); *p*-aminosalicyclic acid (di Lauro, 1954); dimethylsulfoxide (Lebo, 1966); calcium (Moscovitch and Gannon, 1966).

It is customary as well as occasionally useful for review articles to suggest new problems or new regions requiring investigation. Within the governance of cochlear pharmacology many such problems or regions suggest themselves. For example, the nature of afferent transmission between the hair cells and VIII nerve endings is quite unknown. The hair-cell–afferent junction has certain of the aspects of neurohumorally operated synapses, but expert opinion concerning this transmission remains little more than conjecture for want of hard evidence. The problem of the transduction of mechanical energy into nervous impulses is prehaps even more fundamental and more tantalizing. Once again, auditory transduction probably could serve as a model for the transduction processes occurring in some other mechanosensory organs.

The formation and flow of the cochlear fluids has been the subject of great interest among ototlogists. Unfortunately, space and time did not allow discussion of this interesting subject. Elucidation of the formation and flow especially of endolymph and "cortilymph" would undoubtedly be of importance in the understanding of physiological and pathological processes in the cochlea. Exchange between the cochlear fluids across the cochlear partitions and the access of drugs to the cochlear fluids remain to be fully explored.

The incidence of ototoxicity of widely used drugs, such as antibiotics and diuretics, has reached almost epidemic proportions, yet the cause of this toxic effect remains undiscovered. It seems likely that the investigation of ototoxicity would reap not only clinical harvest but could be expected to uncover biochemical processes fundamental to hearing.

Finally, the entire problem of drug interactions with supracochlear structures along the auditory pathway is just beginning to receive proper attention.

VII. Glossary of Cochlear Potentials

Cochlear microphonics (CM) (Fig. 2). As implied by the term "microphonics," this potential faithfully follows the waveform of the input signal, as would a microphone. Sine wave inputs of up to 100,000 Hz produce CM of identical frequencies. The CM amplitude is proportional to the intensity of stimulus within rather wide limits—the upper end is limited by the sound intensities that tend to produce damage, and the lower end is unlimited. There is no threshold amplitude for CM. It has no refractory period and undergoes no adaptation and no fatigue. The hair cells are thought to be the generators of CM.

Sudden blocking of the cochlear blood flow causes CM to decay within seconds to about 10% of its control amplitude; anoxia produced in other

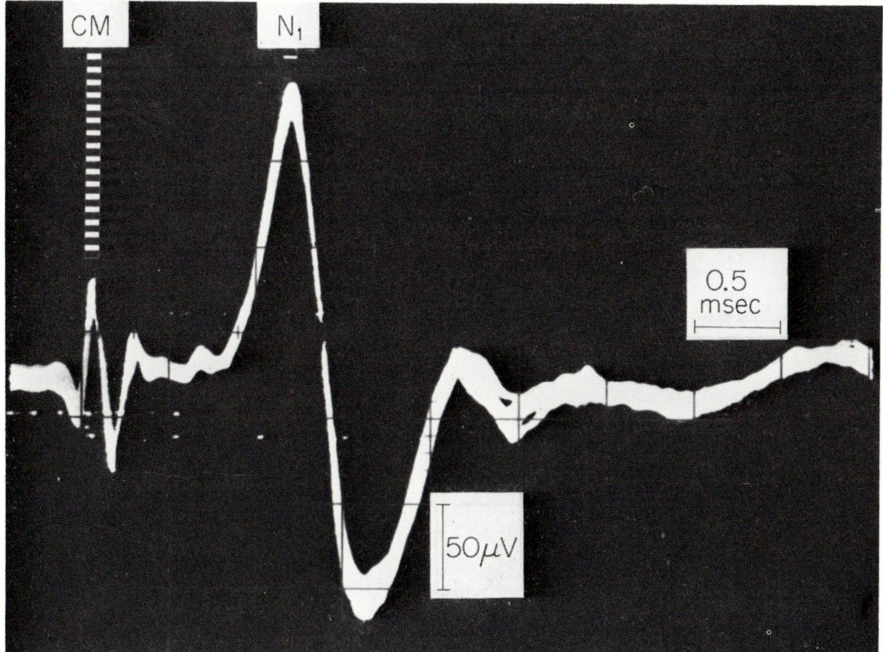

FIG. 2. Cochlear microphonic (CM) and VIII nerve action potential (N_1) evoked by a click and recorded from the round window. Ten traces superimposed.

ways acts similarly. The 10% remaining after anoxia persists even after death.

Integrated VIII nerve action potentials (N_1) (Fig. 2). These potentials may be recorded from the nerve trunk or fibers or, more conveniently, from the round window. Like potentials recorded from other nerve trunks, N_1 potentials are closely related in behavior in regard to all-or-noneness, refractory period, and latency. The integrated response may be synchronized with sound stimulation up to a frequency of about 2000 Hz. The amplitude of N_1 is proportional to stimulus intensity only within very narrow limits. A threshold is seen.

Endolymphatic or Endocochlear Potential (*EP*). This is a dc potential in which the endolymph is positive with reference to perilymph. This potential disappears when the blood or oxygen supply is removed.

Summation potential (summating potential). A change in the EP occurring as a result of sonic or mechanical stimulation. The deviation may be positive or negative. It is proportional to the intensity of stimulus.

Cochlear afterpotential. On cessation of a sound of more than 30 to 40 msec duration, a potential opposite in polarity to the summation potential may be recorded from the cochlea (Stopp, 1967).

Acknowledgments

I wish to thank Dr. Vernon B. Haarstad for the hemicholinium No. 3 and his valued comments on the research done with it. Mrs. Carol Galloway and Miss Margaret Higgins deserve special mention for their devotion to the typing of this review.

References

Adrian, E. D., Bronk, D. W., and Phillips, G. (1931). *J. Physiol.* (*London*) **73,** 2P.

Amaro, J., Guth, P. S., and Wanderlinder, L. (1966). *Brit. J. Pharmacol. Chemother.* **28,** 207.

Ancetti, A. (1956). *Minerva Otorinolaringol.* **6,** 31.

Balazs, E. A., and Jacobson, B. (1966). *In* "The Amino Sugars. Vol. 2B: Metabolism and Interactions" (E. A. Balazs and R. W. Jeanloz, eds.), pp. 361–395. Academic Press, New York.

Beck, C., and Holz, E. (1968). *Acta Oto-Laryngol.* **65,** 327.

Beickert, P., and Terayama, Y. (1965). *Arch. Ohren- Nasen- Kehlkopfheilk.* **185,** 727.

Bishop, P. O. (1967). *Annu. Rev. Physiol.* **29,** 427.

Bobbin, R. P., and Guth, P. S. (1970). *Int. J. Neuropharm.* **9,** 567.

Bobbin, R. P., Gonzalez, G., and Guth, P. S. (1969). *Nature* (*London*) **223,** 70.

Bornschein, H., and Krejci, F. (1950). *Experientia* **6,** 271.

Bornschein, H., and Thalmann, R. (1962). *Experientia* **19,** 413.

Bovero, A. (1914). *Arch. Ital. Otol. Rinol. Laringol.* **25,** 41.

Bredberg, G. (1968). *Acta Oto-Laryngol. Suppl.* **236**.
Brown, R. D., Daigneault, E. A., and Pruett, J. R. (1967). *Fed. Proc. Fed. Amer. Soc. Exp. Biol.* **26,** 324.
Brun, J. P., and Stupp, H. (1969). *Arch. Klin. Exp. Ohren-Nasen-Kehlkopfheilk.* **194,** 566.
Buño, W., Jr., Velluti, R., Handler, P., and Garcia-Ausst, E. (1966). *Physiol. Behav.* **1,** 23.
Butler, R. A., Honrubia, V., Johnstone, B. M., and Fernandez, C. (1962). *Ann. Otol. Rhinol. Laryngol.* **71,** 648.
Chou, J. T. Y. (1970). *Archiv fuer Klinische und Experimentelle Ohren-, Nasen- und Kehlkopfheilkunde* **195,** 246.
Chou, J. T. Y., and Rodgers, K. (1962). *J. Laryngol. Otol.* **76,** 341.
Churchill, J. A., Schuknecht, H. F., and Doran, R. (1956). *Laryngoscope* **66,** 1.
Comis, S. D., and Whitfield, I. C. (1965). *J. Physiol. (London)* **183,** 22.
Comis, S. D., and Whitfield, I. C. (1968). *J. Neurophysiol.* **31,** 62.
Costa, F., and Mazzei, F. (1955). *Arch. Ital. Laringol.* **63,** 451.
Costa, O. A., Thalmann, R., and Covell, W. P. (1966). *Laryngoscope* **76,** 1874.
Crema, A. (1953). *Arch. Sci. Biol. (Bologna)* **37,** 213.
Cutt, R. A. (1963). *Laryngoscope* **73,** 702.
Daigneault, E. A. (1967). Personal communication.
Daigneault, E. A., and Brown, R. D. (1966a). *Arch. Int. Pharmacodyn. Ther.* **162,** 20.
Daigneault, E. A., and Brown, R. D. (1966b). *Pharmacologist* **8,** 273.
D'Angelo, E. P., Patterson, W. C., and Morrow, R. C. (1967). *Arch. Otolaryngol.* **85,** 682.
D'Anna, M. (1965). *Arch. Ital. Laringol.* **73,** 105.
Darrouzet, J., and de Lima Sobrinho, E. (1962). *Rev. Laryngol. Otol. Rinol.* **83,** 781.
Davis, H. (1957). *Physiol. Rev.* **37,** 1.
Davis, H., Derbyshire, A. J., Lurie, M. H., and Saul, L. J. (1934). *Amer. J. Physiol.* **107,** 316.
Dennhardt, H. (1965). *Arch. Ohren- Nasen- Kehlkopfheilk.* **185,** 731.
Desmedt, J. E. (1962). *J. Acoust. Soc. Amer.* **34,** 1478.
Desmedt, J. E., and LaGrutta, V. (1963). *Nature (London)* **200,** 472.
Desmedt, J. E., and Monaco, P. (1960). *Arch. Int. Pharmacodyn. Ther.* **129,** 244.
Desmedt, J. E., and Monaco, P. (1961). *Nature (London)* **192,** 1263.
Desmedt, J. E., and Monaco, P. (1962). *Proc. 1st Int. Pharmacol. Meet., Stockholm,* **8,** 183.
Dewson, J. H. (1968). *J. Neurophysiol.* **31,** 122.
di Lauro, E. (1954). *Valsalva* **30,** 295.
Dittrich, F. L. (1963). "Biophysics of the Ear." Thomas, Springfield, Illinois.
Duggan, D. E., and Noll, R. M. (1965). *Arch. Biochem.* **109,** 388.
Ehmke, O. (1963). *Rev. Paul. Med.* **62,** 109.
Engström, H., Ades, H. W., and Andersson, A. (1966). "Structural Pattern of the Organ of Corti." Williams & Wilkins, Baltimore, Maryland.
Falck, B., Hillarp, N. A., Thieme, G., and Dorp, A. (1962). *J. Histochem. Cytochem.* **10,** 348.
Faltynek, L. (1965). *Bratislav. Lek. Listy* **45,** 292.
Farkashity, J., Black, R. G., and Briant, T. D. R. (1963). *Laryngoscope* **73,** 713.
Fernandez, C., and Alzate, R. (1959). *Arch. Otolaryngol.* **69,** 82.

Fernandez, C., and Brenman, A. (1957). *Amer. J. Physiol.* **188,** 249.
Fex, J. (1962). *Acta Physiol. Scand. Suppl.* **189.**
Fex, J. (1967). *J. Acoust. Soc. Amer.* **41,** 666.
Fex, J. (1968). *In* "Hearing Mechanisms in Vertebrates" (A. V. S. de Reuck and J. Knight, eds.), p. 169. Little, Brown, Boston, Massachusetts.
Fruttero, F., and Sartoris, A. (1966). *J. Fr. Oto-Rhino-Laryngol.* **15,** 805.
Gabrielson, R. M., (1970). *New Engl. J. Med.* **283,** 600.
Galambos, R. (1956). *J. Neurophysiol.* **19,** 424.
Gannon, R. P., and Laszlo, C. A. (1968). *J. Neurophysiol.* **31,** 419.
Gannon, R. P., Laszlo, C. A., and Moscovitch, D. H. (1966). *Acta Oto-Laryngol.* **61,** 536.
Garfield, J. W., Jones, J. M., Cohen, N. L., Daly, J. F., and McClement, J. H. (1966). *Ann. N. Y. Acad. Sci.* **135,** 1039.
Gieldanowski, J. (1963). *Arch. Immunol. Ther. Exp.* **11,** 471.
Gieldanowski, J. (1965). *Med. Pracy* **16,** 448.
Gieldanowski, J., and Prastowsk, W. (1966). *Otolaryngol. Pol.* **20,** 519.
Gisselson, L. (1950). *Acta Oto-Laryngol. Suppl.* **82.**
Gisselson, L. (1952). *Acta Oto-Laryngol.* **42,** 208.
Glynn, I. M. (1957). *J. Physiol. (London)* **136,** 148.
Gold, A., and Wilpizeskie, C. R. (1966). *Laryngoscope* **76,** 674.
Goldbaum, C. R., De Armus, M., and Rodriguez, L. (1965). *Arch. Inst. Farmacol. Exp., Madrid* **17,** 111.
Goldstein, A. J., and Mizukoshi, O. (1967). *Ann. Otol. Rhinol. Laryngol.* **76,** 414.
Goodman, L. S., and Gilman, A. (1970). "The Pharmacologic Basis of Therapeutics." Macmillan (Pergamon), New York.
Gotlib, I. A. L. (1957). *Vestn. Otorinolaringol.* **19**(6), 31.
Gulick, W. L., and Cutt, R. A. (1962a). *Ann. Otol. Rhinol. Laryngol.* **71,** 105.
Gulick, W. L., and Cutt, R. A. (1962b). *Ann. Otol. Rhinol. Laryngol.* **71,** 110.
Guth, P. S (1967). Unpublished observations.
Guth, P. S., and Amaro, J. (1968). *Int. J. Neuropharmacol.* **8,** 49.
Harkins, W. B., and Yanof, H. M. (1967). *Laryngoscope* **77,** 701.
Hart, C. W., and Naunton, R. F. (1964). *Arch. Otolaryngol.* **80,** 407.
Hawkins, J. E., Jr. (1959). *Ann. Otol. Rhinol. Laryngol.* **68,** 698.
Hawkins, J. E., Jr. (1964). *Annu. Rev. Physiol.* **26,** 453.
Hawkins, J. E., Jr. (1970). *In* "Biochemical Mechanisms in Hearing and Deafness" (M. M. Paparella, ed.), p. 323. Thomas, Springfield, Illinois.
Hennebert, D., and Fernandez, C. (1959). *Arch. Otolaryngol.* **70,** 321.
Henriksen, G. F., and Merlis, J. K. (1950). *Proc. Soc. Exp. Biol. Med.* **74,** 882.
Hilding, D. A., and Sugiura, A. (1970). *In* "Biochemical Mechanisms in Hearing and Deafness" (M. M. Paparella, ed.), p. 137. Thomas, Springfield, Illinois.
Holz, E., Strang, G., Soda, T., and Beck, C. (1968). *Arch. Otolaryngol.* **87,** 359.
Honrubia, V., and Ward, P. H. (1966). *Surg. Forum* **17,** 470.
Iinuma, T. (1966). *J. Oto-Rhino-Laryngol. Soc. Jap.* **69,** 1698.
Iinuma, T. (1967). *Laryngoscope* **77,** 141.
Ishii, T., Bernstein, J. M., and Balogh, K. (1967). *Ann. Otol. Rhinol. Laryngol.* **76,** 368.

Iurato, S. (1967). "Submicroscopic Structure of the Inner Ear." Macmillan (Pergamon), New York.
Jankowski, W., Gieldanowski, J., and Birecki, W. (1962a). *Otolaryngol. Pol.* **16,** 321.
Jankowski, W., Gieldanowski, J., and Birecki, W. (1962b). *Otolaryngol. Pol.* **16,** 331.
Jelert, H. (1967). *J. Laryngol. Otol.* **81,** 317.
Johnstone, B. M. (1967). *Curr. Top. Bioenerg.* **2,** 335.
Kahana, L., Rosenblith, W. A., and Galambos, R. (1950). *Amer. J. Physiol.* **613,** 213.
Kaneko, Y. (1965). *Tohoku J. Exp. Med.* **86,** 178.
Kao, C. Y. (1966). *Pharmacol. Rev.* **18,** 997.
Katsuki, Y., Tanaka, Y., and Miyoshi, T. (1965). *Nature (London)* **207,** 32.
Katsuki, Y., Yanagisawa, K., and Kanzaki, J. (1966). *Science* **151,** 1544.
Kluyskens, P. (1953). *Acta Oto-Rhino-Laryngol. Belg.* **7,** 22.
Kohonen, A. (1965). *Acta Oto-Laryngol. Suppl.* **208.**
Koide, Y., Tajima, S., Yoshida, M., and Konno, M. (1960). *Ann. Otol. Rhinol. Laryngol.* **69,** 1083.
Koide, Y., Hata, A., and Hamdo, R. (1966). *Acta Oto-Laryngol.* **61,** 332.
Konishi, T., and Kelsey, E. (1968a). *J. Acoust. Soc. Amer.* **43,** 471.
Konishi, T., and Kelsey, E. (1968b). *J. Acoust. Soc. Amer.* **43,** 462.
Konishi, T., Butler, R. A., and Fernandez, C. (1961). *J. Acoust. Soc. Amer.* **33,** 349.
Küpper, K. (1969). *Archiv fuer Klinische und Experimentelle Ohren-, Nasen- und Kehlkopfheilkunde* **194,** 569.
Kuijpers, W. A. (1969). *Acta Oto-Laryngol.* **67,** 200.
Kuijpers, W. A., Vander Vleuten, A. C., and Bonting, S. L. (1967). *Science* **157,** 949.
LaGrutta, V., and Desmedt, J. E. (1964). *Arch. Int. Pharmacodyn. Ther.* **151,** 289.
Lassman, F. M., and Doyle, T. N. (1969). *In* "Biochemical Mechanisms in Hearing and Deafness" (M. M. Paparella, ed.), p. 115. Thomas, Springfield, Illinois.
Lawrence, M. (1968). *Annu. Rev. Psychol.* **19,** 1.
Lebo, C. P. (1966). *Ann. Otol. Rhinol. Laryngol.* **75,** 208.
Lichtensteiger, W., and Spoendlin, H. (1967). *Life Sci.* **6,** 1630.
Loewenstein, W. R. (1956). *J. Physiol. (London)* **132,** 40.
Lorente de No, R. (1926). *Trab. Inst. Cajal Invest. Biol.* **24,** 53.
Lurie, M. H. (1955). *Trans. Amer. Acad. Ophthalmol. Otolaryngol.* **59,** 111.
McCabe, P. A., and Dey, F. L. (1965). *Ann. Otol. Rhinol. Laryngol.* **74,** 312.
McGee, T. M. (1961). *Trans. Amer. Acad. Ophthalmol. Otolaryngol.* **65,** 222.
McKinstry, D., and Koelle, G. B. (1967). *J. Pharmacol. Exp. Ther.* **157,** 328.
Maher, J. F., and Schreiner, G. E. (1965). *Ann. Intern. Med.* **62,** 15.
Makimoto, K., Takeda, T., Ibusuki, T., and Morimoto, M. (1967). *Ann. Otol. Rhinol. Laryngol.* **76,** 885.
Marseillan, R. F. (1965). *Acta Physiol. Lat. Amer.* **15,** 300.
Martini, V. (1941). *Boll. Soc. Ital. Biol. Sper.* **16,** 70.
Mathog, R. H., and Klein, W. J. (1969). *New Engl. J. Med.* **280,** 1223.
Matschinsky, F. M., and Thalmann, R. (1967). *Laryngoscope* **77,** 292.
Matz, G. J., Beal, D. D., and Krames, L. (1969). *Arch. Otolaryngol.* **90,** 152.
Mazzei, F., and Costa, F. (1954). *Arch. Ital. Laringol.* **62,** 417.
Meuwissen, H. J., and Robinson, G. C. (1967). *Clin. Pediat.* **6,** 262.
Miller, J. D., Popplewell, A. G., Landwehr, A., and Greene, M. E. (1966). *Ann. N.Y. Acad. Sci.* **135,** 1047.

Misrahy, G. A. (1958). *J. Acoust. Soc. Amer.* **30**, 668.

Misrahy, G. A., Spradley, J. F., Dzinovic, S., and Brooks, C. J. (1961). *Ann. Otol. Rhinol. Laryngol.* **70**, 572.

Miyake, H. (1960). *J. Oto-Rhino-Laryngol. Soc. Jap.* **63**, Suppl. 2.

Moretto, G. (1958). *Minerva Otorinolaringol.* **8**(6), 109.

Moscovitch, D. H., and Gannon, R. P. (1966). *J. Acoust. Soc. Amer.* **40**, 583.

Mückter, H. (1961). *Antibiot. Chemother.* (*Basel*) **9**, 83.

Myers, E. M., and Bernstein, J. M. (1965). *Arch. Otolaryngol.* **82**, 483.

Myers, E. M., Bernstein, J. M., and Fostiroupoulas, G. (1965). *New Engl. J. Med.* **273**, 587.

Naumann, H. H. (1964). *Isr. J. Exp. Med.* **11**, 110.

Nowak, R., and Dahl, D. (1966). *HNO* (*Hals- Nasen- Ohrenaerzte*) **14**, 8.

Oka, N. (1929). *Jap. J. Med. Sci. Biol.* **3**, 201.

Oppikofer, E. (1919). *Corresp. Bl. Schweiz. Aerzte* **49**, 161.

Owada, K. (1962). *Chemotherapia* **5**, 227.

Palva, T., and Raunio, V. (1967). *Ann. Otol. Rhinol. Laryngol.* **76**, 23.

Patterson, W. C., and Gulick, W. L. (1963). *Ann. Otol. Rhinol. Laryngol.* **72**, 50.

Perez de Moura, L. F., and Hayden, R. C. (1968). *Arch. Otolaryngol.* **87**, 368.

Perlman, H. B., and Kimura, R. S. (1965). *Ann. Otol. Rhinol. Laryngol.* **69**, 1176.

Permin, P. M. (1957). *Acta Oto-Laryngol.* **47**, 167.

Pierangeli, C. E. (1959). *Clin. Otorinolaringoiat.* **11**, 1.

Pillay, V. K. G., Schwartz, F. D., Aimi, K., and Kark, R. M. (1969). *Lancet* **1**, **77**.

Plester, D. (1963). Discussion of a paper by Musebeck. *Arch. Ohren-Nasen-Kehlkopf-heilk.* **182**, 587.

Pruett, J. R., Daigneault, E. A., and Brown, R. D. (1967). *Pharmacologist* **9**, 253.

Rahm, W. E., Jr., Strother, W. W., Gulick, W. L., and Crump, J. F. (1959). *Ann. Otol. Rhinol. Laryngol.* **68**, 1037.

Rahm, W. E., Jr., Strother, W. W., Gulick, W. L., and Crump, J. F. (1960). *Ann. Otol. Rhinol. Laryngol.* **69**, 969.

Rahm, W. E., Jr., Strother, W. W., Gulick, W. L., and Crump, J. F. (1961). *Ann. Otol. Rhinol. Laryngol.* **70**, 403.

Rahm, W. E., Jr., Strother, W. W., Crump, J. F., and Parker, D. E. (1962). *Ann. Otol. Rhinol. Laryngol.* **71**, 116.

Ransome, J., Ballantyne, J. C., Shaldon, S., Bosher, S. K., and Hallpike, C. S. (1966). *J. Laryngol. Otol.* **80**, 651.

Rasmussen, G. L. (1946). *J. Comp. Neurol.* **84**, 141

Rasmussen, G. L., and Windle, W. F., eds. (1960). "Neural Mechanisms of the Auditory and Vestibular System." Thomas, Springfield, Illinois.

Rauch, S. (1964). *In* "Biochemie de Horogans" (S. Rauch, ed.), pp. 62–64. Thieme, Stuttgart.

Riser, M., Gayral, L., Geraud, J., Coll, J., and Turnin, J. (1959). *Rev. Neurol.* **101**, 610.

Rosenblith, W. A., and Rosenzweig, M. R. (1951). *J. Acoust. Soc. Amer.* **23**, 583.

Roth, D. A. (1918). *South. Med. J.* **11**, 733.

Ruedi, L., Furrer, W., Luthy, F., Nager, G., and Tschirren, B. (1952). *Laryngoscope* **62**, 333.

Savin, V. C., Bustamonte-Gurria, A., and Reyes, E. (1968). *Acta Oto-Laryngol.* **65**, 130.

Scala, N. P., and Spiegel, E. A. (1950). *Confin. Neurol.* **10,** 285.
Schueler, F. W. (1960). *Int. Rev. Neurobiol.* **2,** 77.
Schuknecht, H. F., Churchill, J. A., and Doran, R. (1959). *Arch. Otolaryngol.* **69,** 549.
Schwartz, G. H., David, P. S., Riggio, R. R., Stenzel, K. H., and Rubin, A. L. (1970). *New Engl. J. Med.* **282,** 1413.
Schwartzkopf, J. (1967). *Annu. Rev. Physiol.* **29,** 485.
Silverstein, H., Bernstein, J. M., and Davies, D. G. (1967). *Ann. Otol. Rhinol. Laryngol.* **76,** 118.
Simmons, F. B. (1967). *Laryngoscope* **77,** 171.
Simmons, F. B., and Beatty, D. L. (1962). *Ann. Otol. Rhinol. Laryngol.* **71,** 767.
Sohmer, H., and Feinmesser, M. (1963). *Arch. Int. Pharmacodyn. Ther.* **144,** 446.
Spoendlin, H. (1966). "The Organization of the Cochlear Receptor." Karger, Basel.
Stopp, P. E. (1967). *Nature (London).* **215,** 1400.
Strother, W. F., Parker, D. E., Rahm, W. E., Jr., and Crump, J. F. (1964). *Ann. Otol. Rhinol. Laryngol.* **73,** 141.
Stupp, H., Rauch, S., Sous, H., Brun, J. P., and Lagler, F. (1967). *Arch. Otolaryngol.* **86,** 515.
Tanaka, Y. (1963). *J. Oto-Rhino-Laryngol. Soc. Jap.* **66,** 999.
Tanaka, Y., and Katsuki, Y. (1966). *J. Neurophysiol.* **29,** 94.
Tasaki, I. (1954). *J. Neurophysiol.* **16,** 97.
Tasaki, I. (1957). *Annu. Rev. Physiol.* **19,** 417.
Tasaki, I., Davis, H., and Legouix, J. P. (1952). *J. Acoust. Soc. Amer.* **24,** 502.
Tasaki, I., Davis, H., and Eldredge, D. H. (1954). *J. Acoust. Soc. Amer.* **26,** 765.
Terayama, Y., Holz, E., and Beck, C. (1966). *Ann. Otol. Rhinol. Laryngol.* **15,** 64.
Tonndorf, J., and Tabor, J. R. (1962). *Ann. Otol. Rhinol. Laryngol.* **71,** 5.
Tschirren, B. (1957). *Pract. Oto-Rhino-Laryngol.* **19(5),** 416.
Tsunao, M., and Perlman, H. B. (1965). *Acta Oto-Laryngol.* **59,** 437.
Varga, G., Miriszlai, E., and Szabo, L. Z. (1966). *J. Laryngol. Otol.* **80,** 270.
Vinnikov, Y. A., and Titova, L. K. (1964) "The Organ of Corti." Consultants Bureau, New York.
von Békésy, G. (1952). *J. Acoust. Soc. Amer.* **24,** 72.
von Békésy, G. (1960). "Experiments in Hearing" (E. G. Wever, ed.). McGraw-Hill, New York.
Vosteen, K. H. (1961). *Arch. Ohren- Nasen- Kehlkopfheilk.* **178,** 1.
Vrabec, D. P., Cody, D. T. R., and Ulrich, J. A. (1965). *Ann. Otol. Rhinol. Laryngol.* **74,** 688.
Warner, W. A., and Saunders, E. (1971). *J. Amer. Med. Ass.* **215,** 1153.
Watanabe, Y. (1963). *J. Oto-Rhino-Laryngol. Soc. Jap.* **66,** 657.
Welles, J. S., Harris, P. N., Small, R. M., Worth, H. M., and Anderson, R. C. (1966). *Ann. N.Y. Acad. Sci.* **135,** 960.
Wersäll, J., and Flock, A. (1964). *Life Sci.* **3,** 1151.
Wersäll, J., and Lundquist, P. G. (1968). *In* "Drugs and Sensory Functions" (A. Herxheimer, ed.), p. 142. Little, Brown, Boston, Massachusetts.
Wever, E. G. (1949). "Theory of Hearing," Wiley, New York.
Wever, E. G., and Lawrence, M. (1955). *J. Acoust. Soc. Amer.* **27,** 853.

Wever, E. G., Lawrence, M., Hemphill, R. W., and Straut, C. B. (1949). *Amer. J. Physiol.* **159,** 199.
Wing, K. G. (1959). *Acta Oto-Laryngol. Suppl.* **148.**

Biochemical Mechanisms of Transferable Drug Resistance

WILLIAM V. SHAW

Departments of Medicine and Biochemistry
University of Miami School of Medicine
Miami, Florida

I. Introduction

Whereas a review of the biochemical mechanisms of extrachromosomal antibiotic resistance might have seemed premature only a few years ago, the rapidity with which information has accumulated recently has made a preliminary appraisal necessary. Since the advent of antimicrobial therapy, the "emergence" of drug-resistant bacteria has been a problem of interest to clinicians, microbial geneticists, and pharmacologists. An unanticipated benefit from an initially adverse development has been the insights which certain types of resistance have provided for a better understanding of the mechanisms of action of agents such as streptomycin and related inhibitors of ribosome function (Weisblum and Davies, 1968).

Although early studies of drug resistance stressed the mechanisms observed in random clinical isolates and strains isolated in the laboratory as a result of spontaneous or induced mutation (Moyed, 1964), the recognition of novel genetic mechanisms for clinically important resistance prompted a number of laboratories to examine the expression of drug resistance determinants from different points of view. There is now little doubt that the conventional view of the spread of drug-resistant bacteria by the mechanism of mutation and selection must be revised to include a consideration of those resistance genes that reside on extrachromosomal elements which, in the most general sense, are best described as "plasmids" (Hayes, 1969) to connote their autonomous existence and replication apart from the bacterial chromosome. A number of outstanding reviews have appeared recently which serve to define the importance of such elements and stress their mechanism of transfer and expression (Watanabe, 1963; Meynell *et al.*, 1967; Richmond, 1968; Anderson, 1968; Novick, 1969). The analogies of the resistance transfer factor (RTF) of enteric bacteria with the fertility factor (F factor) of *Escherichia coli* have led to its inclusion in the group of "episomes" (Meynell and Datta, 1969) harbored by the Enterobacteriaceae. As pointed out by Hayes (1969) and others (Novick, 1969), however, the exclusion of certain extrachromosomal elements from the family of episomes may in certain instances be quite arbitrary and at least premature because of their inability to promote conjugation or apparent lack of association with the bacterial chromosome. The importance of extrachromosomal determinants of drug resistance rests with their ease of transmissibility, either by conjugation or by phage-mediated transduction. In the overall view, the latter mechanism may ultimately prove to be at least as important as conjugation since plasmid-mediated drug resistance genes in pathogenic staphylococci are transferred solely by transduction (Novick, 1967; Richmond, 1968).

The commonly observed plasmid and episomal determinants of drug resistance are clearly dispensable genetic elements in that they are readily lost irreversibly under varying conditions which include growth at elevated temperature (May *et al.*, 1964) and exposure to chemical agents and mutagens (Hirota, 1960; Tomoeda *et al.*, 1968; Bouanchaud *et al.*, 1969). The resulting drug-sensitive derivative strains do not appear to be at a selective disadvantage apart from their lack of resistance to antibiotics or other agents specified by the extrachromosomal element in question. It is clear, however, that the RTF episomes and their counterpart, staphylococcal plasmids, do indeed contain more genetic information than can be accounted for by the observable resistance determinants (Falkow *et al.*, 1966). As will be discussed later, the size of the extrachromosomal deoxyribonucleic acid (DNA) isolated from plasmids of various enteric bacteria and staphylococci correlates with their complexity but may exceed that estimated from the apparent phenotypes in certain instances (Falkow *et al.*, 1966; Rush *et al.*, 1969). It is apparent that much work remains to be done to explore the nature of the DNA which is unaccounted for, either by hybridization experiments with DNA from plasmid-negative variants or by direct detection of other phenotypic differences between sensitive and resistant species. It seems likely that the "silent" regions of extrachromosomal DNA in drug-resistant plasmids will be found to represent nutritional genes or to specify resistance to inhibitors and antibiotics which have not yet been employed or isolated. The demonstration of R factor-mediated resistance to certain aminoglycoside agents which have not been used clinically (Smith, 1967a) and the construction of hybrid episomes carrying colicinogenic, resistance, and nutritional determinants (Fredericq, 1969) are cases in point. The spectrum of unsuspected resistance determinants may be quite broad in view of the evidence that many RTF episomes and penicillinase plasmids of staphylococci contain genes mediating resistance to a variety of metal ions (Smith, 1967b, Novick, 1967). Phage susceptibility, bacteriocin sensitivity, antigenic constitution, nutritional characteristics, and toxin production are examples of possible plasmid-linked functions which may be found to coexist with the commonly observed antibiotic resistance genes (Novick, 1967).

The origin of drug resistance genes carried by various bacterial episomes and plasmids remains uncertain but constitutes an area of possibly fruitful investigation. Table I summarizes the information currently available

TABLE I

COMPARISON OF OBSERVED MECHANISMS OF RESISTANCE[a]

Drug	Chromosomal	Extrachromosomal
Penicillins[b]	β-Lactamase ? Other mechanisms (methicillin resistance)	β-Lactamase
Tetracyclines	Permeability	Permeability
Chloramphenicol	Permeability Enzymatic acetylation	Enzymatic acetylation ? Other mechanisms
Aminoglycosides	Decreased ribosomal affinity	Enzymatic inactivation Acetylation (kanamycin) Phosphorylation (streptomycin) Adenylylation (streptomycin)
Sulfonamides	Altered folate-synthesizing enzyme Permeability	Unknown

[a] For a detailed discussion of each type the appropriate sections of the text should be consulted. The examples chosen are from those bacterial species in which transferable or extrachromosomal resistance genes have been demonstrated (enteric bacteria and staphylococci).

[b] The term "penicillins" is taken to include all antibiotics of the β-lactam type (penicillins and cephalosporins), including those prepared by semisynthetic methods. The examples of methicillin resistance and penicillin tolerance (Barber, 1962) have not yet been explained adequately but probably do not involve β-lactamases (see Section III, B).

concerning the biochemical mechanisms underlying the resistance observed with extrachromosomal elements and those observed for classic chromosomal mutants with similar phenotypes. A cursory examination of the summarized results leads to the conclusion that there is an obvious lack of concordance between the two genetic types of resistance and that multiple mechanisms may underlie the observed phenotypes in both categories. The most striking discrepancy exists for the aminoglycoside group of antibiotics wherein ribosomal resistance to such inhibitors of protein synthesis is commonly observed in the chromosomal type of resistance but has never been implicated in extrachromosomal resistance of enteric bacteria or staphylococci (see Section III, E). The converse is also true in that enzymatic inactivation by adenylylation, phosphorylation, or acetylation of aminoglycosides has not been noted among resistant isolates which do not bear plasmid-linked loci of resistance. As will be discussed later in connection with individual antibiotics, such findings suggest that the attractive theory of "gene pickup" of resistance determinants from the chromosome by various bacterial sex factors and plasmids may be inadequate to explain their emergence. The experimental isolation of augmented sex factors (F′) such as F′ (lac) by recombination of wild-type sex factors with homologous regions of bacterial chromosome is a satisfactory precedent for such a mechanism (Jacob and Adelberg, 1959). However, the lack of demonstrable allelic chromosomal determinants for a number of plasmid-linked resistance genes suggests that a more complicated process must be implicated in certain instances. Multistep mutations of a chromosomal gene for a polyfunctional protein after its acquisition by an episome or plasmid is at best an unwieldy hypothesis. An alternative explanation is that the chromosomal alleles to observed plasmid resistance genes arise at a very low frequency and are thereby undetected by conventional techniques of mutagenesis and selection. The experimental difficulties in substantiating such a mechanism are formidable, however, since the isolation of random and induced mutants with typical chromosomal genotypes would be expected at frequencies several orders of magnitude greater than for the proposed rare mutants being sought.

Some years prior to the advent of more detailed techniques for the genetic and biochemical mechanisms of drug resistance, Davis and Maas (1952) summarized the general types of resistance mechanisms which should be considered for any given determinant. Their outline continues to be a useful means of approaching the problem and serves to accommodate a number of apparently conflicting proposed mechanisms for a given resistance phenotype (Table II). The lack of evidence for one of the possible resistance mechanisms in a given case may in most instances merely mean

TABLE II

POSSIBLE BIOCHEMICAL MECHANISMS OF DRUG RESISTANCE[a]

1. Drug inactivation
2. Altered enzyme or target structure (with decreased affinity for drug and/or increased activity)
3. Decreased accumulation of drug by resistant cells
4. New pathway bypassing inhibited reaction
5. Increased concentration of metabolite antagonizing inhibitor
6. Decreased requirement for product of inhibited reaction

[a] The above outline is adapted from an earlier discussion by Davis and Maas (1952) which was elaborated upon by Moyed (1964). The concept of drug inactivation is best exemplified by the β-lactamases. Examples in category (2) would be the case of sulfonamide (Section III, F) and ribosomal resistance to streptomycin (Section III, E). Decreased accumulation has been documented for tetracycline (Section III, D). The last three types of mechanisms have received little support in studies of resistance to clinically important antibiotics. Categories (5) and (6) were conceived with special reference to competitive inhibitors such as sulfonamides. They have little attraction as possible resistance mechanisms for antibiotics which inhibit major classes of reactions (ribosomal protein synthesis and cell wall transpeptidation) rather than single enzymatic steps in biosynthetic sequences.

that it has not been looked for or that selection techniques are not adequate to identify it. A further complexity in attempting to differentiate between alternative possible modes of resistance has arisen at the level of the experimental design of mechanism studies. A case in point from the author's experience is that of R factor-mediated chloramphenicol resistance in *E. coli*. Early studies (Unowsky and Rachmeler, 1966) with chloramphenicol-^{14}C demonstrated that less radioactivity could be recovered in cell pellets of resistant bacteria as compared with their episome-free sensitive counterparts. The tentative conclusion drawn from these experiments was that the R factor-mediated mechanism of resistance was one of relative impermeability to chloramphenicol. This hypothesis was noted to be incompatible with the observation in other laboratories that R factor-mediated chloramphenicol resistance was due to inactivation of the antibiotic (Okamoto and Suzuki, 1965) which subsequently was shown to be due to enzymatic acetylation by acetyl coenzyme A (CoA) (Shaw, 1967a; Suzuki and Okamoto, 1967). The apparent conflict was resolved by the realization that the radioactivity measurements did not discriminate between free chloramphenicol and its acetylated products. The subsequent demonstration that ^{14}C-labeled chloramphenicol-3-acetate does not bind to *E. coli* ribosomes argued that the uptake experiments were in fact measuring the facilitated diffusion of labeled chloramphenicol into the bacterial cells when the antibiotic was reversibly bound to intracellular ribosomes (Shaw and Unowsky, 1968). Because of the above observations one should interpret "permeability" experiments on antibiotic resistance with caution unless the experimental design has taken into account possible further metabolism of the drug in question. A case in point which deserves further study in the light of such considerations is the sulfonamide resistance gene of R factors which has been reported to involve decreased permeability of resistant cells (Kata *et al.*, 1962). The high resolution of current chromatographic techniques should in most instances permit decisions on the identity of radioactive material present in resistant cells.

An important and relatively simple technique which is useful in preliminary assessments of the mode of resistance to antimicrobial agents is worthy of note since it is so frequently omitted. Cells which owe their resistance to inactivating enzymes will enter the exponential phase of growth only after the concentration of the inhibitor is reduced to subinhibitory levels. The latter is a function of the number of bacterial cells present in the test inoculum and the initial antibiotic concentration. An inoculum effect has been documented for the familiar case of resistance to the penicillin group of drugs mediated by β-lactamases (Barber, 1957) and for enzymatic inactivation of chloramphenicol (Shaw and Brodsky, 1968a). A useful point to be noted in such studies is that resistant bacterial strains possessing an inactivating system often show a pronounced lag phase before the control rate of growth is achieved. Although other interpretations of an augmented lag are possible, such as induction of a specific permeability block, a search for this obvious characteristic may simplify studies aimed toward a more detailed explanation of the resistance mechanism. In the author's laboratory it has been possible to differentiate at least three probably different phenotypes of chloramphenicol resistance in clinical isolates of *E. coli* on the basis of an analysis of growth curves in the presence of the antibiotic (Shaw, unpublished experiments). Strains with R factors demonstrated by conjugal transfer of the resistance determinant invariably show a prolonged lag before assuming the exponential rate of growth seen in uninhibited control cultures, whereas chloramphenicol-resistant strains without demonstrable R factors show no such lag but do exhibit either (*a*) normal exponential growth following addition of the antibiotic or (*b*) exponential growth with doubling times substantially less than that noted in controls. The biochemical bases of the latter types of resistance remain obscure but may represent examples of chromosomal loci identical with those described for mutants isolated *in vitro* (Reeve, 1968).

The regulatory aspects of resistance gene expression have not yet received the attention they deserve when one considers the elegant analyses achieved for certain biosynthetic and catabolic enzyme systems (Martin, 1969). This is especially true for the more thoroughly studied extrachromosomal determinants. The only possible exception which will be dealt with subsequently is β-lactamase synthesis dictated by the pencillinase plasmids of staphylcocci (Section II, B, 1). Early reviews of R factor-mediated drug resistance in enteric bacteria stressed the fact that such episome-mediated characteristics are usually constitutive properties of the resistant strains (Watanabe, 1963). To the author's knowledge the only probable exception is tetracycline resistance which appears to be due to an inducible decrease in permeability in R factor strains (Franklin, 1967). In contrast, all of the plasmid-linked staphylococcal resistance determinants thus far examined in any detail appear to be inducible by growth in the presence of subinhibitory concentrations of the antibiotic in question (Novick, 1967; Shaw and Brodsky, 1968b; Novick and Roth, 1968; Hashimoto *et al.*, 1968). Current concepts of the genetic control of inducible enzyme synthesis would predict that such inducible enzymes or permeation defects would be subject to control by a locus dictating the synthesis of a substrate-specific repressor and that constitutive mutants of such plasmids or episomes could be isolated which either lack a repressor or possess an aporepressor that no longer recognizes the inducing antibiotic (Martin, 1969). Only in the cases of plasmid-mediated staphylococcal β-lactamase (Novick, 1967) and macrolide resistance (Saito *et al.*, 1970) has the isolation of constitutive strains been accomplished. Apart from their interest to microbial geneticists, such constitutive isolates have special epidemiologic significance since they are fully resistant prior to contact with the antibiotic in question and may possess special survival characteristics in an antibiotic-rich environment. The inducibility loci appear to be highly specific since induction of a given plasmid determinant fails to induce resistance to associated markers on the same plasmid. Staphylococci bearing multiple compatible elements such as the penicillinase and chloramphenicol plasmids also show independent control of synthesis of their respective inactivating enzymes (Shaw, unpublished observations). It is clear, however, that repressor control of a single resistance gene is not plasmid-specific since it can operate when the inducibility locus is in the trans position. Richmond (1965a) has shown that when a diploid strain of *Staphylococcus aureus* bearing both a constitutive and an inducible plasmid is induced, the enzyme types specific for each plasmid are synthesized in equal amounts.

II. Replication of R Factors and Other Resistance Plasmids

The recognition of transmissable drug resistance determinants in enteric bacteria led to obvious comparisons of their structure and replication with the classic fertility factors and episomes of *Escherichia coli*. Although important biologically, a detailed summary of these analogies is outside the scope of the present review and has been presented in detail elsewhere (Meynell *et al.*, 1967; Novick, 1969). Only selected aspects which are relevant to an understanding of the expression of resistance determinants will be discussed.

The methodology used for the demonstration of episomal and plasmid DNA of the drug resistance elements has in large measure been similar to that employed for more conventional extrachromosomal structures. Most investigators have taken advantage of the preliminary biological separation which takes place when one transfers sex factors such as F′ (lac) or R factors from their "natural" host *E. coli* to hosts with different chromosomal DNA characteristics. The buoyant density of episomal DNA (F factor or R factor) has been found to correlate with that of *E. coli* and closely related species in having nucleotide base characteristics typical of approximately 50% guanosine plus cytosine (G + C), whereas the observed buoyant densities for chromosomal DNA of *Serratia marcescens* and *Proteus mirabilis* are compatible with G + C contents of approximately 58 and 39%, respectively (Schildkraut *et al.*, 1962). Where studied in analytical or preparative ultracentrifugation in cesium chloride gradients the DNA from R factor-bearing strains of the latter species was shown to contain smaller satellite bands of the DNA with clearly different average base compositions than the host DNA (Falkow *et al.*, 1966; Rownd *et al.*, 1966). Such experiments represented the first demonstrations by physical means of the nonchromosomal properties of R factor DNA. An important early correlation was the disappearance of such satellite DNA from strains of *Serratia* or *Proteus* which had lost their resistance determinants either spontaneously or following treatment with acridine dyes. These preliminary studies also attempted to analyze the detail of the satellite DNA profiles by means of a prior purification of the extrachromosomal DNA by chromatography. The fine structure of such peaks suggested a lack of homogeneity which was initially interpreted as due to specific DNA regions attributable to the antibiotic resistance determinants per se (Falkow *et al.*, 1966). More recent studies from a number of laboratories now suggest that the conclusion drawn from the earlier studies may not be justified and that a far more complicated interpretation must be invoked. Whereas DNA profiles of R factor DNA from variant episomes lacking in certain determinants suggested that specific G + C contents were typical for each resistance marker, it now appears that the early results can be attributed to the growth conditions employed (Rownd, 1969a). These were not, however, artifacts but probably due to quite unexpected variations in episome synthesis in *P. mirabilis.* It would appear that R factor replication in this species is under a "relaxed" form of control which permits the synthesis of multiple episome copies when essential nutrients are limiting or when cultures approach the stationary phase of growth (Rownd, 1969b; Falkow *et al.*, 1969). Rownd (1969b) has also shown that the satellite DNA may increase to values as high as 60% of the chromosomal DNA during stationary phase. Based on the relative sizes of R factor and host chromosomal DNA, it was estimated that approximately 10 R factors were present throughout the exponential phase of growth and that up to sixty copies could be harbored by viable cells in stationary phase. Experiments with ^{14}N- and ^{15}N-labeling of replicating DNA have suggested that copy selection is a random process in *P. mirabilis* in the sense that a given R factor can be replicated more than once during a given generation (Rownd, 1969b). This phenomenon of relaxed control has now been amply confirmed and extended with the demonstration that the increased gene dose of R factor DNA is transcribed and translated since the readily measured levels of inactivating enzymes for penicillin and chloramphenicol increase proportionately with the extrachromosomal DNA (Falkow *et al.*, 1969; Rownd *et al.*, 1970). Studies with *P. mirabilis* have also suggested a physical dissociation between the DNA-bearing drug resistance genes and those regions conferring the property of conjugal fertility. The genetic evidence of the existence of such transfer elements lacking resistance markers has been reviewed by Anderson (1968). Rownd and co-workers (1970) observed that with R factor NR 1, three species of DNA having different buoyant sensitivities were observed in *P. mirabilis* and that they appeared to be interconvertible. The hypothesis presented to explain the experimental data is that the material of lowest density (1.712 gm/cm^3) represents the simple transfer element (RTF) under relaxed control, whereas the most dense (1.718 gm/cm^3) material is made up of the RTF element plus multiple copies of the resistance determinants. It has been suggested that the DNA of intermediate density should be attributed to a complete R factor bearing only a single copy of each resistance gene.

In view of the known circularity of the chromosome of *E. coli* and from the genetic analysis of segregants of wild-type R factors, it was initially suggested that R factors might exist within the cell in a circular form (Watanabe, 1963). Such has proved to be the case since it is abundantly clear that all of the extrachromosomal resistance elements thus far examined (Nisioka *et al.*, 1969; Cohen and Miller, 1969; Rush *et al.*, 1969) exist as closed, covalently linked circles of double-stranded DNA. This property is apparently shared by other sex factors such as colicinogenic factors (Hickson *et al.*, 1967) and prophage P1 (Ikeda and Tomizawa, 1968). The electron microscopic size estimates in most cases agree well with the estimates of extrachromosomal DNA based on earlier ultracentrifugation measurements. A newer technique which has simplified the physical study of R factors and other plasmids has been the use of ultracentrifugation in the presence of ethidium bromide—a dye which intercalates with double stranded DNA (Vinograd *et al.*, 1965; Bauer and Vinograd, 1968). Special use has been made of the resistance of closed circular DNA to alkali denaturation combined with the ethidium bromide technique which produces different buoyant density changes for such closed duplex DNA as compared with nicked circular or linear DNA. Thus it is now possible to isolate and demonstrate R factor DNA in duplex circular form from its "natural" host *E. coli* (Cohen and Miller, 1969). Such measurements have led to the conclusions that more stringent control of R factor replication occurs in *E. coli* than in *P. mirabilis* and that less than two copies of R factor DNA exist per copy of the chromosome (Nisioka *et al.*, 1970). The ethidium bromide technique has also led to a gratifying confirmation of the hypothesis that direct recombination of segregant R factors does in fact occur. By using various segregant R factors with sizable deletions of resistance determinants, Clowes and his collaborators have shown that when recombinant factors arise from matings between cells bearing each of two segregants the size of circular DNA duplexes of the recombinants is the same as that observed for the original wild-type R factor (Nisioka *et al.*, 1970). A similar approach has been used to demonstrate the physical basis of the so-called "SΔ" R factor originally isolated in *Salmonella typhimurium* (Anderson, 1968) which confers transferable resistance to streptomycin and sulfonamides and can dissociate into segregants with only the transfer locus (Δ^+) or the resistance genes (S^+). Centrifugation and electron microscopic studies of SΔ and its segregants in *E. coli* have revealed three species of covalently closed circular DNA which correlate with the SΔ, S^+, and Δ^+ elements (Smith *et al.*, 1970).

It is appropriate to stress, however, that the physical characterization of R factor DNA is producing interesting discrepancies and exceptions as rapidly as it is clarifying the genetic hypotheses. An example is the anomalous behavior of an R factor-mediating penicillinase in *E. coli* which appears to be under relaxed control reminiscent of earlier studies in *P. mirabilis* (Kontomichalou *et al.*, 1970). It is apparent, therefore, that plasmid-specific replication control may be as important as host-mediated mechanisms and that the design of future studies should take both factors into account.

For the sake of completeness it should be emphasized that progress has been reported in analyzing the physical properties of extrachromosomal DNA in plasmid-bearing strains of *Staphylococcus aureus*. Although the species specificity of transmissible staphylococcal plasmids has precluded their transfer to cells with different (G + C) ratios of the chromosomal DNA, it has been possible to distinguish between plasmid and host DNA by the ethidium bromide technique (Rush *et al.*, 1969) and by polylysine kieselguhr column chromatography (Cannon and Dunican, 1970). The former study demonstrated the covalently closed, circular nature of penicillinase plasmid DNA and revealed circular duplexes of varying sizes that correlated with size estimates obtained from deletional mapping of the plasmids in question. In all cases examined the staphylococcal, plasmid, DNA circles were substantially smaller than those noted for most R factors.

III. Biochemical Expression of Extrachromosomal Drug Resistance

A. General Considerations

The present discussion attempts to take into account the preliminary nature of much of the information currently available. In certain instances, most notably the penicillinase plasmids of staphylococci, the genetic and biochemical mechanisms of resistance have been demonstrated rigorously. For other systems, such as staphylococcal resistance to chloramphenicol, the biochemical aspects of resistance are clearer than the genetic aspects of its apparent extrachromosomal nature. Still less certain are the biochemical mechanisms of resistance to sulfonamides mediated by R factors or the genetic distinctions between tetracycline resistance observed in R factor-bearing strains of *Escherichia coli* and those of chromosomal origin. Some consideration will also be given to resistance to agents which are not usually thought of as "drugs" in the sense that they are not clinically useful. Resistance to the heavy metal ions is such a case since these determinants are frequently observed in association with conventional drugs such as antibiotics and the sulfonamides and since a better understanding of their function may shed some light on more general properties of drug resistance plasmids.

B. Penicillin Resistance

1. *Penicillinase Plasmids of Staphylococci*

The hydrolytic cleavage of the β-lactam ring of the penicillin group of antibiotics is the best known and most intensively studied example of antibiotic resistance mediated by an inactivating enzyme. Although properly referred to as β-lactamase to stress the range of susceptible substrates, this activating enzyme has been referred to as penicillinase for two decades. In most instances the author has elected to use the latter trivial designation which has the virtue of wide recognition and continuing common usage.

The history of the recognition of penicillin resistance among staphylococci and its subsequent explanation by the demonstration of penicillinase production by such strains is well known (Chain, 1962; Pollock, 1962; Richmond, 1965b) and will not be recounted. For the present discussion the important points noted by early workers are that (*1*) penicillinase production and penicillin resistance of staphylococci are lost concurrently as frequencies in excess of expected mutation rates, and (*2*) mutation to penicillin resistance mediated by penicillinase has never been conclusively demonstrated in staphylococci (Barber, 1957). These facts and a number of other observations led Novick (1963) to the hypothesis that the genes for penicillinase synthesis in *S. aureus* are not located on the bacterial chromosome but rather exist as part of an autonomous genome best described as a "plasmid" (Lederberg, 1952). The more restrictive term of "episome" was not chosen since its definition (Jacob and Wollman, 1958) presupposes the existence of an alternative state of chromosomal integration.

The most convincing evidence for the extrachromosomal location of penicillinase genes in *S. aureus* comes from transduction studies and has been discussed by Novick (1967) and Richmond (1968). Briefly stated, the simultaneous exponential decrease in plaque-forming activity and frequency of transduction on treatment of transducing phage with ultraviolet radiation is a most compelling argument for a plasmid location of the penicillinase gene in most strains. An apparently rare exception is *S. aureus* PS 80 which has been studied by Asheshov (1969). When phage 80 was propagated on its host strain and the resulting lysate subjected to ultraviolet irradiation, phage survival and transduction of extrachromosomal mercury resistance decreased exponentially whereas an increased frequency of transduction of penicillin resistance was observed. The finding that ultraviolet irradiation increases the frequency of transduction for chromosomal markers but reduces such frequencies for episomal determinants was first reported by Arber (1960) in *E. coli* and has proved to be a useful tool for the analysis of gene location in *S. aureus*.

The genetics of the penicillinase plasmids of *S. aureus* have been summarized recently (Novick, 1969; Richmond, 1968) and will not be reviewed in detail. For the purposes of the present discussion, however, it should be noted that at least three types (A, B, and C) of immunologically distinct penicillinases have been described and that two such species of enzymes can be detected in cells made diploid by introducing two compatible plasmids mediating the synthesis of different penicillinases (Richmond, 1965a). The construction of such diploid genotypes has led to a second interesting observation which may have more general significance (Richmond, 1967a). There appears to be a restriction to the expression of the structural genes for penicillinase in such diploid strains in that the total synthesis of each of the specific penicillinases is approximately one-half that observed in fully induced or constitutive haploid cells. In other words, the double gene dose is not accompanied by a proportional increment in enzyme synthesis, as has been observed for *E. coli* diploid for β-galactosidase by virtue of the presence of an F′ (lac) episome (Jacob and Monod, 1961). This interesting observation should be confirmed and extended with other plasmids and host strains of staphylococci. In any case, the availability of such relatively stable diploid cells has permitted a test of the control of penicillinase synthesis from a more conventional point of view. Since plasmids constitutive (i^-) for penicillinase production have been isolated and introduced into cells carrying compatible inducible (i^+) plasmids, it has been possible to test for dominance. As expected, i^+ is active in the trans position since i^+/i^- diploids are fully inducible. Somewhat anomalous positional effects have been noted by Asheshov and Dyke (1968) in a diploid of *S. aureus* PS 80 when the i^+ determinant is chromosomal and the plasmid is i^-. This genotype showed incomplete repression of penicillinase synthesis in the absence of inducer (methicillin) and markedly enhanced induction in its presence. There is no information available on the nature or mode of action of the presumed repressor product of the i region. The reciprocal genotype with a plasmid i^+ locus gave a more conventional phenotype showing adequate repression and normal inducibility. Sweeney and Cohen (1968) have independently observed the same phenomenon in isolates of *S. aureus* and have shown that the penicillinase synthesized by the plasmid and chromosomal linkage groups in their strains is immunologically Type A. It is of interest that Richmond (personal communication) has observed that the chromosomal penicillinase of PS 80 is also Type A.

An interpretation of these findings is not yet available, but it is clear that control of expression of the penicillinase structural gene is more complicated than anticipated. Richmond (1967b) has presented evidence for a second regulatory region involved in plasmid-mediated penicillinase synthesis, and Cohen's laboratory has recently described the influence of maintenance-compatability type on the derepressibility of various plasmids by the chromosomal constitutive locus (Cohen *et al.*, 1970). A final decision on the number and interactions of penicillinase-controlling linkage groups will have to await further studies.

In addition to the immunological differences between staphylococcal penicillinases noted above, there is ample evidence that such naturally occurring enzymes have distinguishing catalytic properties. Immunological Types A and C have been associated with staphylococci from Groups I or III, whereas the less common Type B has thus far been implicated only in phage Group II. The penicillinase type can also be correlated with plasmid compatibility types (Richmond, 1965b). In any event, there are detectable substrate preferences among the three types of penicillinase. All three share the characteristic of a low apparent dissociation constant (K_m) for benzyl penicillin, phenoxymethylpenicillin, and phenoxyethylpenicillin, but the Type B enzyme has a lower specific activity against all penicillins. All three penicillinases have a low affinity and show markedly diminished rates of hydrolysis for the semisynthetic penicillins and cephalosporins. It is clear from their approximately identical molecular weights (29,500) and similar amino acid analyses (Richmond, 1965c) that they are closely related from an evolutionary point of view and may differ only in a few amino acid substitutions that critically affect immunological reactivity or catalytic properties. As will be discussed later, there is no evidence that subsequent mutational events have occurred to permit inactivation of methicillin and the related semisynthetic penicillins. Although the latter group is hydrolyzed at a slow rate by so-called "methicillin-resistant" staphylococci, there is much information to suggest that mechanisms other than a "new" penicillinase are involved.

Throughout the above discussion the concept of inducibility has been used fully to define the genetic aspects of penicillinase synthesis. It should be pointed out that the various natural and semisynthetic penicillins probably differ widely in their capacity to induce penicillinase synthesis in *S. aureus*. Data on the inducing potential of penicillin analogs are available (Pollock, 1962) but are difficult to interpret because of the various methods of assay and the inherent susceptibility of certain penicillins to hydrolysis by the enzyme being synthesized. Reproducible and meaningful values are most likely to be obtained for compounds approaching conditions of "gratuitous" induction wherein minimal toxic effects on the host cell are likely and the inducer itself is relatively stable in the presence of penicillinase. In practice, induction is usually carried out with low concentrations of a suitable penicillinase-resistant penicillin, such as methicillin or oxacillin. In theory, an approach to the therapy of infections due to penicillinase producing staphylococci with penicillins would be the use of an analog which is an effective antibiotic but incapable of inducing penicillinase synthesis. The search for such a compound is, however, not likely to be given a high priority in view of the degree of control of such infections by the penicillinase-resistant penicillins and cephalosporins.

For the sake of completeness, it should be pointed out that penicillinase-producing staphylococci other than *S. aureus* have been isolated from diverse sources (Corse and Williams, 1968). The ubiquity of coagulase-negative staphylococci (*Staphylococcus epidermidis*) and the frequency with which they have been found to be multiply resistant to antibiotics suggest that they may be of considerable importance as a gene pool for the inter-species spread of resistance. In this connection it is of interest that Baldwin and co-workers (1969) have partially characterized the penicillinase found in *S. epidermidis* and have isolated several phages from this species which are active for *S. aureus*. Considerable comparative work needs to be done in order to interpret these findings and clarify possible transfer mechanisms and genetic homologies among the micrococci.

The development of penicillinase-resistant semisynthetic penicillins was a remarkable achievement in the control of infections by penicillin-resistant staphylococci, but there is now ample reason to believe that resistance to the newer agents is a real clinical problem (Barrett *et al.*, 1968) and that such strains are resistant to semisynthetic penicillins other than methicillin as well as the cephalosporins (Barber, 1962; Parker and Hewitt, 1970). Early studies of so-called "methicillin resistance" stressed the point that such cultures are heterogeneous in that only a small fraction of bacterial cells in a given culture are capable of expressing resistance (Sutherland and Rolison, 1964). Seligman (1966) has shown that, although significant destruction of methicillin may occur in such cultures, there is no evidence that penicillinase is involved per se. Derivative strains of methicillin-resistant *S. aureus* which have lost the penicillinase plasmid are still resistant to methicillin and also to benzyl penicillin (Dyke *et al.*, 1966). Methicillin resistance should, therefore, be considered as a case of intrinsic resistance to the β-lactamase family of antibiotics and may bear some relationship to penicillin "tolerance" of the type described by Barber (1957, 1962) in earlier studies. At the present time the genetic basis of methicillin resistance is poorly understood and the biochemical mechanism is not yet clear (Dyke, 1969). Evidence has been presented that methicillin resistance may be extrachromosomal (Dornbusch *et al.*, 1969), but the data are not yet convincing and further confirmation is necessary. Seligman (personal communication) has not been able to transduce methicillin resistance under conditions favorable for plasmid transduction and has uniformly found that plasmid "curing" of other markers in such resistant strains is not accompanied by loss of methicillin resistance. Dyke (1969) has also been unable to transduce methicillin resistance in a single highly resistant strain and has offered possible explanations for nontransducibility.

Several approaches have been taken to explore the biochemical basis of methicillin resistance in *S. aureus*. An electron microscopic study of a single strain of methicillin-resistant *S. aureus* grown in the presence of the antibiotic revealed a morphologically normal cell wall both for the normal clones and the small-colony variants (Bulger and Bulger, 1967). Cocci from the small-colony variant appeared slightly larger than those from the normal-size colonies when both were grown in the presence of methicillin and were seen more often with a complete cell wall septum. It is not yet apparent whether these subtle differences are the consequence of resistance and, therefore, trivial or are of primary importance. Potentially more revealing physiological and biochemical studies have demonstrated that phenotypic methicillin resistance is (*a*) expressed more effectively at lower incubation temperatures (Dyke, 1969) and (*b*) is enhanced by increasing the salt content of the growth medium (Barber, 1964; Dyke, 1969). Both of these observations are of great importance in improving routine methods for detecting methicillin-resistant strains of *S. aureus* and suggest that subtle changes in the function of the cell wall may be involved. Chemical analyses of mucopeptide amino acids from sensitive and resistant strains have revealed no gross differences (Dyke, 1969; Sabath *et al.*, 1970), but the latter group of investigators has observed that cultures with a large proportion of highly resistant cells are lysed by lysostaphin more slowly than either fully sensitive strains or methicillin-resistant variants with few resistant cells. Although several interpretations of this phenomenon are possible, it may provide a promising approach and should be confirmed and extended to take into account the morphological data cited earlier and the pronounced effects of temperature and salt concentration.

2. *Penicillin Resistance of Enteric Bacteria*

A discussion of the biochemistry of extrachromosomal resistance in gram-negative bacteria should take into account not only the specific increments in resistance attributable to R factors but also the inherent decreased sensitivity of such species compared with gram-positive bacteria. In certain instances the interactions between these factors are likely to be complex. It is also apparent that the finding of various types of β-lactamases in gram-negative species has complicated an interpretation of a number of studies purporting to show specific R factor-mediated mechanisms of resistance. Because of the above considerations the author has been forced to be selective in reviewing the current status of penicillin resistance and has stressed those studies that, in his judgment, seem to provide a basis for meaningful future investigations.

Although the first reports (reviewed by Watanabe, 1963) of R factor resistance stressed the determinants for resistance to sulfonamides (Su), streptomycin (Sm), tetracycline (Tc), and chloramphenicol (Cm), it became apparent that resistance to ampicillin (aminobenzylpenicillin, Amp) was frequently mediated by extrachromosomal elements with one or more other resistance markers and was due to a specific penicillin-inactivating enzyme (Anderson and Datta, 1965). Subsequent studies confirmed the suspicion that R factor-mediated ampicillin resistance was, indeed, due to a β-lactamase and pointed to possible differences in substrate specificity between the episomal enzyme and the basal activity found in wild-type sensitive strains and in isolates "cured" of the (Amp) R factor (Datta and Kontomichalou, 1965). The activity of specific episomal β-lactamase correlated well with the observed degree of resistance, was not inducible by growth in the presence of penicillins, and appeared to be cell-bound rather than extracellular. The low rates of hydrolysis for benzyl penicillin and ampicillin by whole cell suspensions pointed to a relative impermeability which may in part explain the failure of earlier workers to demonstrate penicillinase activity in isolates of ampicillin-resistant *E. coli* (Ayliffe, 1963). The first hint of the complexity of R factor-mediated β-lactamase synthesis was apparent in the work of Datta and Kontomichalou (1965) wherein different R factors appeared to dictate the synthesis of enzymes with varying absolute rates of hydrolysis and different substrate profiles. A more detailed investigation of an R factor-mediated penicillinase was carried out with one of the isolates (*E. coli* TEM) used in the above study which produced large amounts of enzyme (Datta and Richmond, 1966). Penicillinase from broken cell preparations was purified by conventional techniques to yield material of constant specific activity which was clearly very different from previously reported purified enzymes obtained from *S. aureus*, *Bacillus cereus*, and *Bacillus licheniformis*. Estimates of the molecular weight (16,700) and apparent sedimentation velocity ($S_{20,w}$ = 1.85 S) suggested that the *E. coli* enzyme was the size of the penicillinases of gram-positive species. Subsequent studies on two independent R factor isolates (Yamagishi *et al.*, 1969) have yielded $S_{20,w}$ values for purified penicillinases of 2.66 S and 1.43 S, suggesting that the R factor-mediated enzymes are, in fact, a family of β-lactamases with quite divergent physical properties. Confirmation of the complexity of the question of size of the catalytic protein has come from recent reports on episomal β-lactamases in *E. coli* (Lindqvist and Nordström, 1970) and *Salmonella typhimurium*

(Neu and Winshell, 1970) which yielded values of approximately 22,000 and 31,000, respectively. At the present time it seems to be pertinent to inquire whether the discrepancies reflect more than merely differences in the analytical techniques employed by various laboratories. An alternative unitary hypothesis worthy of consideration is the existence of a fundamental β-lactamase polypeptide of minimal size which has evolved into a larger enzyme with somewhat different catalytic properties. For the purpose of provoking further studies, it might also be well to consider whether subunit considerations might be invoked to explain the variety of values obtained. Variable degrees of association of catalytically active subunits, perhaps induced by specific host functions or the techniques of purification, might be expected to explain such widely discordant results. In spite of the apparent universality of the genetic code, there is now preliminary evidence that host-induced modifications may alter the characteristics of episomal enzymes. In a recent study of naturally occurring transmissible F′ (lac) elements from *Salmonella* strains, the β-galactosidase activity in crude lysates was found to be markedly more heat resistant when examined in *E. coli* and *Salmonella typhosa* than in their original *Salmonella* hosts (Easterling *et al.*, 1969). Although the above experiments are subject to other interpretations, it will be important to characterize a number of different R factors mediating penicillinase activity in the same host under identical conditions before a final decision is possible.

Apart from considerations of molecular size, it is apparent that R factor penicillinases fall into at least two categories on the basis of their catalytic properties and substrate specificities (Egawa *et al.*, 1967). Studies by Yamagishi and his collaborators (Yamagishi *et al.*, 1969, 1970) and by Jack and Richmond (1970) suggest that the most common R factor penicillinase is the so-called Type I enzyme which is a general-purpose β-lactamase active against benzyl penicillin, ampicillin, and the cephalosporins. The Type I enzymes are acidic proteins which share immunological similarities, are resistant to inhibition by *p*-mercuribenzoate, and are inhibited by cloxacillin. It now appears that R factors mediating Type I β-lactamase have found their way into hosts which are genetically remote from *E. coli*. Reporting independently but using the same strains of *Pseudomonas aeruginosa*, two groups of investigators have characterized an enzyme with both penicillinase and cephalosporinase activity and general properties similar to the Type I lactamase. The penicillinase structural gene is lost with other resistance markers on treatment with acridines and linked to these determininants in conjugal transfer experiments using *E. coli* as the recipient (Sykes and Richmond, 1970; Fullbrook *et al.*, 1970).

The Type II enzyme which is apparently less widely distributed is also resistant to organic mercurials but has a net positive charge at neutral pH, fails to react with anti-Type I sera, has generally higher apparent affinities for a wide range of substrates, and is apparently inhibited by simple univalent anions (Yamagishi *et al.*, 1970). It seems likely, however, that structural genes other than the above two types can be found on R factors. Jack and Richmond (1970) have found two other episomal β-lactamases which show very different substrate profiles from either Type I or Type II. Although both enzymes hydrolyze benzyl penicillin, one has high cephalosporinase activity but no activity toward ampicillin, whereas the other R factor-mediated β-lactamase has reciprocal substrate preferences. It should be stressed that although the ampicillin resistance determinant first directed attention to episome-mediated penicillinase synthesis, there is evidence that R factor enzymes similar to Types I and II have been found in bacteria isolated some 5 years before ampicillin was first synthesized (Evans *et al.*, 1968).

Throughout the above discussion the emphasis has been on those instances in which the synthesis of specific β-lactamases has been mediated by R factors. A number of reports have now appeared which point to the wide occurrence of β-lactamases in enteric bacteria of all species. More often than not such activity is not transferable by conjugation and the determinants are presumed to be chromosomal. Although more rigorous evidence of their nonepisomal state would be more convincing (transductional analysis, elimination studies, absence of plasmid DNA), the determinants appear in most cases to have substrate profiles and catalytic properties which distinguish them from the R factor β-lactamases (Yamagishi *et al.*, 1970; Jack and Richmond, 1970). Although there may be important similarities between the common Type I β-lactamase and a species-specific enzyme of *Klebsiella*, the data are preliminary and to date there is no convincing evidence for the identity of an R factor β-lactamase with a chromosomal counterpart.

Most of the studies cited above have attempted to characterize the transferability and enzymatic properties of β-lactamase in random isolates of enteric bacteria. A different approach is illustrated by the work of Nordström and Boman and their collaborators in which an effort has been made to (a) define the characteristics of mutation to ampicillin in *E. coli* K-12 and (*b*) compare the genetic and enzymatic properties of a chromosomal penicillinase with the R factor-mediated system. Two cooperative but unlinked mutations have been described to account for high level (50μg/ml of ampicillin) resistance (Boman *et al.*, 1967). The Amp A locus is a regulatory gene for a penicillinase that has low activity in wild-type K-12 but is increased 10-fold in Amp A mutants, sufficient to permit resistance to 10 μg/ml. A second unlinked mutation at a site designated "Amp B" confers a further increase in resistance. The Amp B appeared to be a pleiotropic mutation affecting surface properties of the cell since such mutants showed increased sensitivity to osmotic shock and cycloserin, had lost the ability to grow on succinate, showed delayed chromosome transfer in mating experiments, and had altered kinetics of lysis in the presence of high concentrations of ampicillin (summarized in Nordström *et al.*, 1968). More recent studies with a mutant of this class have revealed a number of other properties which are best considered as the consequence of a change in the cell envelope (Nordström *et al.*, 1970). Such Amp B strains (or Class II mutants in their new nomenclature) show increased extracellular proportions of either episomal or chromosomal penicillinase, are more sensitive to osmotic shock and lysis by sodium cholate, and are defective in phage adsorption. The Amp B mutation is also capable of promoting modest increases in R factor-mediated resistance to the aminoglycosides and chloramphenicol.

The above discussion of transmissible ampicillin resistance has stressed what is known with some degree of certainty, but there are large gaps in our knowledge of the controls of R factor β-lactamase synthesis in bacteria possessing allelic or nonallelic genes on the chromosome. There is also reason to inquire further into the wide variations in R factor-promoted synthesis of β-lactamase in various hosts (Smith, 1969; Jack and Richmond, 1970). The possible importance of episomal, nonlactamase, inactivation mechanisms should also be explored, especially that of penicillin acylase in *E. coli* (Cole, 1969). Finally, the relationship of β-lactamase in enteric bacteria to the transpeptidation reactions of cell wall biosynthesis remains to be clarified. The periplasmic location of the former and the interaction of penicillins with both enzymatic systems suggest that a unifying hypothesis may yet emerge and receive experimental support.

C. Chloramphenicol Resistance

1. Gram-Negative Bacteria and R Factors

As noted earlier in this review (Section I), the early studies of R factor-mediated chloramphenicol resistance favored the view that permeability considerations might account for the observed phenotype (Watanabe, 1963; Okamoto and Mizuno, 1964; Unowsky and Rachmeler, 1966). It became clear from the studies of Okamoto and Suzuki (1965) that inactivation of chloramphenicol occurred in cell-free extracts of R factor strains of *Escherichia coli* if acetate was included in the incubation medium.

More recent studies have shown conclusively that inactivation occurs via enzymatic acetylation with acetyl CoA as the acetyl donor (Shaw, 1967a; Suzuki and Okamoto, 1967). The overall reaction appears to proceed by several steps:

$$\text{chloramphenicol} + \text{acetyl-S-CoA} \rightarrow \text{chloramphenicol-3-acetate} + \text{HS-CoA} \quad (1)$$

$$\text{chloramphenicol-3-acetate} \rightleftarrows \text{chloramphenicol-1-acetate} \quad (2)$$

$$\text{chloramphenicol-1-acetate} + \text{acetyl-S-CoA} \rightarrow \text{chloramphenicol-1, 3-diacetate} + \text{HS-CoA} \quad (3)$$

The formation of the monoacetyl derivative proceeds rapidly and is sufficient to account for resistance since chloramphenicol-3-acetate is inactive as an antibiotic. As the 1-hydroxyl is apparently unreactive the formation of chloramphenicol 1,3-diacetate probably occurs via a nonenzymatic pH-dependent rearrangement [Eq. (2)] and subsequent attack again at the 3-hydroxyl position. Chloramphenicol acetyltransferase is synthesized constitutively in all enteric bacteria carrying the R factor determinant for chloramphenicol resistance and has been purified to a state of homogeneity by conventional techniques of protein fraction (Shaw and Brodsky, 1968b; Shaw, 1970). Unlike R factor-mediated β-lactamase, the acetylating enzyme is not periplasmic since it is not liberated by osmotic shock from protoplasts (Suzuki and Okamoto, 1967; Shaw, unpublished experiments). Earlier estimates of the size of the native enzyme were consistent with a molecular weight of 78,000. More recent gel filtration studies have yielded a value of approximately 80,000 and sedimentation studies have provided a figure of $S_{20,w}$ of 5.2 S which is compatible with this estimate (Shaw, unpublished experiments).

An early observation which may be of great interest in terms of the possible origin of R factor-mediated resistance genes was the finding that low but detectable levels of acetylating enzyme can be found in numerous gram-negative bacteria which do not harbor R factors and which are phenotypically sensitive (Shaw, 1967b; Okamoto *et al.*, 1967). *Proteus mirabilis* yielded sufficient material for preliminary comparative studies, and experiments with crude enzyme showed it to be quite similar to that found in R^+ cultures (Shaw and Brodsky, 1968c). More recent experiments have extended these observations by demonstrating that single-step highly resistant strains of *P. mirabilis* can be isolated which possess chloramphenicol acetyltransferase activity comparable to that seen in R factor-containing strains (Jacobsen and Shaw, 1970). The presumed chromosomal enzyme is similar to that of episomal origin in all respects except for a threefold higher K_m for chloramphenicol. Of special interest was the observation that polyacrylamide electrophoresis in sodium dodecyl sulfate revealed a single polypeptide of 20,000 molecular weight. Although evidence for the identity of the presumed subunits is not yet available, it is apparent that the native enzyme of chromosomal or episomal origin is a tetramer. Important correlations of these findings have been made with chloramphenicol-resistant staphylococci and will be discussed below.

Although the findings of trace amounts of chloramphenicol acetyltransferase in sensitive (R^-) bacteria suggested that the drug resistance episomes might function by specifically derepressing a chromosomal determinant (Shaw, 1967a), it is now clear that the structural gene for the acetylating enzyme is episomal in location. Hashimoto and Hirota (1966) isolated several point mutants of an R factor mediating chloramphenicol resistance. One of these mutants has been shown to produce normal amounts of an enzyme which is catalytically deficient but immunologically identical with the normal transacetylase (Wadzinsky and Shaw, unpublished experiments). More convincing data have come from the work of Mise and Suzuki (1968) in which temperature-sensitive mutants of the R factor chloramphenicol resistance gene were isolated. The temperature sensitivity was specific for chloramphenicol resistance and did not affect the expression of resistance to streptomycin or tetracycline, nor did the mutation alter the stability of the R factor per se. Since the heat lability of the enzyme was independent of the host strain in which the R factor resided, it was concluded that the observed phenotype was the result of a structural gene mutation for the acetylating enzyme.

One of the present enigmas of chloramphenicol resistance in enteric bacteria is the infrequency with which the chloramphenicol acetylating enzyme can be invoked to explain the resistance of *E. coli* mutants isolated spontaneously or following mutagenesis. A detailed study of single-step mutations to chloramphenicol resistance in *E. coli* K-12 has revealed a chromosomal locus (cmlA) which mediates low-level (10 μg/ml) resistance (Reeve, 1966; Reeve and Suttie, 1968). Such mutants fail to synthesize chloramphenicol acetyltransferase (Reeve, personal communication). Similar results were obtained by Sompolinsky and Samra (1968) in that no drug inactivation was observed in single-step low-level or multistep high-level mutants of *E. coli* K-12. The latter authors were able to isolate single-step mutants of *E. coli* B which were resistant to 100 μg/ml of chloramphenicol and which were rapid inactivators of the antibiotic. Although an interpretation of this discrepancy is not yet available, it is clear that searches for the chromosomal allele of R factor-mediated chloramphenicol will not only have to take into account species-specific differences but also variations in the substrain genotypes of enteric bacteria.

Mention has already been made of the ease with which single-step mutants of *P. mirabilis* can be isolated which synthesize large quantities of chloramphenicol acetyltransferase and are phenotypically resistant to high concentrations of the antibiotic. If R factor-linked genes have, in fact, arisen by recombination between sex factors and bacterial chromosomes, it is obvious that such interactions must have occurred in hosts that have both the gene in question and a reasonable degree of homology in DNA sequence. The examples of enzyme-mediated chloramphenicol resistance and penicillin resistance induced by R factors offer attractive experimental models to test this hypothesis.

Although enzymatic acetylation accounts for chloramphenicol resistance in a very high proportion of clinical isolates of gram-negative bacteria (Shaw, 1967b; Sompolinsky *et al.*, 1968; Piffaretti and Pitton, 1970), it may well be that other mechanisms will be detected. Iyer and Iyer (1969) have described an apparently novel situation in *Klebsiella* wherein two distinct phenotypes of chloramphenicol resistance have been found in substrains derived from a highly resistant R factor-bearing parent. The data suggest that both high and low resistance determinants exist and that they are episomal and unlinked since they are independently eliminated by acridines and ethidium bromide. Since only the highly resistant derivatives contain the acetylating enzyme (Shaw and Iyer, unpublished experiments), it is possible that the low-level resistance phenotype is genetically related to the chromosomal mutants of *E. coli* K-12 described above.

It is apparent from the structure of chloramphenicol that modes of attack other than *O*-acetylation could be responsible for drug inactivation. Reduction of the aromatic nitro group (Merkel and Steers, 1953), cleavage of the amide linkage (Holt, 1967), and oxidation of the propanediol side chain represent plausible mechanisms since the expected products are all inactive as antibiotics (Brock, 1961). To date, however, there is no evidence that such reactions are responsible for clinically important resistance of either the chromosomal or episomal types. By contrast with the success achieved in determining the mechanism of inhibition seen with the aminoglycoside drugs, it is of interest that there are no examples of resistance to chloramphenicol which can be attributed to decreased ribosomal affinity for the antibiotic (Weisblum and Davies, 1968).

2. Plasmid-Mediated Chloramphenicol Resistance of Staphylococci

The analogies between the penicillinase plasmids of *Staphylococcus aureus* and R factor-linked penicillinase production in enteric bacteria have been described in some detail (Section II). Although the genetic analysis of staphylococcal chloramphenicol resistance has not yet appproached the refinement of that for penicillin resistance, there are clear indications that a similar pattern may emerge. In certain respects the enzymology of chloramphenicol resistance is better understood than its genetic basis and for that reason the former area will be discussed in more detail.

Although early experiments showed that drug inactivation was likely in chloramphenicol-resistant isolates of *S. aureus* (Dunsmoor *et al.*, 1964; Miyamura, 1964), the work of Suzuki and co-workers (1966) demonstrated that enzymatic acetylation was the likely mechanism and pointed to its similarity to the R factor-mediated system in enteric bacteria. More recent work from several laboratories has defined the characteristics of staphylococcal chloramphenicol resistance in more detail (Shaw and Brodsky, 1968b; Winshell and Shaw, 1969). Unlike the constitutive synthesis of chloramphenicol acetyltransferase observed in R^+ enteric bacteria, the *S. aureus* enzyme is induced by the presence of chloramphenicol and certain analogs. The kinetics of induction are complicated since the parent antibiotic is an inhibitor of induced enzyme synthesis and is rapidly converted by the acetylating enzyme to products (chloramphenicol-acetate and chloramphenicol-1,3-diacetate) which are ineffective as inducers. A partial solution to this problem was achieved by the observation that 3-deoxychloramphenicol is ineffective as an antibiotic, is not susceptible to acetylation, but is still a potent inducer. Conditions of "gratuitous" induction can, therefore, be achieved and permit the preparation of cell-free extracts with high specific activity for chloramphenicol acetyltransferase. The staphylococcal enzyme has been shown to be identical with the R factor-mediated *E. coli* enzyme as regards pH optimum, catalytic properties, and molecular weight (approximately 80,000), but striking differences have been observed with regard to heat stability, substrate specificity and affinities, electrophoretic mobility, and immunological reactivity. Although a general picture has emerged for the structural properties of the molecule which are required for induction and susceptibility to acetylation, it is noteworthy that no analog has been found that has been shown conclusively to be an effective antibiotic but which either fails to induce the acetylating enzyme or is not a substrate for it (Shaw and Winshell, 1969). Although a recent report (Mitsuhashi *et al.*, 1969) suggested that the 1,3-dichloro analog of chloramphenicol (which lacks the hydroxyl groups which are essential for acetylation) has significant antibiotic activity, the author's laboratory has not been able to confirm this observation (Shaw, unpublished experiments.). Mitsuhashi's group has also reported that a series of chloramphenicol analogs lacking the C-3-hydroxyl and containing a keto function at C-1, are effective antibiotics against resistant *S. aureus* (Kono *et al.*, 1969). These observations are difficult to reconcile with the apparent importance of an intact 1,3-propanediol side chain for antibiotic activity (Brock, 1961).

A recent study of chloramphenicol resistance in clinical isolates of *Staphylococcus epidermidis* has revealed the presence of chloramphenicol acetyltransferase in resistant cultures and its absence in strains rendered sensitive by growth at elevated temperatures or treatment with acridine dyes (Shaw *et al.*, 1970). The enzyme found in resistant *S. epidermidis* has been purified to a state of homogeneity and compared with the homologous protein of *S. aureus* with the conclusion that they are identical in most important respects but differ in electrophoretic behavior and sensitivity to inhibition by mercuric ion. An important derivative product of this study was the observation that both staphylococcal enzymes are tetramers consisting of four subunits of 20,000 molecular weight. The smaller polypeptides are catalytically inactive and appear to be identical. A similar observation has already been mentioned in connection with the chromosomal and episomal types of acetylating enzyme found in *P. mirabilis*.

A critical analysis of the genetic basis of chloramphenicol resistance observed in resistant staphylococci cannot be made with certainty at the present time. In common with the finding noted above for *S. epidermidis*, it has been commonly observed that chloramphenicol-sensitive variants can be obtained from resistant cultures at rates which are typical of plasmid-mediated determinants (Chabbert *et al.*, 1964; Kono *et al.*, 1968; Sabath *et al.*, 1968). The segregation of resistance markers from multiply resistant strains and the results of transduction experiments suggest that the chloramphenicol resistance gene is not linked with either that for penicillinase production or other known plasmid genotypes.

There is clearly a need for a more detailed genetic study of chloramphenicol resistance in staphylococci in which attention is given to the effects of ultraviolet irradiation on the frequency of transduction and the possible interspecies transduction of chloramphenicol between *S. aureus* and *S. epidermidis*. Experiments of the latter type have been reported (Goto *et al.*, 1965) and deserve to be confirmed and extended. The most compelling evidence for the extrachromosomal state of chloramphenicol resistance in *S. aureus* is the recent finding that circular duplex DNA can be isolated from cells carrying only the chloramphenicol resistance determinant (Novick, personal communication). Its size (2.5×10^6) is considerably smaller than that reported for penicillinase plasmids ($16–18 \times 10^6$) by Rush and his co-workers (1969). Since three nucleotide pairs of a molecular weight of 1800 are needed for each amino acid, it is apparent that the chloramphenicol plasmid contains sufficient information for approximately 1390 amino acids of which only approximately 170 would be necessary for the structural gene for the acetylating enzyme subunit (20,000 molecular weight; see above). It is clear, therefore, that even this small element must contain DNA sufficient for the expression of other plasmid functions such as replication enzymes and compatibility determinants.

The information currently available on enzyme-mediated chloramphenicol resistance suggests that the enteric (R factor and chromosomal) and staphylococcal (plasmid) transacetylases represent a "family" of closely related proteins of probable common origin. The specific properties and function of their common ancestor remains obscure, but its delineation should provide important information on the origin and mode of acquisition of other extrachromosomal determinants.

D. Tetracycline Resistance

1. Gram-Negative Bacteria and R Factors

The widespread use of tetracyclines in clinical medicine and veterinary practice and the frequent appearance of transferable resistance to this group of antibiotics (Anderson, 1968), make it imperative that the mechanisms of tetracycline resistance be understood in biochemical terms. Although preliminary experiments with R factor-containing strains(cited by Watanabe, 1963) pointed toward permeability considerations, subsequent studies provided only negative data arguing against other mechanisms. Okamoto and Mizuno (1964) showed that the cell-free protein-synthesizing system prepared from *E. coli* carrying an R factor for tetracycline resistance was as sensitive as that obtained from sensitive strains. Izaki and Arima (1963) were the first investigators to demonstrate directly that episomal resistance was accompanied by decreased cellular uptake of oxytetracycline. Similar observations were reported subsequently by Franklin and Godfrey (1965) for a mutant of *E. coli* isolated after serial passage in the presence of chlortetracycline and by Unowsky and Rachmeler (1966) for *E. coli* bearing R factors for tetracycline resistance. It was clear that analogous mechanisms probably existed for both R factor-mediated tetracycline resistance and that observed with conventional variants selected from wild-type *E. coli*. Independent studies from several laboratories have pointed to the complexity of tetracycline uptake by sensitive bacteria and the probable course to be pursued for studies with resistant strains. The overall process in normal cells appears to require an energy source and magnesium ion, and is sensitive to agents that uncouple oxidative metabolism (Izaki and Arima, 1965). Further studies by De Zeeuw (1968) implicated a biphasic uptake process in which, at subinhibitory concentrations, the uptake appeared to be explicable in terms of physical adsorption, whereas, at higher concentrations, an azide-sensitive active transport process seemed likely. The above general observations were confirmed and extended by Franklin and Higginson (1970) who pointed out that net tetracycline uptake at low concentrations was reversed rapidly by incubation of the cells in drug-free medium and showed that the efflux of antibiotic was temperature-dependent. An anomalous finding was the observation that cells preloaded in the presence of high concentrations of tetracycline showed markedly decreased loss of antibiotic when the exit phase was examined. Although the authors suggest several theoretical hypotheses to account for this important observation, there is as yet no clear explanation.

In view of the uncertainties surrounding the normal process of tetracycline accumulation in sensitive cells, it is not surprising that the mechanism of resistance is still poorly understood. In contrast to resistance mediated by β-lactamases and chloramphenicol acetyltransferase which are constitutive (see later discussion), the R factor tetracycline resistance phenotype is an inducible property of such strains (Franklin, 1967). The R factor-resistant *E. coli* cells cultured in the absence of antibiotic showed relatively low-level resistant (50% inhibition of protein synthesis at 50 μg/ml) when challenged with tetracycline, whereas bacteria preincubated with subinhibitory concentrations required 200 μg/ml of tetracycline for a comparable degree of inhibition. High-level resistance under these conditions was accompanied by an uptake of tetracycline which was six- to tenfold less than that observed with resistant cells which had not been preincubated with the antibiotic. The induction process may require macromolecule synthesis since inhibitors of protein (chloramphenicol) and DNA-dependent ribonucleic acid (RNA) synthesis (proflavin) diminished the preincubation effects noted by Franklin. Although penicillin spheroplasts prepared from the resistant strain showed a qualitatively similar response, the rate of the preinduction-promoted fall in uptake was lower than that seen in intact cells. More recent studies have succeeded in demonstrating that (*1*) tetracycline uptake by purified membrane preparations is temperature- and divalent cation-dependent, and (*2*) there is a depression in the level of resistance of *E. coli* exposed to osmotic shock (Franklin, personal communication). The evidence available at present suggests that R factor-mediated resistance can be viewed as the result of the induced synthesis of an inhibitor of transport which is periplasmic in location. Such an inhibitor would appear to be a protein due to the effect noted with chloramphenicol but could equally well be a small molecular weight effector, the synthesis of which requires the induction of a specific enzyme.

A preliminary observation which requires further study is the apparent activity of minocycline, an alkylated tetracycline analog, against R factor strains of tetracycline-resistant enteric bacteria (Jarolmen *et al.*, 1970). One could surmise that minocycline fails to induce this hypothetical R factor-specific inhibitor of transport or gain access to the cell independently of the energy-dependent accumulation system.

2. Tetracycline Resistance in Staphylococcus aureus

Studies of tetracycline resistance in staphylococci have progressed sufficiently to state that extrachromosomal determinants distinct from the penicillinase plasmids seem likely in certain strains (May *et al.*, 1964; Poston, 1966; Asheshov, 1966) but may be chromosomal in others (Kasuga *et al.*, 1965, 1968). There has been no study of the mechanism of tetracycline resistance in a strain of *S. aureus* with a well-documented plasmid locus for resistance. Such experiments would be welcome in view of the recent observations with tetracycline-resistant staphylococci of uncertain genetic status. Two groups have reported independently that the mechanism in *S. aureus* is strikingly similar to that described for *E. coli* (Sasaki *et al.*, 1970; Inoue *et al.*, 1970). Accumulation studies revealed a sigmoidal concentration dependence for sensitive cells and indicated that resistance was induced by preincubation in the presence of antibiotics, was prevented by inhibitors of protein synthesis, and was accompanied by a one-hundred-fold reduction in uptake of tetracycline. Some insight into the structural specificity of either the induction process or the transport mechanism may come from studies with tetracycline analogs. Minocycline has been shown to be effective *in vitro* against tetracycline-resistant *S. aureus* of unstated genetic type (Nakazawa *et al.*, 1970).

Although the above discussion stresses the importance of decreased tetracycline accumulation in resistant bacterial cells, it should be pointed out that most studies have failed to rule out drug inactivation conclusively. The ease with which tetracyclines can be epimerized at the 4-dimethylamino position of the A ring (reviewed by Boothe, 1962) suggests that the possibility of enzyme-catalyzed reactions of this type should be kept in mind. Such conversions might lead to an apparent decrease in accumulation if the resultant epitetracyclines failed to participate in the proposed energy-dependent transport process.

E. Resistance to Aminoglycoside Antibiotics

In contrast to the observed similarities between chromosomal and extrachromosomal mechanisms of resistance to penicillins, chloramphenicol, and tetracyclines, there is less evidence for allelic or homologous mechanisms of resistance to the aminoglycoside group of antibiotics. In spite of the pleiotropic effects of streptomycin and related drugs on sensitive bacteria, there is ample reason to believe that their effects on the bacterial ribosome are of paramount importance (reviewed by Weisblum and Davies, 1968). The associated properties of aminoglycoside-induced inhibition of protein synthesis and misreading of natural or artificial messenger RNA ("ambiguity") are clearly related to the sensitivity of one or more ribosomal proteins (Ozaki *et al.*, 1969). There are qualitative and quantitative differences in the effects of the streptomycin, neomycin, and kanamycin groups of antibiotics on ribosomal function and genetic evidence that resistance to each group is specified by independent loci determining various ribosomal proteins (see above references). By way of contrast the R factor-mediated mechanisms of aminogycoside resistance thus far described do not involve alterations in ribosomal structure or assembly but are examples of drug inactivation by specific episome-promoted enzymes.

The first clear evidence implicating an inactivating mechanism for the aminoglycoside antibiotics was the observation by Okamoto and Suzuki (1965) that cell-free extracts of *E. coli* bearing an R factor for dihydrostreptomycin and kanamycin were capable of inactivating these drugs in the presence of ATP and acetyl CoA, respectively. These observations have been confirmed and extended by several independent groups of investigators. There is now evidence that the inactivating enzymes are quite specific with respect to the antibiotic substrate and function by at least three mechanisms.

The same R factor strain of *E. coli* described by Okamoto and Suzuki was employed by Umezawa and co-workers (1967a) in a study that showed that the sole product of inactivation of kanamycin A by a soluble enzyme was the *N*-acetyl derivative of the amino group of the 6-amino-6-deoxyglucose moiety. The specificity of the reaction was striking since kanamycin C (containing D-glucosamine) was not acetylated. In subsequent reports the same group reported experiments with another R factor conferring resistance to kanamycins A and C, paromomycin, and neomycin (Kondo *et al.*, 1968; Okanishi *et al.*, 1968). Rather than acetylation they observed an absolute requirement for ATP and Mg^{2+} and demonstrated that the products of the reaction were phosphoryl derivatives of the C-3 hydroxyl group of 6-amino-6-deoxy-D-glucose (in kanamycin) and D-glucosamine (in paromamine). The same crude enzyme preparation was capable of phosphorylating dihydrostreptomycin (Umezawa *et al.*, 1967b), but the product was not characterized save for its conversion to an active form by alkaline phosphatase. Subsequent studies (Ozanne *et al.*, 1969) have shown that phosphorylating activity for the aminoglycosides could be separated into an enzyme specific for streptomycin and a more labile fraction capable of phosphorylating the kanamycin–neomycin group. The structure of the product of inactivation by the former enzyme was shown to be consistent with phosphorylation of streptomycin at the C-3 hydroxyl of the 2-deoxy-2-methylamino-L-glucose moiety by the following reaction:

$$\text{streptomycin} + \text{ATP} \rightarrow \text{streptomycin-3}'\text{-P} + \text{ADP} \tag{4}$$

Additional evidence for two distinct phosphorylating systems came from genetic experiments in which single-step mutants were isolated which had lost their ability to phosphorylate either streptomycin or the kanamycin–neomycin group in parallel with their loss of resistance. Both phosphorylating enzymes were judged to be periplasmic in location by their liberation by osmotic shock.

From a comparative point of view it is of interest that phosphorylation of aminoglycosides has been reported in resistant strains of *S. aureus* (Doi *et al.*, 1968a) and *Pseudomonas aeruginosa* (Doi *et al.*, 1968b). Although genetic studies are lacking concerning the sites of the loci for resistance in these strains, it is of interest that two distinct enzymes have been described which resemble those mediated by R factors. Both *Pseudomonas* and *S. aureus* inactivate the kanamycin–neomycin group by the same mechanism as R^+ *E. coli*, whereas only the former species contains the streptomycin-phosphorylating enzyme. Since the kanamycin-inactivating enzyme has been purified in high yield from *Pseudomnoas* (Doi *et al.*, 1969), it will be important to compare its properties with enzymes of comparable purity from R factor strains of *E. coli*.

A second mode of R factor-promoted inactivation of aminoglycosides also involves enzymatic attack by ATP at the C-1 hydroxyl of the *N*-methyl-L-glucosamine but the reaction mechanism is quite different. The products are the adenylate derivative of streptomycin and pyrophosphate (PPi) rather than the phosphoryl product and adenosine diphosphate (ADP) (Yamada *et al.*, 1968; Harwood and Smith, 1969; Takasawa *et al.*, 1968; Benveniste *et al.*, 1970). The overall reaction is

$$\text{streptomycin} + \text{ATP} \rightarrow \text{streptomycin-3}'\text{-AMP} + \text{PPi} \tag{5}$$

The R factors mediating resistance to streptomycin via adenylylation were found to specify resistance to spectinomycin as well. Spectinomycin resistance was accompanied by enzymatic adenylylation at one of the hydroxyl groups of the actinamine moiety. Davies' group has purified the adenylylating enzyme to a considerable degree and has shown that the activities toward streptomycin and spectinomycin copurify as expected for a single enzyme (Benveniste *et al.*, 1970). The identity of the mechanism of resistance to streptomycin and spectinomycin was further substantiated by the constant ratio of adenylylating activities for both antibiotics observed for seven different R factors. Substrate specificity studies have revealed no significant adenylylation of other aminoglycosides including the kanamycin–neomycin group and gentamicin. A possibility that the adenylation mechanism can be circumvented is suggested by recent studies showing that mannosidostreptomycin (D-mannose on adjacent C-4 hydroxyl of *N*-methyl-L-glucosamine) is less readily adenylylated (Schwartz and Perlman, 1970; Smith, 1970).

At the present time it seems clear that multiple inactivation mechanisms can be invoked to explain aminoglycoside resistance mediated by R factors. Progress has been made in characterizing the reactions and purifying the enzymes responsible. It is not certain, however, which mechanisms account for resistance most often. It is no longer sufficient to characterize an R factor as conferring streptomycin resistance or kanamycin resistance. Although screening R factors for determinants of resistance to other aminoglycosides, such as spectinomycin and gentamicin, will reduce the uncertainties as to correct genotype, it will be necessary to assay for each inactivating enzyme under conditions which will discriminate between alternatives. Taking into account the information currently available, the situation regarding R factor-specific inactivating enzymes can be summarized as follows.

Transferable streptomycin resistance can be due to phosphorylation or adenylylation. The additional finding of spectinomycin resistance in a given strain argues for adenylylation since the streptomycin-phosphorylating enzyme reacts only with streptomycin and, to a lesser extent, with gentamicin A. Kanamycin resistance of the R factor type can be due to phosphorylation or acetylation. A choice between these alternatives can be made by checking for neomycin sensitivity since the acetylating enzyme will not inactivate this aminoglycoside.

F. Sulfonamide Resistance

Of all the commonly observed resistance determinants mediated by R factors, that of sulfonamide resistance is the least well understood biochemically. The failure to describe adequately episomal sulfonamide resistance is in marked contrast to the success achieved in other bacterial systems possessing chromosomal determinants. The ability of *p*-aminobenzoic acid (PABA) to reverse sulfonamide inhibition (Woods, 1940) and the subsequent demonstration that such antagonism was related to the participation of PABA in folic acid synthesis (Lascelles and Woods, 1952) have provided the framework in which resistance has been studied. A clear understanding of the complexities of sulfonamide resistance was not available until the studies with resistant *E. coli* (Brown, 1962; Pato and Brown, 1963) and pneumococci (Wolf and Hotchkiss, 1963; Ortiz and Hotchkiss, 1966; Ortiz, 1970) pointed to genetic alterations in the condensing enzymes forming dihydropteroic acid from the PABA and dihydropteridines. Altered sensitivity of the pneumococcal enzymes is reflected in a tenfold increase in K_i (decrease in affinity) for sulfonamide. Similar observations were made in *E. coli* where sulfathiazole-resistant mutants were shown to be capable of synthesizing folate activity in the presence of a number of different sulfonamides. The latter studies also pointed to the possibility of alternative mechanisms of resistance since folate synthesis in extracts of certain sulfonamide-resistant strains was inhibited to the same degree as in wild-type sensitive bacteria. Pato and Brown suggested that permeability considerations might be involved in such mutants—a conclusion reached by Japanese investigators working with strains of *E. coli* bearing R factor determinants for sulfonamides (Kato *et al.*, 1962). It should be pointed out that these observations were limited to a single R factor isolate and have not been confirmed or extended and that other mechanisms of episomal resistance, such as drug inactivation or altered folate-synthesizing enzymes, have not been excluded rigorously. It should be stressed that the sulfonamide locus is the only determinant thus far associated with R factors which confers resistance to an inhibitory substance not likely to be present in nature. If altered permeability should subsequently be demonstrated to be the underlying biochemical event, it would be pertinent to inquire as to the specificity of the exclusion mechanism. The possibility should be entertained that impermeability to sulfonamides represents one facet of a more general permeation defect having an as yet undefined importance in microbial ecology. The further demonstration that certain chromosomal mutants and R factor strains have a common defect in sulfonamide accumulation would be a major step in unifying current views of the origin of episomal determinants.

G. Resistance to Macrolide Antibiotics in *Staphylococcus aureus*

The intrinsic resistance or tolerance of most gram-negative bacteria to erythromycin and related antibiotics of the macrolide group is apparently the result of drug impermeability. Since biologically active erythromycin can be recovered from cultures of *E. coli* and *Proteus vulgaris* (Haight and Finland, 1952) and because the cell-free protein-synthesizing system of *E. coli* is as susceptible to erythromycin inhibition as *S. aureus* (Mao and Putterman, 1968), it is apparent that whole cells of the gram-negative bacteria are incapable of accumulating the antibiotic. Direct evidence favoring this view has come from experiments showing the sensitivity of stable L-forms of *Proteus mirabilis* to the macrolide group (Taubeneck, 1962) and from direct measurements of erythromycin uptake in *E. coli* as compared with gram-positive species (Mao and Putterman, 1968). Although the latter studies indicate that active transport of the macrolides is unlikely in *S. aureus*, it is fair to state that an explanation for impaired accumulation in gram-negative bacteria is not at hand.

Since there is no evidence for R factor-mediated resistance over and above the naturally occurring tolerance of enteric bacteria to the macrolide group, the present discussion will be concerned with acquired erythromycin and macrolide resistance in staphylococci. The genetic locus for such resistance is extrachromosomal and is usually linked with penicillinase production in view of the high frequency of their cotransduction and the simultaneous loss of both determinants following growth at elevated temperatures (Novick, 1967; Mitsuhashi, 1966). The occasional appearance of erythromycin-resistant and penicillin-sensitive isolates can best be understood by noting the variety of deletion mutants which can be obtained from a single, complex penicillinase plasmid (Novick, 1967). There is no evidence suggesting that macrolide resistance is linked to other plasmids such as those mediating tetracycline or chloramphenicol resistance.

In contrast to the progress which has been made in understanding the genetics of erythromycin resistance in staphylococci, there is considerable confusion as to the number and types of biochemical mechanisms operating and the extent to which they can be identified as corresponding to well-characterized plasmid genotypes. Prior to the development of the concept of plasmid-linked macrolide loci, Garrod (1957) described cultures with so-called "dissociated" resistance to erythromycin that were characterized by their ability to grow in the presence of other macrolides following exposure to subinhibitory concentrations of erythromycin only. Weaver and Pattee (1964) confirmed this observation and suggested that the synthesis of a specific protein or enzyme was involved. Subsequent studies from another laboratory (Kono *et al.*, 1966) revealed that at least three distinct phenotypes of macrolide resistance may exist—the inducible type of cross-resistance described by Garrod (Group C) plus inducible resistance to erythromycin and oleandomycin only (Group B) and constitutive coresistance to erythromycin and all other macrolides (Group A). The complexities of the situation were compounded by the observation that mutants of Group C could be isolated which possessed the Group A phenotype. Subsequent studies confirmed the likelihood of a closely linked regulatory locus for macrolide resistance which, when rendered nonfunctional by mutation, can give rise to constitutive cross-resistance (Hashimoto *et al.*, 1968). A broadening of the range of resistance was noted in certain mutants which were also observed to be resistant to lincomycin—an agent distinct from the macrolide group from a chemical point of view but which has a similar spectrum of activity and resistance characteristics (Barber and Waterworth, 1964).

The first indications of the mechanism of resistance to erythromycin in *S. aureus* were the experiments by Nakajima *et al.* (1968) which demonstrated reduced accumulation of erythromycin by cells of constitutive and induced resistant strains. More recent studies along similar lines have confirmed the apparent permeability defect but have focused on diminished ribosomal binding of macrolides as the mechanism of resistance (Saito *et al.*, 1970). The search for altered ribosomal affinities was prompted by their inhibitory effects on protein synthesis and the fact that the macrolides and lincomycin appear to compete for a common site on the 50 S ribosomal subunit (Vazquez, 1966; Weisblum and Davies, 1968). The studies of Saito and co-workers demonstrated that all resistant strains examined (constitutive and induced) shared the common property of diminished ribosomal binding of erythromycin-^{14}C as compared with sensitive controls or uninduced resistant strains. They also isolated a temperature-sensitive mutant of the inducible type which was phenotypically resistant at 42°C in the absence of inducer. Ribosomes prepared from cells grown at 42°C were deficient in erythromycin binding, suggesting that such inducible resistance is due to substrate- or temperature-induced inactivation of a hypothetical repressor of a regulatory gene. As pointed out by this group of investigators, the data pose a novel question. How can one account for changes in ribosomal affinity within minutes after the addition of inducer and before changes in the composition of structural ribosomal proteins can be expected to occur? An answer to this dilemma would be the demonstration of an inducible soluble protein or enzyme product which directly interacts with ribosomes to interfere with macrolide binding. However neat such an answer might seem, the larger question of the specificity of inducer structure remains unanswered since one must envision a family of receptors among inducible strains responding to one, a few, or all of the macrolide antibiotics.

H. Other Extrachromosomal Resistance Determinants

In addition to those already discussed there are several other resistance genes which have been reported to occur on R factors or staphylococcal plasmids and which have not been adequately studied. The most striking of these are the determinants for resistance to heavy metal ions such as lead, cadmium, mercury, zinc, and arsenate (Smith, 1967b; Novick, 1967; Dyke *et al.*, 1966).

The demonstration by Novick and Roth (1968) that arsenate resistance in *S. aureus* is inducible is consistent with the inducibility of all resistance determinants thus far described for staphylococcal plasmids. Recent studies have confirmed this observation and defined certain features of the biochemical mechanism (Hammond and Shaw, unpublished experiments). Arsenate appears to compete with phosphate for at least two pH and energy-dependent transport systems in *S. aureus*. The induction of resistance to arsenate is (*a*) prevented by inhibitors of protein synthesis, such as chloramphenicol and puromycin, and (*b*) accompanied by selective decrease in uptake of arsenate at pH 8. Although no studies have been reported for R factor systems, it should be noted that chromosomal mutants of *E. coli* have been isolated which show similar arsenate transport defects (Bennett and Malamy, 1970).

Numerous studies have attempted to define conditions favoring the selective loss of bacterial episomes and plasmids. Mention has already been made of the use of the acridine dyes and ethidium bromide. In the course of screening cultures for the loss of antibiotic resistance, at least two instances have been reported of presumed plasmid-mediated resistance to such agents. Ericson (1969) has described a strain of *S. aureus* in which penicillinase production, cadmium resistance, and resistance to acriflavin were simultaneously lost following growth at 42°C. It will be of interest to compare the mechanism in *S. aureus* with that reported by Silver (1965) for *E. coli* with phage-mediated acriflavin resistance.

Johnston and Dyke (1969) have studied a strain of *S. aureus* resistant to ethidium bromide as well as penicillin, tetracycline, chloramphenicol, and oleandomycin. Elimination and cotransduction experiments suggest that ethidium bromide resistance is linked to penicillinase production and is independent of the other antibiotic resistance determinants. Studies of the inducibility and mechanism of resistance to both acriflavin and ethidium bromide will be awaited with great interest.

Fusidic acid is a steroid antibiotic that inhibits protein synthesis at the translocation step (Tanaka *et al.*, 1968). In the course of clinical studies with this drug, Evans and Waterworth (1966) noted two resistant cultures of *S. aureus* in which fusidic acid resistance was unstable. Resistance was lost simultaneously with reversion to penicillin sensitivity in one case and was associated with the loss of resistance to tetracycline and kanamycin in the other. Although a plasmid location for fusidic acid resistance was not proven rigorously and no suggestion was made as to possible mechanisms, this interesting observation deserves further study. The recent isolation of a fusidic acid-resistant mutant of *E. coli* which possesses a resistant, soluble G factor for translocation offers a possible approach to the resistance mechanism in *S. aureus* (Leder *et al.*, 1969).

IV. Comments and Predictions

Most of the studies described in this review were carried out during the latter half of a decade that spans our knowledge of extrachromosomal drug resistance. The measure of success which has been achieved in describing the biochemical mechanisms is a tribute to improved techniques in the chemistry and characterization of antibiotics and advances in enzymology and molecular genetics. There is little doubt, however, that several areas are ripe for further detailed study and that even a general notion of the mechanisms of resistance are lacking for certain antibiotics. The author would like to make a plea that the design, execution, and reporting of future studies take into account not only the biochemical features of each system but the site of the genetic loci that determine the phenotype under study. A full understanding of topics such as β-lactamase production in enteric bacteria or macrolide resistance in staphylococci will not be forthcoming unless the biochemical studies are carried out on well-characterized strains. As one reviews the literature on this fast growing area of interest, it is apparent that results tend to appear in fragmentary form and lead to conclusions which lack conviction. The reviewer relishes those studies which seem to have had a clear point of origin and a satisfying conclusion.

During the next decade the study of antibiotic resistance should continue to draw heavily on collateral advances in molecular biology and its many subdisciplines. It seems likely that we shall see considerable progress in defining the chromosomal alleles (or at least the genes for homologous functions) of several episomal resistance determinants. One should not be surprised if, as some of the preliminary data suggest, the chromosomal counterparts of R factor-mediated β-lactamase or chloramphenicol acetyltransferase are found more frequently in *Klebsiella* and *Proteus* sp. rather than in *E. coli*. Another area which will be under intensive study is the comparative biochemistry of extrachromosomal elements. The various immunological types of β-lactamases and other inactivating enzymes with properties which may be episome-specific offer unique tools for correlating resistance genes with the structure and function of their protein products.

One could also single out the area of control of R factor expression as one of the more fruitful topics for study. Why are most of the R factor-mediated resistance systems of the constitutive type whereas plasmid-linked determinants of staphylococci are almost invariably inducible? What of the phenotypic variabilities in the level of resistance seen for certain episomal genes when they are examined in different hosts? How does the synthesis of multiple constitutive enzymes affect the energy economy of the host cell both in the absence as well as the presence of antibiotics? The phenomenon of catabolite repression has now appeared on the R factor scene (Harwood and Smith, 1971), and the apparent involvement of the ubiquitous effector, cyclic AMP (adenosine 3′, 5′-cyclic monophosphate), suggests that the latter will turn out to be as important in the induction of staphylococcal resistance as it appears to be in so many other biological systems.

Addendum

This account of the biochemical aspects of drug resistance was based upon information available prior to August 1, 1970. The author would like to alert the reader to the rapidity with which information continues to accumulate in the field covered by this review. A useful compendium of current developments and more recent references may be found in the proceedings of a conference on the "The Problems of Drug-Resistant Pathogenic Bacteria," held under the auspices of the New York Academy of Sciences in New York City, October 12–14, 1970, and published (1971) in the *Annals of the New York Academy of Sciences,* Vol. 182.

References

Anderson, E. S. (1968). *Annu. Rev. Microbiol.* **22,** 131.

Anderson, E. S., and Datta, N. (1965). *Lancet* **1,** 407.

Arber, W. (1960). *Virology* **11,** 273.

Asheshov, E. H. (1966). *J. Gen. Microbiol.* **42,** 403.

Asheshov, E. H. (1969). *J. Gen. Microbiol.* **59,** 289.

Asheshov, E. H., and Dyke, K. G. H. (1968). *Biochem. Biophys. Res. Commun.* **30,** 213.

Ayliffe, G. A. (1963). *J. Gen. Microbiol.* **30,** 339.

Baldwin, J. N., Strickland, R. H., and Cox, M. F. (1969). *Appl. Microbiol.* **18,** 628.

Barber, M. (1957). *In* "Drug Resistance in Microorganisms" (G. E. W. Wolstenholme and C. M. O'Connor, eds.), p. 262. Little, Brown, Boston, Massachusetts.

Barber, M. (1962). *In* "Resistance of Bacteria to the Penicillins" (A. V. S. de Reuck and M. P. Cameron, eds.), p. 89. Little, Brown, Boston, Massachusetts.

Barber, M. (1964). *J. Gen. Microbiol.* **35,** 183.

Barber, M., and Waterworth, P. M. (1964). *Brit. Med. J.* **ii,** 603.

Barrett, F. F., McGehee, R. F., and Finland, M. (1968). *New Engl. J. Med.* **279,** 441.

Bauer, W., and Vinograd, J. (1968). *J. Mol. Biol.* **33,** 141.

Bennett, R. L., and Malamy, M. H. (1970). *Bacteriol. Proc.* p. 131.

Benveniste, R., Yamada, T., and Davies, J. (1970). *Infec. Immunity* **1,** 109.

Boman, H. G., Eriksson-Grennberg, K. G., Földes, J., and Lindström, E. B. (1967). *In* "Regulation of Nucleic Acid and Protein Synthesis" (V. V. Koningsberger and L. Bosch, eds.), p. 366. Elsevier, Amsterdam.

Boothe, J. H. (1963). *Antimicrob. Ag. Chemother. 1962*, p. 213.

Bouanchaud, D. H., Scarrizzi, M. R., and Chabbert, Y. A. (1969). *J. Gen. Microbiol.* **54,** 417.

Brock, T. D. (1961). *Bacteriol. Rev.* **25,** 32.

Brown, G. M. (1962). *J. Biol. Chem.* **237,** 536.

Bulger, R. J., and Bulger, R. E. (1967). *J. Bacteriol.* **94,** 1244.

Cannon, M. C., and Dunican, L. K. (1970). *Biochem. Biophys. Res. Commun.* **39,** 423.

Chabbert, Y. A., Baudens, J. G., and Gerbaud, G. R. (1964). *Ann. Inst. Pasteur* **107,** Suppl. 678.

Chain, E. B. (1962). *In* "Resistance of Bacteria to the Penicillins" (A. V. S. de Rueck and M. P. Cameron, eds.), p. 3. Little, Brown, Boston, Massachusetts.

Cohen, S., and Miller, C. A. (1969). *Nature (London)* **224,** 1273.

Cohen, S., Vernon, E. G., and Sweeney, H. M. (1970). *J. Bacteriol.* **103,** 616.

Cole, M. (1969). *Biochem. J.* **115,** 733.

Corse, J., and Williams, R. E. O. (1968). *J. Clin. Pathol.* **21,** 722.

Datta, N., and Kontomichalou, P. (1965). *Nature (London)* **208,** 239.

Datta, N., and Richmond, M. H. (1966). *Biochem. J.* **98,** 204.

Davis, B. D., and Maas, W. K. (1952). *Proc. Nat. Acad. Sci. U.S.* **38,** 775.

De Zeeuw, J. R. (1968). *J. Bacteriol.* **95,** 498.

Doi, O., Miyamoto, M., Tanaka, N., and Umezawa, H. (1968a). *Appl. Microbiol.* **16,** 1282.

Doi, O., Ogura, M., Tanaka, N., and Umezawa, H. (1968b). *Appl. Microbiol.* **16,** 1276.

Doi, O., Kondo, S., Tanaka, N., and Umezawa, H. (1969). *J. Antibiot.* **22,** 273.

Dornbusch, K., Hallander, H. O., and Löfquist, F. (1969). *J. Bacteriol.* **98,** 351.

Dunsmoor, C. L., Pim, K. L., and Sherris, J. C. (1964). *Antimicrob. Ag. Chemother. 1963*, p. 500.

Dyke, K. G. H. (1969). *J. Med. Microbiol.* **2,** 261.

Dyke, K. G. H., Jevons, M. P., and Parker, M. T. (1966). *Lancet* **i,** 835.

Easterling, S. B., Johnson, E. M., Wohlhieter, J. A., and Baron, L. S. (1969). *J. Bacteriol.* **100,** 35.

Egawa, R., Sawai, T., and Mitsuhashi, S. (1967). *Jap. J. Microbiol.* **11,** 173.

Ericson, C. (1969). *Acta Pathol. Microbiol. Scand.* **76,** 333.

Evans, J., Galindo, E., Olarte, J., and Falkow, S. (1968). *J. Bacteriol.* **96,** 1441.

Evans, R. J., and Waterworth, P. M. (1966). *J. Clin. Pathol.* **19,** 555.

Falkow, S., Citarella, R. V., Wohlhieter, J. A., and Watanabe, T. (1966). *J. Mol. Biol.* **17,** 102.

Falkow, S., Haapala, D. K., and Silver, R. P. (1969). *In* "Bacterial Episomes and Plasmids" (G. E. W. Wolstenholme and M. O'Connor, eds.), p. 136. Churchill, London.

Franklin, T. J. (1967). *Biochem. J.* **105,** 371.

Franklin, T. J., and Godfrey, A. (1965). *Biochem. J.* **94,** 54.

Franklin, T. J., and Higginson, B. (1970). *Biochem. J.* **116,** 287.

Fredericq, P. (1969). *In* "Bacterial Episomes and Plasmids" (G. E. W. Wolstenholme and M. O'Connor, eds.), p. 163. Churchill, London.

Fullbrook, P. D., Elson, S. W., and Slocombe, B. (1970). *Nature (London)* **226,** 1054.

Garrod, L. P. (1957). *Brit. Med. J.* **ii,** 57.

Goto, S., Niwa, C., and Kuwahara, S. (1965). *Jap. J. Microbiol.* **9,** 15.
Haight, T. H., and Finland, M. (1952). *Proc. Soc. Exp. Biol. Med.* **81,** 175.
Harwood, J. H., and Smith, D. H. (1969). *J. Bacteriol.* **97,** 1262.
Harwood, J. H., and Smith, D. H. (1971). *Biochem. Biophys. Res. Commun.* **42,** 57.
Hashimoto, H., and Hirota, Y. (1966). *J. Bacteriol.* **92,** 1351.
Hashimoto, H., Oshima, H., and Mitsuhashi, S. (1968). *Jap. J. Microbiol.* **12,** 321.
Hayes, W. (1969). *In* "Bacterial Episomes and Plasmids" (G. E. W. Wolstenholme and M. O'Connor, eds.), p. 4. Churchill, Londo
Hickson, F. T., Roth, T. F., and Helinski, D. R. (1967). *Proc. Nat. Acad. Sci. U.S.* **58,** 1731.
Hirota, Y. (1960). *Proc. Nat. Acad. Sci. U.S.* **46,** 57.
Holt, R. (1967). *Lancet* **i,** 1259.
Ikeda, H., and Tomizawa, J. (1968). *Cold Spring Harbor Symp. Quant. Biol.* **33,** 791.
Inoue, M., Hashimoto, H., and Mitsuhashi, S. (1970). *J. Antibiot.* **23,** 68.
Iyer, R. V., and Iyer, V. N. (1969). *J. Bacteriol.* **100,** 605.
Izaki, K., and Arima, K. (1963). *Nature (London)* **200,** 384.
Izaki, K., and Arima, K. (1965). *J. Bacteriol.* **89,** 1335.
Jack, G. W., and Richmond, M. H. (1970). *J. Gen. Microbiol.* **61,** 43.
Jacob, F., and Adelberg, E. A. (1959). *C. R. Acad. Sci.* **249,** 189.
Jacob, F., and Monod, J. (1961). *J. Mol. Biol.* **3,** 318.
Jacob, F., and Wollman, E. L. (1958). *C. R. Acad. Sci.* **247,** 154.
Jacobsen, H. W., and Shaw, W. V. (1970). *Bacteriol. Proc.* p. 60.
Jarolmen, H., Hewel, D., and Kain, E. (1970). *Infect. Immunity* **1,** 321.
Johnston, L. H., and Dyke, K. G. H. (1969). *J. Bacteriol.* **100,** 1413.
Kasuga, T., Hashimoto, H., Oshima, H., Kawaharada, U., and Mitsuhashi, S. (1965). *Nippon Saikingaku Zasshi* **20,** 374.
Kasuga, T., Hashimoto, H., and Mitsuhashi, S. (1968). *J. Bacteriol.* **95,** 1764.
Kato, T., Akiba, T., Yokota, T., Kimura, S., Mizuno, T., Niijima, K., Koyama, T., Kuwahara, S., and Arai, T. (1962). *Igaku To Seibutsugaku* **64,** 9.
Kondo, S., Okanishi, M., Utahara, R., Maeda, K., and Umezawa, H. (1968). *J. Antibiot.* **21,** 22.
Kono, M., Hashimoto, H., and Mitsuhashi, S. (1966). *Jap. J. Microbiol.* **10,** 59.
Kono, M., Ogawa, K., and Mitsuhashi, S. (1968). *J. Bacteriol.* **95,** 886.
Kono, M., O'hara, K., Houda, M., and Mitsuhashi, S. (1969). *J. Antibiot.* **22,** 603.
Kontomichalou, P., Mitani, M., and Clowes, R. C. (1970). *J. Bacteriol.* **104,** 34.
Lascelles, J., and Woods, D. D. (1952). *Brit. J. Exp. Pathol.* **33,** 288.
Leder, P., Bernardi, A., Livingston, D., Loyd, B., Roufa, D., and Skogerson, L. (1969). *Cold Spring Harbor Symp. Quant. Biol.* **34,** 411.
Lederberg, J. (1952). *Physiol. Rev.* **32,** 403.
Lindqvist, R. C., and Nordström, K. (1970). *J. Bacteriol.* **101,** 232.
Mao, J. C.-H., and Putterman, M. (1968). *J. Bacteriol.* **95,** 1111.
Martin, R. G. (1969). *Annu. Rev. Genet.* **3,** 181.
May, J. W., Houghton, R. H., and Perret, C. J. (1964). *J. Gen. Microbiol.* **37,** 157.
Merkel, J. R., and Steers, E. (1953). *J. Bacteriol.* **66,** 389.
Meynell, E., and Datta, N. (1969). *In* "Bacterial Episomes and Plasmids" (G. E. W. Wolstenholme and M. O'Connor, eds.), p. 120. Churchill, London.
Meynell, E., Meynell, G. G., and Datta, N. (1967). *Bacteriol. Rev.* **32,** 55.
Mise, K., and Suzuki, Y. (1968). *J. Bacteriol.* **95,** 2124.
Mitsuhashi, S. (1966). *Jap. J. Microbiol.* **2,** 49.

Mitsuhashi, S., Kono, M., Sagawa, M., and Mori, H. (1969). *Jap. J. Microbiol.* **13,** 177.

Miyamura, S. (1964). *J. Pharm. Sci.* **53,** 604.

Moyed, H. S. (1964). *Annu. Rev. Microbiol.* **18,** 347.

Nakajima, Y., Inoue, M., Oka, Y., and Yamagishi, S. (1968). *Jap. J. Microbiol.* **12,** 248.

Nakazawa, S., Ono, H., Nishino, T., Kuwahara, S., and Goto, S. (1970). *In* "Progress in Antimicrobial and Anticancer Chemotherapy," Vol. 1, p. 353. Univ. of Tokyo Press, Tokyo.

Neu, H. C., and Winshell, E. B. (1970). *Arch. Biochem. Biophys.* **139,** 278.

Nisioka, T., Mitani, M., and Clowes, R. (1969). *J. Bacteriol.* **97,** 376.

Nisioka, T., Mitani, M., and Clowes, R. C. (1970). *J. Bacteriol.* **103,** 166.

Nordström, K., Eriksson-Grennberg, K. G., and Boman, H. G. (1968). *Genet. Res.* **12,** 157.

Nordström, K., Burman, L. G., and Eriksson-Grennberg, K. G. (1970). *J. Bacteriol.* **101,** 659.

Novick, R. P. (1963). *J. Gen. Microbiol.* **33,** 121.

Novick, R. P. (1967). *Fed. Proc. Fed. Amer. Soc. Exp. Biol.* **26,** 29.

Novick, R. P. (1969). *Bacteriol. Rev.* **33,** 210.

Novick, R. P., and Roth, C. (1968). *J. Bacteriol.* **95,** 1335.

Okamoto, S., and Mizuno, D. (1964). *J. Gen. Microbiol.* **35,** 125.

Okamoto, S., and Suzuki, Y. (1965). *Nature (London)* **208,** 1301.

Okamoto, S., Suzuki, Y., Mise, K., and Nagaya, R. (1967). *J. Bacteriol.* **94,** 1616.

Okanishi, M., Kondo, S., Utahara, R., and Umezawa, H. (1968). *J. Antibiot.* **21,** 13.

Ortiz, P. J. (1970). *Biochemistry* **9,** 355.

Ortiz, P. J., and Hotchkiss, R. D. (1966). *Biochemistry* **5,** 67.

Ozaki, M., Mizushima, S., and Nomura, M. (1969). *Nature (London)* **222,** 333.

Ozanne, B., Benveniste, R., Tipper, D., and Davies, J. (1969). *J. Bacteriol.* **100,** 1144.

Parker, M. T., and Hewitt, J. H. (1970). *Lancet* **i,** 800.

Pato, M. L., and Brown, G. M. (1963). *Arch. Biochem. Biophys.* **103,** 443.

Piffaretti, J. C., and Pitton, J. S. (1970). *Chemotherapia* **15,** 84.

Pollack, M. R. (1962). *In* "Resistance of Bacteria to the Penicillins" (A. V. S. de Rueck and M. P. Cameron, eds.), p. 56. Little, Brown, Boston, Massachusetts.

Poston, S. M. (1966). *Nature (London)* **210,** 802.

Reeve, E. C. R. (1966). *Genet. Res.* **7,** 281.

Reeve, E. C. R. (1968). *Genet. Res.* **11,** 303.

Reeve, E. C. R., and Suttie, D. R. (1968). *Genet. Res.* **11,** 97.

Richmond, M. H. (1965a). *J. Bacteriol.* **90,** 370.

Richmond, M. H. (1965b). *Brit. Med. Bull.* **21,** 260.

Richmond, M. H. (1965c). *Biochem. J.* **94,** 584.

Richmond, M. H. (1967a). *Nature (London)* **216,** 1191.

Richmond, M. H. (1967b). *J. Mol. Biol.* **26,** 357.

Richmond, M. H. (1968). *In* "Advances in Microbial Physiology" (A. H. Rose and J. F. Wilkinson, eds.), Vol. 2, p. 43. Academic Press, New York.

Rownd, R. (1969a). *In* "Symposium on Infectious Multiple Drug Resistance" (S. Falkow, ed.), p. 17. U.S. Govt. Printing Office, Washington, D. C.

Rownd, R. (1969b). *J. Mol. Biol.* **44,** 387.

Rownd, R., Nakaya, R., and Nakamura, A. (1966). *J. Mol. Biol.* **17,** 376.

Rownd, R., Watanabe, H., Mickel, S., Nakaya, R., and Gargan, B. (1970). *In* "Progress in Antimicrobial and Anticancer Chemotherapy," Vol. 2, p. 535. Univ. of Tokyo Press, Tokyo.

Rush, M. G., Gordon, C. N., Novick, R. P., and Warner, R. C. (1969). *Proc. Nat. Nat. Acad. Sci. U.S.* **63,** 1304.

Sabath, L. D., Gerstein, D. A., Lode, P. B., and Finland, M. F. (1968). *Antimicrob. Ag. Chemother.* p. 264.

Sabath, L. D., Leaf, C. D., Gerstein, D. A., and Finland, M. (1970). *Nature* (*London*) **225,** 1074.

Saito, T., Oshima, H., Shimizu, M., Hashimoto, H., and Mitsuhashi, S. (1970). *In* "Progress in Antimicrobial and Anticancer Chemotherapy," Vol. 2, p. 572. Univ. of Tokyo Press, Tokyo.

Sasaki, K., Suzue, G., Ishimara, K., Odani, S., and Tanaka, S. (1970). *J. Gen. Appl. Microbiol.* **16,** 145.

Schildkraut, C. L., Marmur, J., and Doty, P. (1962). *J. Mol. Biol.* **4,** 430.

Schwartz, J. L., and Perlman, D. (1970). *J. Antibiot.* **23,** 254.

Seligman, S. J. (1966). *Nature* (*London*) **209,** 994.

Shaw, W. V. (1967a). *J. Biol. Chem.* **242,** 687.

Shaw, W. V. (1967b). *Antimicrob. Ag. Chemother.* p. 221.

Shaw, W. V. (1970). *In* "Progress in Antimicrobial and Anticancer Chemotherapy," Vol. 2, p. 552. Univ. of Tokyo Press, Tokyo.

Shaw, W. V., and Brodksy, R. F. (1968a). *Antimicrob. Ag. Chemother. 1967,* p. 257.

Shaw, W. V., and Brodsky, R. F. (1968b). *J. Bacteriol.* **95,** 28.

Shaw, W. V., and Brodsky, R. F. (1968c). *Bacteriol. Proc.* p. 32.

Shaw, W. V., and Unowsky, J. (1968). *J. Bacteriol.* **95,** 1976.

Shaw, W. V., and Winshell, E. (1969). *Antimicrob. Ag. Chemother. 1968,* p. 7.

Shaw, W. V., Bentley, D. W., and Sands, L. (1970). *J. Bacteriol.* **104,** 1095.

Silver, S. (1965). *Proc. Nat. Acad. Sci. U.S.* **53,** 24.

Smith, C., Anderson, E. S., and Clowes, R. (1970). *Bacteriol. Proc.* p. 60.

Smith, D. H. (1967a). *Lancet* **1,** 252.

Smith, D. H. (1967b). *Science* **156,** 1114.

Smith, J. T. (1969). *J. Gen. Microbiol.* **55,** 109.

Sompolinsky, D., and Samra, Z. (1968). *J. Gen. Microbiol.* **50,** 55.

Sompolinsky, D., Ziegler-Schlomowitz, R., and Herezog, D. (1968). *Can. J. Microbiol.* **14,** 891.

Sutherland, R., and Rolinson, G. N. (1964). *J. Bacteriol.* **87,** 887.

Suzuki, Y., and Okamoto, S. (1967). *J. Biol. Chem.* **242,** 4722.

Suzuki, Y., Okamoto, S., and Kono, M. (1966). *J. Bacteriol.* **92,** 798.

Sweeney, H. M., and Cohen, S. (1968). *J. Bacteriol.* **96,** 920.

Sykes, R. B., and Richmond, M. H. (1970). *Nature* (*London*) **226,** 952.

Takasawa, S., Utahara, R., Okanishi, M., Maeda, K., and Umezawa, H. (1968). *J. Antibiot.* **21,** 477.

Tanaka, N., Kinoshita, T., and Masukawa, H. (1968). *Biochem. Biophys. Res. Commun.* **30,** 278.

Taubeneck, U (1962). *Nature* (*London*) **196,** 195.

Tomoeda, M., Inuzuka, M., Kubo, N., and Nakamura, S. (1968). *J. Bacteriol.* **95,** 1078.

Umezawa, H., Okanishi, M., Utahara, R., Maeda, K., and Kondo, S. (1967a). *J. Antibiotic., Ser. A* **20,** 136.

Umezawa, H., Okanishi, M., Kondo, S , Hamana, K., Utahara, R., Maeda, K., and Mitsuhashi, S. (1967b). *Nature (London)* **157,** 1559.

Unowsky, J., and Rachmeler, M. (1966). *J. Bacteriol.* **92,** 358.

Vazquez, D. (1966). *In* "Biochemical Studies of Antimicrobial Drugs" (B. A. Newton and P. E. Reynolds, eds.), p. 169. Cambridge Univ. Press, London and New York.

Vinograd, J., Lebowitz, J., Radloff, R., Watson, R., and Laipis, P. (1965). *Proc. Nat. Acad. Sci. U.S.* **57,** 1514.

Watanabe, T. (1963). *Bacteriol. Rev.* **27,** 87.

Weaver, J. R., and Pattee, P. A., (1964). *J. Bacteriol.* **88,** 574.

Weisblum, B., and Davies, J. (1968). *Bacteriol. Rev.* **32,** 493.

Winshell, E., and Shaw, W. V. (1969). *J. Bacteriol.* **98,** 1248.

Wolf, B., and Hotchkiss, R. D. (1963). *Biochemistry* **2,** 145.

Woods, D. D. (1940). *Brit. J. Exp. Pathol.* **21,** 74.

Yamada, T., Tipper, D., and Davies, J. (1968). *Nature (London)* **219,** 288.

Yamagishi, S., O'hara, K., Sawai, T., and Mitsuhashi, S. (1969). *J. Biochem. (Tokyo)* **66,** 16.

Yamagishi, S., Sawai, T., O'hara, K., Takahashi, K., and Mitsuhashi, S. (1970). "Progress in Antimicrobial and Anticancer Chemotherapy," Vol. 2, p. 579. Univ. of Tokyo Press, Tokyo.

The Pharmacology of Propanediol Carbamates

B. J. LUDWIG AND J. R. POTTERFIELD

Wallace Laboratories, Division of Carter-Wallace, Inc., Cranbury, New Jersey

I. Introduction

The introduction of meprobamate as a tranquilizing agent in 1955 inaugurated a new era of clinical medicine. This era was characterized by a growing realization in the medical community of the value of tranquilizers and psychopharmacology and the contributions that these make to the understanding and treatment of emotional illness. Acceptance of the concept that meprobamate specifically counteracted anxiety without decreasing awareness and without impairing physical and intellectual performance led to a better understanding of the nature of anxiety and made it possible to treat this condition more effectively.

The intensive interest generated in the pharmacology of meprobamate represented a departure from previous emphasis on more complex and more sophisticated chemical substances as potential therapeutic agents.

Investigations stimulated by this interest led to the accumulation of a vast volume of knowledge concerning the pharmacology of carbamate compounds. It is the purpose of this review to discuss and compare the pharmacological properties of meprobamate, the related carbamates (mebutamate, carisoprodol, and tybamate), and a large number of chemically similar compounds synthesized and evaluated in the development of these useful therapeutic agents.

The introduction of meprobamate as a tranquilizing agent came about as a result of knowledge gained with the muscle relaxant drug, mephenesin. Mephenesin was originally introduced as a centrally acting muscle relaxant by Berger and Bradley (1946), and in their original publication these investigators called attention to its tranquilizing activity. Publications describing the usefulness of mephenesin in psychiatric disorders appeared within a few years after the original description of the drug. The failure of this promising drug to find a prominent place in clinical medicine was due to its low potency and short duration of activity.

The finding by Riley and Berger (1949) that the short duration of action of mephenesin was due to the rapid oxidation of its primary hydroxyl group prompted the investigation of chemical variations having a terminal hydroxyl group less susceptible to enzymatic attack. Various ester derivatives were synthesized, and these were found to have substantially greater duration of action than mephenesin but were weaker in their paralyzing activity. At about this same time, it was shown that certain simple, 2-substituted 1,3-propanediols had properties similar and, in some cases, superior to those of mephenesin (Berger, 1949). The activity of these diol compounds was interesting in several respects, but they had little practical interest because of their similar short duration of action. Esterification of the free hydroxyl groups of mephenesin was carried out in an effort to prolong its action. These mephenesin esters showed little advantage over the parent compound (Berger and Ludwig, 1950). The carbamate esters of mephenesin exhibited a stronger paralyzing action than mephenesin, but they did not produce paralysis of significantly longer duration (Berger, 1952a). The dicarbamates derived from the 2-substituted 1,3-propanediols, however, were outstanding in having potent anticonvulsant and muscle relaxant properties. In addition, they exhibited a markedly prolonged duration of action. Among these compounds was 2-methyl-2-propyl-1,3-propanediol dicarbamate which was unique in that it possessed a muscle relaxant and sedative action of an unusual type (Berger, 1952b). This compound became commercially available as meprobamate and soon achieved a prominent position as a tranquilizing and antianxiety agent.

In the course of clinical investigations with meprobamate, several clinicians reported that this drug exerted a mild hypotensive action in some patients suffering from essential hypertension. These findings prompted the investigation of the mechanism of the hypotensive action of meprobamate. The evaluation of a large number of compounds of this series led to the selection of 2-methyl-2-*sec*-butyl-1,3-propanediol dicarbamate as a centrally acting, pressure lowering agent which produced its hypotensive effect by direct action on the brainstem vasomotor centers.

Meprobamate produces both tranquilization and muscle relaxation in suitable patients. Since separation of these two actions not only could yield a new and more useful drug but might also shed some light on the interrelation between anxiety and muscular tension, numerous compounds chemically related to meprobamate were synthesized and subjected to pharmacological evaluation. A series of compounds derived from 2-substituted 1,3-propanediol dicarbamates having an alkyl substituent in place of a hydrogen atom on one of the carbamyl nitrogen atoms appeared of unusual interest. This relatively simple substitution yielded compounds surprisingly unlike meprobamate in their pharmacological activity. One

TABLE I

PROPANEDIOL DICARBAMATE DRUG COMPOUNDS

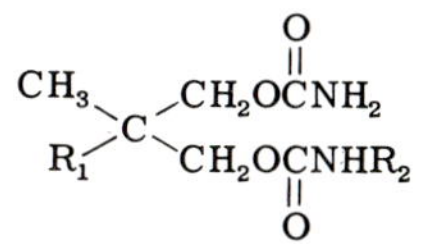

$$\begin{array}{l} CH_3 \\ R_1 \end{array} \!\!>\! C \!<\! \begin{array}{l} CH_2OC(=O)NH_2 \\ CH_2OC(=O)NHR_2 \end{array}$$

Drug	R_1	R_2
Meprobamate	$CH_3CH_2CH_2—$	H
Mebutamate	$CH_3CH_2CH(CH_3)—$	H
Carisoprodol	$CH_3CH_2CH_2—$	$—CH(CH_3)_2$
Tybamate	$CH_3CH_2CH_2—$	$—CH_2CH_2CH_2CH_3$

of these derivatives, *N*-isopropyl-2-methyl-2-propyl-1,3-propanediol dicarbamate, carisoprodol, not only had an entirely different profile of effects on the central nervous system but unexpectedly exhibited analgesic properties of an unusual type. Another derivative of this type, *N*-*n*-butyl-2-methyl-2-propyl-1,3-propanediol dicarbamate, tybamate, was found to exhibit neuropharmacological, relaxant, and taming properties generally similar to those of meprobamate but which differed from that drug in several significant respects. This compound has found usefulness as a tranquilizing agent.

In these four chemically related compounds (Table I), muscle relaxant and anticonvulsant properties are disassociated and independent of each other. From a chemical standpoint, the sharp differences in properties observed in comparisons among these compounds stress the uncertainty encountered in attempting to establish structure–activity relationships. It should be apparent that a careful evaluation of compounds having similar chemical structures can lead to the discovery of interesting and important pharmacological differences which, in turn, can result in the development of valuable therapeutic agents.

II. Chemical Structure and Biological Activity

In the search for compounds that would possess more potent muscle relaxant and tranquilizing activity than mephenesin, compounds were evaluated primarily for their ability to produce reversible paralysis of voluntary muscles in laboratory mice. A compound was considered to have potential when it produced loss of righting reflex without causing significant excitement prior to the onset of paralysis. Compounds were also assayed for their ability to counteract pentylenetetrazole convulsions, a characteristic which was considered an index of supraspinal center, nervous depressant action. In these investigations, modifications in chemical structure were explored not only to delineate their biological activities but also to determine the duration of their effectiveness in laboratory animals.

A. Propanediols and Propanediol Esters

Evidence was obtained (Berger and Ludwig, 1950) indicating that 2,2-diethyl-1,3-propanediol (DEP) was in part conjugated in the body as an ether-type glucuronide. Another portion was oxidized to α, α-diethylhydracrylic acid. These investigators subsequently evaluated a large number of 2-substituted 1,3-propanediols modified chemically to render their primary hydroxyls less susceptible to metabolic oxidation and conjugation. Typical of the results obtained by such chemical modifications were the findings reported for various esters of DEP. The effectiveness and duration of action of these compounds were tested by their ability to elevate the threshold to persistent convulsions produced by pentylenetetrazole in mice. 2,2-Diethyl-1,3-propanediol itself produced a very marked elevation of threshold within 30 minutes after oral administration. The effect then decreased rapidly, and 2 hours later the threshold returned to normal. The monoacetate of DEP behaved similarly. The diacetate of DEP produced a moderate increase of threshold within 30 minutes after administration, but this threshold then decreased more gradually than that of DEP. The acid succinate and dibenzoate esters of this diol produced only insignificant elevation of threshold and were practically ineffective.

B. Propanediol Carbamates

On the hypothesis that these esters were too resistant toward enzymatic hydrolysis to generate the free diol, the cyclic carbonate, monocarbamate, and dicarbamate esters were prepared (Ludwig and Piech, 1951). The cyclic carbonate esters of 2-substituted 1,3-propanediols resembled their parent diols in having a low intensity and short duration of action. Most of the monocarbamates also resembled the unesterified compounds from which they were derived in exhibiting a short duration of activity. The relatively short action of these cyclic carbonates and monocarbamates was probably due to rapid metabolism of the free primary alcohol group present in the latter compounds and readily generated by hydrolysis of the

TABLE II

Anticonvulsant Activity of Esters of 2-Methyl-2-Propyl-1, 3-Propanediol[a]

Compound	Electroshock protective dose (EED_{50} ±SE) in mice (mM/kg p.o.)[b]	
	30 min	150 min
Diol	2.0 ± 0.1	Ineff. at 4.8
Cyclic carbonate	2.5 ± 0.32	Ineff. at 4.8
Monocarbamate	1.5 ± 0.14	Ineff. at 4.8
Dicarbamate	0.76 ± 0.04	1.4 ± 0.04

[a] Data from Berger (1952b) and Berger (unpublished).

[b] EED_{50} = dose (mg/kg) preventing appearance of extensor tonic phase of electroshock seizures in 50% of animals; p.o. = orally. Data show mean ± standard error of mean.

former type. Only the dicarbamate derivatives were effective in protecting animals from electroshock seizures 150 minutes after administration (Berger, 1952b). The data summarized in Table II compare the mean protective doses of 2-methyl-2-propyl-1,3-propanediol dicarbamate, the diol from which it is derived, and the intermediate cyclic carbonate and monocarbamate compounds. The activity of the various compounds is expressed as the dose required to prevent electroshock seizures in mice 30 and 150 minutes after oral administration. The muscle-paralyzing activity of this same series of compounds showed a similar pattern. Of these, only the dicarbamate was capable of paralyzing 100% of the treated animals when the drug was administered intraperitoneally in a dose of 420 mg/kg. The duration of paralysis under these conditions was 90 minutes. These studies, which demonstrated that many of the dicarbamate esters of 2-substituted 1,3-propanediols when administered on an equimolar

TABLE III

ACTIVITY OF 2-SUBSTITUTED PROPANEDIOL DICARBAMATES IN MICE[a]

$$\begin{matrix} R_1 & & CH_2OCONH_2 \\ & C & \\ R_2 & & CH_2OCONH_2 \end{matrix}$$

R_1	R_2	PD_{50},[b] i.p.	EED_{50},[c] p.o.	LD_{50},[d] i.p.
H	Propyl	660	140	1100
H	*n*-Hexyl	1725	1400	3200
H	Phenyl	2200	52	4000
Methyl	Propyl	215	165	800
Methyl	*sec*-Butyl	175	290	460
Methyl	1-Ethylpropyl	175	280	490
Methyl	Phenyl	380	102	620
Isopropyl	Isopropyl	900	670	770
Phenyl	Phenyl	>3200	1400	4700
Propylidene		1060	[e]	160
Tetramethylene		1570	490	2400

[a] Data from Ludwig *et al.* (1969).

[b] PD_{50} = dose (mg/kg) producing loss of righting reflex for a duration of more than 1 min in 50% of animals; i.p. = intraperitoneally.

[c] EED_{50} = dose (mg/kg) preventing appearance of extensor tonic phase of electroshock seizures in 50% of animals; p.o. = orally.

[d] LD_{50} = lethal dose 50% (mg/kg) calculated from the mortality occurring up to 7 days after administration of the compound.

[e] Data not available.

basis possess a stronger action than the corresponding diol, show that the activity of the dicarbamate is a function of the whole molecule and not a consequence of release of the diol in the body prior to onset of action.

The nature of the 2-substituent in substituted 1,3-propanediol dicarbamates has a striking effect on muscle-paralyzing and anticonvulsant activity. Ludwig *et al.* (1969) reported the activities of 66 compounds of this type. The muscle-paralyzing and anticonvulsant activities and the acute toxicity of representative members of this series are summarized in Table III.

None of the compounds with a single 2-substituent possessed strong paralyzing action, but of these the 2-propyl and 2-*sec*-butyl compounds were the most potent. On the other hand, many of the 2,2-dialkyl-1,3-propanediol dicarbamates possessed strong paralyzing action. Of these, the 2-methyl-2-*sec*-butyl and 2-methyl-2-(1-ethylpropyl) derivatives had the strongest action and, in this respect, were equal or superior to meprobamate. The greatest muscle-paralyzing activity was generally shown by compounds having alkyl groups in the 2-position containing a total of 5 to 7 carbon atoms.

Introduction of an aromatic group failed to enhance paralyzing activity, but anticonvulsant activity was increased in compounds having such a substituent. The most potent anticonvulsant compound was the 2-phenyl derivative followed closely by the 2-methyl-2-phenyl compound. Variations of this structure having substituents in the 2-position containing nitrogen, sulfur, and chlorine and derivatives having alkylene, alkyne, alkoxy, and aryloxy substituents possessed insignificant paralyzing and anticonvulsant activity. Modification in structure in which the alkyl groups in the 2-position are fused into a ring were likewise uninteresting in their activity.

Delga *et al.* (1962) also noted that certain additional 2,2-dialkyl-1,3-propanediol dicarbamates had less activity than meprobamate. According to these investigators, this decrease was not due to a more rapid elimination of these compounds from the body. Witkin *et al.* (1962) studied the neuropharmacology of 2-cyclopentyl-2-methyl-1,3-propanediol dicarbamate and found this compound to possess many properties in common with meprobamate and to show a greater degree of specificity in obtunding hyperemotional states in animals at doses which produced minimal neurological impairment. Ferrari and Casagrande (1963) studied the relaxant action of several 2-methyl-2-aryl- and 2-methyl-2-aralkyl-1,3- propanediol dicarbamates and noted that a number of these compounds were equal to meprobamate in their effectiveness.

Stewart *et al.* (1962) prepared a short series of 1,3-propanediol dicarbamates substituted in the 2-position with halogenated alkyl groups and found these compounds to have an action qualitatively similar to that of meprobamate. Halogenation and minor alteration in the length of the side chain generally resulted in a decrease in muscle relaxant potency. Pallos (1963) has reported that 2,2-bis (chloromethyl)-1,3-propanediol dicarbamate exhibits stimulatory activity in laboratory animals.

C. Isomers of Meprobamate

Meprobamate is one of seven possible structural isomers having the basic 2-substituted trimethylene glycol dicarbamate structure. Of these, four are the isomeric 2-butyl derivatives; the remaining three are the 2,2-diethyl-, 2-methyl-2-propyl-, and 2-methyl-2-isopropyl-1,3-propanediol dicarbamates. In addition to these seven isomers, there are a total of twenty-seven structural isomers having alkyl substitution on 1 or more of each of the 3 carbon atoms of the trimethylene glycol nucleus. These dicarbamates differ from meprobamate in that they are derived from mixed primary, secondary, and tertiary glycols, whereas the seven isomers described above, including meprobamate, are all dicarbamates of diprimary glycols. The seven primary glycol isomers and two of the compounds with substitution on the 1 and 3 carbon atoms of trimethylene glycol were prepared and evaluated in a study reported by Berger *et al.* (1956). These were the dicarbamates of the primary–secondary glycol, 2-propyl-1,3-butanediol, and the disecondary glycol, 2,4-heptanediol. In addition, the cyclic compound, 1, 1-bis(carbamoxymethyl)cyclopentane was evaluated. This compound differs from meprobamate in having the 2-methyl and 2-propyl groups fused into the five-member ring.

Alkyl substitution on the 1 and 3 carbon atoms resulted in compounds having decreased muscle-paralyzing activity and a narrower margin between paralyzing and lethal doses. The anticonvulsant activity of these compounds approached that of meprobamate. A more detailed comparison of the seven 2-substituted trimethylene glycol dicarbamate isomers reveals an interesting pattern of activities. In paralyzing action, meprobamate was more than twice as active as the next best compound and substantially more active than the remaining isomers. When compared to meprobamate for their ability to protect from convulsions or death produced by pentylenetetrazole, larger amounts of the isomers were required. The order of potency of the isomers as pentylenetetrazole antagonists was similar to the order of their paralyzing effectiveness. When evaluated for their ability to modify maximal electroshock seizures, the isomeric compounds differed much less in potency from each other. The toxicity of the isomers generally paralleled their paralyzing action, but meprobamate had a greater margin between the median paralyzing and median toxic doses than any of its isomers. Figure 1 depicts graphically the relationships among these various activities possessed by the 2-substituted isomers of 2-methyl-2-propyl-1,3-propanediol dicarbamate. Included in this figure are the activities of the nonisomeric cyclic derivative, 1,1-bis (carbamoxymethyl)cyclopentane.

Berger (1952b) computed the ratio of the median paralyzing dose to the median electroshock seizure modifying dose as a measure of the ability of a compound to prevent seizure in nonparalytic

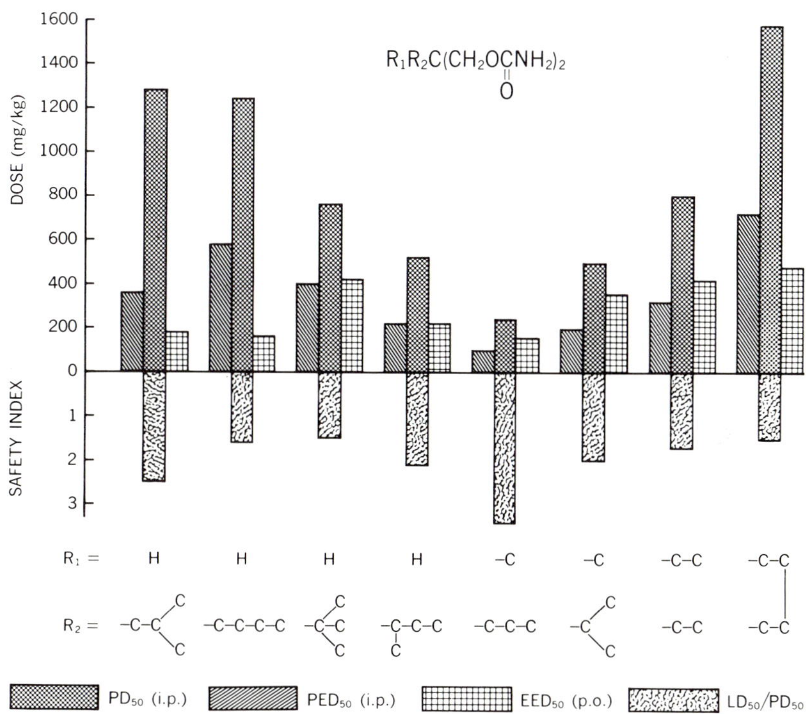

FIG. 1. Muscle-paralyzing and anticonvulsant activity of meprobamate isomers in mice. PD_{50} = dose (mg/kg) producing loss of righting reflex for a duration of more than 1 min in 50% of animals; PED_{50} = dose (mg/kg) preventing appearance of extensor tonic phase of pentylenetetrazole seizures in 50% of animals; EED_{50} = dose (mg/kg) preventing appearance of extensor tonic phase of electroshock seizures in 50% of animals; LD_{50} = lethal dose (mg/kg) calculated from the mortality occurring up to 7 days after intraperitoneal administration of the compound; i.p. = intraperitoneally; p.o. = orally. (From data of Berger *et al.*, 1956.)

TABLE IV

ACTIVITY OF SULFUR ANALOGS OF MEPROBAMATE IN MICE[a]

$$\begin{matrix} CH_3 & & CH_2XR_1 \\ & C & \\ C_3H_7 & & CH_2YR_2 \end{matrix}$$

Compound	X	Y	R_1	R_2	PD_{50} ±SE,[b] i.p.	EED_{50} ±SE,[c] p.o.	LD_{50} ±SE,[d] i.p.
I	S	S	$CONH_2$	$CONH_2$	212 ± 10.2	225 ± 12.2	410 ± 37
II	O	O	$CSNH_2$	$CSNH_2$	235 ± 18.7	235 ± 24.6	460 ± 22.8
III	O	O	$CONH_2$	$CSNH_2$	138 ± 8.5	[e]	345 ± 71
IV	O	S	$CONH_2$	$CONH_2$	173 ± 24.2	[e]	720 ± 64
V	O	O	H	$CSNH_2$	205 ± 14.7	[e]	530 ± 29
Meprobamate					235 ± 7.0	166 ± 8.7	800 ± 15

[a] Data from Ludwig *et al.*, (1964), Leaffer *et al.* (1965), and Berger (unpublished). Data show mean ± standard error of mean.

[b] PD_{50} = dose (mg/kg) producing loss of righting reflex for a duration of more than 1 min in 50% of animals; i.p. = intraperitoneally.

[c] EED_{50} = dose (mg/kg) preventing appearance of extensor tonic phase of electroshock seizures in 50% of animals; p.o. = orally.

[d] LD_{50} = Lethal dose 50% (mg/kg) calculated from the mortality occurring up to 7 days after administration of the compound.

[e] Data not available.

doses. This ratio was lowest for meprobamate, whereas 2-*n*-butyl-1,3-propanediol dicarbamate was remarkable in having a wide margin between the two doses. These same investigators made a comparison of the physical and pharmacological properties of the various meprobamate isomers. Water solubility did not appear to account for the observed differences in pharmacological action. All of the isomers were largely insoluble in water, and, of the two most soluble compounds of the series, one was the most potent and the other the least potent.

D. SULFUR ANALOGS

By replacing one or more of the 4 oxygen atoms of meprobamate with sulfur, it is possible to obtain two mono, four di-, two tri-, and one tetrathio analogs. Four of these—2-methyl-2-propyl-1,3-propanedithioldicarbamate (I), 2-methyl-2-propyl-1,3-propanediol bis (thioncarbamate) (II), 2-

methyl-2-propyl-1,3-propanediol monothiondicarbamate (III), and 3-carbamoxy-2-methyl-2-propylpropylthiolcarbamate (IV)—have been synthesized and studied (Ludwig *et al.*, 1964; Leaffer *et al.*, 1965). Wasson and Parker (1959) had earlier reported the synthesis and activity of a compound identified by them as II. Subsequent chemical studies by Ludwig and co-workers led the latter authors to conclude that Wasson and Parker's compound was the monothioncarbamate, 2-methyl-2-propyl-3-hydroxypropylthioncarbamate (V). The thiocarbamates, when evaluated for muscle-paralyzing action and lethality in white mice of the CF-1 strain, were found to possess activity comparable to that of meprobamate. Only the monothiondicarbamate (III) possessed paralyzing activity significantly greater in intensity than that of meprobamate, and all the sulfur analogs were somewhat more toxic than meprobamate (Table IV).

Wasson and Parker reported that their compound, presumably V, was more rapid in its action than the corresponding oxygen analog and yet produced muscle relaxation and sedation of similar duration. This finding was unexpected since this compound contains a primary hydroxyl group vulnerable to rapid metabolism. It would be expected to be comparable to 2-methyl-2-propyl-3-hydroxypropyl carbamate in having a short duration of action. It may be postulated that the substitution of oxygen by sulfur in the adjacent carbamate moiety renders the compound less susceptible to enzymatic degradation. An interesting observation reported by Wasson and Parker is the complete absence of a bitter taste for compound V. Meprobamate and its closely related homologs and the other thiocarbamates available for examination are all extremely bitter substances.

E. Miscellaneous Compounds

A broad selection of compounds having a chemical relationship to meprobamate have been studied by Berger and Ludwig (1960) for their potential muscle-paralyzing and anticonvulsant activities (Table V). Several of these compounds which resemble the cyclic carbonate esters of 1,3-propanediols in their structure were found to be virtually inactive in these tests. 5-Methyl-5-propyl-1,3,2-dioxathiane 2-oxide (VI), a sulfur analog of the cyclic carbonate ester, was not only inactive in these tests but exhibited potent convulsant activity when administered to mice in low doses. Potassium 2-methyl-2-propyl-1,3-propylene dithiophosphate (VII) displayed insignificant activity. The alleged sedative-hypnotic and hypothermic activity of 5-methyl-5-propyl-2-*p*-tolyl-1,3,2-dioxaborinane (VIII) (Caujolle *et al.*, 1960) could not be confirmed (Berger and Ludwig, 1960). 5-Methyl-5-propyl-3,4,5,6-tetrahydro-2H-1,3-oxazin-2-one

TABLE V

STRUCTURAL FORMULAS OF MEPROBAMATE-LIKE COMPOUNDS

CH_3 CH_2O C $S{=}O$ C_3H_7 CH_2O (VI)	CH_3 CH_2O S C P C_3H_7 CH_2O SK (VII)	CH_3 CH_2O C B—C_6H_4—CH_3 C_3H_7 CH_2O (VIII)
CH_3 CH_2O C $C{=}O$ C_3H_7 CH_2NH (IX)	O CH_3 $CH_2OCNHNH_2$ C C_3H_7 $CH_2OCNHNH_2$ O (X)	O O CH_3 $CH_2OCNHCNH_2$ C C_3H_7 $CH_2OCNHCNH_2$ O O (XI)
O CH_3 CH_2OCNH_2 C C_3H_7 $CH_2OCNHNH_2$ O (XII)	O CH_3 CH_2OCNH_2 Si C_3H_7 CH_2OCNH_2 O (XIII)	R O R $CHOCNH_2$ C R $CHOCNH_2$ R O (XIV)
O CH_2OCNH_2 $(RCR)_n$ CH_2OCNH_2 O (XV)	O CH_2 CH_2OCNH_2 $(CH_2)_n$ C CH_2 CH_2OCNH_2 O (XVI)	O CH_2OCNH_2 C $(CH_2)_n$—$CHOCNH_2$ O (XVII)

(IX), a cyclic carbamate derivative isosteric with the cyclic carbonate, was also found to possess minimal activity. 2-Methyl-2-propyl-1,3-propanediol dicarbazate (X) and 2-methyl-2-propyl-1,3-propanediol diallophanate (XI) possessed interesting pharmacological activities. This dicarbazate and the mixed carbamate–carbazate compound (XII) produced mild muscle relaxant activity in mice and, in addition, elicited a hypotensive response in these test animals. The allophanate derivative possessed anticonvulsant and paralyzing activities which resembled, in some respects, those of meprobamate.

In a study comparing a number of silicon-containing analogs of pharmaceutically active drug compounds, Fessenden and Coon (1965) found silameprobamate (XIII)—a meprobamate bioisotere, comparable to meprobamate in its activity but considerably shorter acting. Fessenden attributed this short duration of activity to its more rapid metabolism in the animal body. Other variations explored by Berger and Ludwig (1960) for their potential therapeutic usefulness were a series of 1-, 2-, and 3-substituted propanediol dicarbamates (XIV), dicarbamates of butane-, pentane-, and hexanediol (XV), bis(hydroxymethyl)cycloalkane dicarbamates (XVI), and hydroxymethylcycloalkanol dicarbamates (XVII). None of the representatives of these types synthesized and evaluated in this study possessed more than minimal paralyzing and anticonvulsant activity.

Yamamoto *et al.* (1960) prepared a series of camphane mono- and dicarbamates, and found 2,10-dihydroxycamphane dicarbamate, the camphane analog corresponding to XVII, less effective as an anticonvulsant than some of the monocarbamates of the same series.

The numerous syntheses carried out in an attempt to discover a compound that would be more desirable than meprobamate have been exhaustive. It is unlikely that a compound superior to meprobamate will be found among this class of aliphatic carbamate compounds.

F. Hypotensive Propanediol Dicarbamates

A number of clinical investigators reported that meprobamate exerted a mild hypotensive action in some patients suffering from essential hypertension (Dunsmore *et al.*, 1957; Boyd *et al.*, 1959). It was also noted that ingestion of large quantities of the drug with suicidal intent or due to inadvertent overdosage often produced marked hypotension (Shane and Hirsch, 1956; Charkes, 1958; Aitchison, 1960). These findings led to the investigation of the mechanism of the hypotensive action of meprobamate and to a study to establish whether other members of this series would have a more prominent hypotensive action (Berger *et al.*, 1961).

A number of meprobamate-like compounds were screened for their antihypertensive activity in rabbits. Systolic and diastolic arterial blood pressure was determined in male albino rabbits according to the method of McGregor (1928). The blood pressure in the abdominal aorta was measured with a standard sphygnomanometer cuff applied around the lower half of the body of the animal. The drugs were given intraperitoneally as aqueous suspensions, and blood pressure readings were taken at 15-minute intervals for 3 to 4 hours following the injection of the drug. Only a small fraction of the 2-substituted 1,3-propanediol dicarbamates

TABLE VI

ANTIHYPERTENSIVE ACTIVITY OF SUBSTITUTED PROPANEDIOL DICARBAMATES[a]

$$R_1R_2C(CH_2O\overset{\overset{O}{\|}}{C}NH_2)_2$$

R_1	R_2	Activity[b]
Methyl	Methyl	>100
Methyl	Propyl	77
Methyl	Isopropyl	>100
Methyl	Isobutyl	60
Methyl	*sec*-Butyl	40
Ethyl	Ethyl	>100
Ethyl	Phenyl	75
Propyl	Propyl	75
Phenyl	Phenyl	>100

[a] Data from Berger (unpublished).

[b] Dose required (mg/kg i.p.) for 25 mm Hg lowering of systolic pressure in rabbits.

evaluated in this test had a significant effect on the blood pressure. The dose required for 25 mm Hg lowering of systolic pressure for the more active compounds of this series is tabulated in Table VI. Two derivatives, 2-methyl-2-isobutyl-1,3-propanediol dicarbamate and 2-methyl-2-*sec*-butyl-1,3-propanediol dicarbamate, were more potent than meprobamate in this assay. The latter compound, mebutamate, has been evaluated extensively in normotensive and hypertensive rabbits and rats by Berger and his associates.

G. *N*-SUBSTITUTED PROPANEDIOL CARBAMATES

The replacement of one hydrogen on one of the carbamyl nitrogen atoms of meprobamate with a short-chain alkyl group yielded compounds possessing muscle relaxant activity of substantially greater intensity than that of the parent compound.

1. N-Substituted Monocarbamates

Ludwig *et al.* (1969) synthesized and investigated the activity of forty-seven *N*-monosubstituted and *N*-disubstituted 3-hydroxypropyl carbamates. Attaching a single alkyl group to the carbamate nitrogen produced compounds with appreciable paralyzing activity, and ethyl and propyl substitution in this manner yielded compounds of greatest activity. It was of interest that N-CH_3 and N-C_2H_5 derivatives of 2,2-diphenyl-3-hydroxypropyl carbamate resulted in compounds having strong paralyzing activity. This activity contrasts with the low paralyzing action of the corresponding N-unsubstituted monocarbamate. N-Substitution with a higher alkyl group generally resulted in loss of activity. Introduction of a single allyl group improved activity, but this enhancement in activity did not occur when substitution was made with higher alkylene or alkyne groups. The N,N-dimethyl analogs possessed good paralyzing action, but this activity was lost when substituents larger than methyl were used.

2. N-Substituted Dicarbamates

The paralyzing activity of propanediol dicarbamates in which only one of the hydrogens on one of the carbamyl nitrogen atoms was replaced by a short-chain alkyl group was outstanding. Ludwig *et al.* (1969) reported the synthesis and muscle-paralyzing activity of eighty-three of these unsymmetrical N-substituted dicarbamate derivatives. An examination of the paralyzing activity of these compounds disclosed some interesting relationships. Of the seventeen compounds possessing a PD_{50} value* of less than 160 mg/kg, fifteen have a 3-carbon substituent attached to the carbamate nitrogen. In addition, fifteen of these seventeen potent compounds contain a total of either 7 or 8 carbon atoms attached to the carbamate nitrogen and substituted at the 2-position of the propanediol chain. The paralyzing activity of these compounds is presented schematically in Fig. 2.

In this study there were included a large number of N-polysubstituted dicarbamate derivatives. These were compounds in which two or more hydrogens attached to carbamate nitrogen atoms were replaced by various substituents and included N,N-disubstituted, N,N'-disubstituted, N,N,N'-trisubstituted, and N,N,N',N'-tetrasubstituted variations. The introduction of two alkyl groups on one nitrogen or a single alkyl group on each nitrogen failed to yield compounds of significant effectiveness. The use of bulky substituents, such as xanthyl, likewise did not increase effectiveness. Attaching three or four alkyl substituents to the carbamate nitrogens, as a rule, did not yield compounds having appreciable activity, although one such compound, N,N,N',N'-tetramethyl-2-methyl-2-propyl-1,3- pro-

* Dose producing loss of righting reflex for a duration of more than 1 minute in 50% of animals.

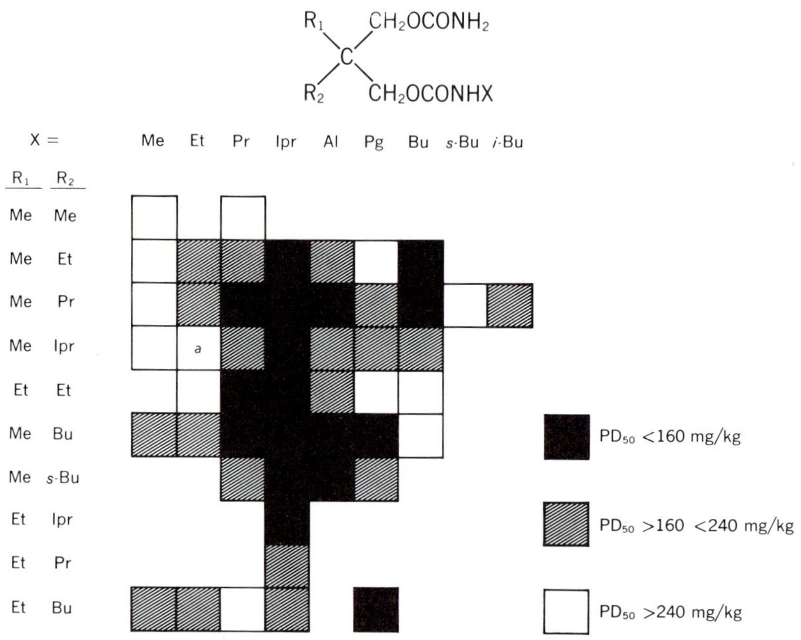

FIG. 2. Paralyzing activity of *N*-substituted propanediol dicarbamates in mice. PD_{50} = dose (mg/kg) producing loss of righting reflex for a duration of more than 1 min in 50% of animals. Al = allyl; Pg = propargyl; *a* = data not available. (From data of Ludwig *et al.*, 1969.)

panediol dicarbamate was active. *N*-Acylated derivatives of both *N*-substituted and *N*-unsubstituted dicarbamate compounds were invariably inactive. Compounds wherein the carbamate nitrogen was substituted with hydroxy-, carboxy-, or haloalkyl possessed insignificant activity. 2-Methyl-2-propyl-1,3-propanediol-*N*-isopropylamino dicarbamate and 3-hydroxypropyl-2-methyl-2-propyl-*N*-isopropylamino carbamate exhibited significant paralyzing activity. With the exception of these carbazate derivatives, none of the *N*-amino, *N*-alkoxy, *N*-hydroxy, *N*-carbamyl, *N*-nitro, and *N*-sulfonyl carbamates displayed significant paralyzing or anticonvulsant activity.

Leaffer *et al.* (1965) prepared for pharmacological study two monothioncarbamate analogs of carisoprodol, 3-carbamoxy-2-methyl-2-propylpropyl *N*-isopropylthioncarbamate (XVIII) and 2-methyl-2-propyl-3-thioncarbamoxypropyl *N*-isopropylcarbamate (XIX). When evaluated for their muscle-paralyzing activity in CF-1 strain white mice, these

TABLE VII

PARALYZING ACTIVITY OF SULFUR ANALOGS OF CARISOPRODOL IN MICE[a]

$$\begin{array}{l} \qquad\qquad\qquad Y_1 \\ \qquad\qquad\qquad \| \\ CH_3 \diagdown \quad \diagup CH_2OCNH_2 \\ \qquad\quad C \\ C_3H_7 \diagup \quad \diagdown CH_2OCNHCH(CH_3)_2 \\ \qquad\qquad\qquad \| \\ \qquad\qquad\qquad Y_2 \end{array}$$

Compound	Y_1	Y_2	PD_{50} ±SE,[b] i.p.	LD_{50} ±SE,[b] i.p.
XVIII	O	S	130 ± 12.2	482 ± 40.5
XIX	S	O	130 ± 20.2	448 ± 60.5
Carisoprodol			165 ± 78	980 ± 78

[a] Data from Leaffer *et al.* (1965) and Berger (unpublished).

[b] PD_{50} = dose (mg/kg) producing loss of righting reflex for a duration of more than 1 min in 50% of animals; LD_{50} = lethal dose 50% (mg/kg) calculated from mortality occurring up to 7 days after administration of the compound; i.p. = intraperitoneally. Data show mean ± standard error of mean.

compounds were found to be somewhat more potent than carisoprodol but considerably more toxic than the parent compound (Table VII).

III. Metabolism of Propanediol Dicarbamates

A. ABSORPTION AND DISTRIBUTION

1. *N-Unsubstituted Carbamates*

The propanediol dicarbamate compounds possess limited water solubility, but their favorable lipid–water partition coefficient promotes their prompt and efficient absorption from the gastrointestinal tract. Walkenstein *et al.* (1958) confirmed the ready absorption of meprobamate from the gastrointestinal tract of animals and humans and showed that the distribution of the drug in the body took place rapidly, with higher concentrations of the drug occurring in the visceral tissues of the rat and substantially lower quantities in the brain and fat.

More extensive studies of the absorption and distribution of meprobamate were made by Ewaldsson (1963) and van der Kleijn (1969a) using ^{3}H- and ^{14}C-labeled meprobamate, respectively. Ewaldsson concluded that it was not possible to demonstrate any specific localization in the brain which could be related to the mode of action of meprobamate. In a detailed whole-body radioautographic study, van der Kleijn found that shortly after intravenous or oral administration of meprobamate-^{14}C to mice, the brain, thymus, and body fat showed a lower concentration of radioactivity than blood, lungs, and skeletal muscles, while myocardium, liver, hypophysis, and adrenal cortex demonstrated a higher concentration. A slow penetration of meprobamate into the central nervous system was observed with a maximum concentration of radioactivity occurring 10–15 minutes after intravenous administration. Within 5 minutes after oral administration, high concentrations were present in the liver and kidney. After 30 minutes, a rather uniform pattern of distribution throughout the body was observed, and the brain showed a lower intensity of labeling than the blood, soft organs, and skeletal muscle.

Emmerson *et al.* (1960) studied the metabolic state of meprobamate in the rat brain using meprobamate-^{14}C administered intraperitoneally. These workers found that the peak activity in all areas of the brain occurred within 1 hour after drug administration and that distribution within the brain was uniform. They also demonstrated that the metabolites of meprobamate are not present in the brain of the rat.

Blood meprobamate levels of a large number of human subjects reported by several investigators indicate that peak concentrations occur 1–2 hours after oral administration. A steady decline in concentration occurs thereafter with a half-life of approximately 10 hours. In a typical study, a 70-kg adult, taking 800 mg of meprobamate, exhibits a peak concentration of about 16 $\mu g/ml$ of blood. At this concentration, it can be estimated that approximately 15% of the ingested dose is present in the bloodstream (Hoffman and Ludwig, 1959).

Maddock and Bloomer (1967) have correlated plasma meprobamate concentrations in humans with the state of consciousness. Deep coma is associated with concentrations over 100 $\mu g/ml$, and light coma with values between 60 and 120 $\mu g/ml$. At concentrations below 50 $\mu g/ml$, all patients were awake.

Chambon (1959) has reported evidence that meprobamate ingested by pregnant women a few hours preceding delivery is transmitted to the fetus. His findings indicate that the newborn infant's blood usually contains from one-fourth to about one-half of the concentration of meprobamate found in the blood of the mother. This value is substantially lower than the range of 57 to 98% transplacental passage of meprobamate from the rabbit mother to fetus reported by Palmieri (1964) and the essentially uniform distribution of this compound throughout the organs of rat mother and fetus observed by Chiesara and Conti (1964).

Mebutamate also achieves a maximum blood concentration in adult humans 1 to 2 hours after oral administration (Douglas *et al.*,1962a). Studies in the rat using mebutamate-^{14}C revealed a pattern of distribution comparable to that observed for meprobamate (Douglas, 1962). More extensive distribution studies have not been reported for mebutamate. Because of the close chemical similarity of these two drug compounds, however, it can be anticipated that the pharmacokinetics of their absorption, body distribution, and elimination would be similar.

2. N-Substituted Carbamates

The *N*-alkyl carbamates, carisoprodol and tybamate, are also rapidly absorbed and reach peak blood concentrations within 1 to 2 hours following oral administration to dogs and humans (Douglas *et al.*, 1962b; 1966). Because of their lipophilic character, these compounds are rapidly taken up in the central nervous system. van der Kleijn (1969a) noted the rapid uptake of carisoprodol-^{14}C and tybamate-^{14}C in several regions of the mouse brain within 1 minute after intravenous injection. A similar rapid uptake was observed in the adipose tissue of these animals. Unquestionably, the differences between the pharmacological properties of these homologous *N*-alkyl carbamate compounds and those of meprobamate can be attributed in part to differences in their ability to penetrate the blood–brain barrier.

Douglas *et al.* (1964) investigated the binding of carbamate drug compounds by the proteins of human plasma using the equilibrium dialysis technique. They demonstrated a correlation between the extent of binding and the partition coefficient of these compounds between cottonseed oil and water. van der Kleijn (1969b) conducted a more extensive study of the influence of protein binding on the penetration rate into the central nervous system and on the elimination rate from the bloodstream. They concluded that the inhibiting influence of protein binding is compensated for by the lipid solubility of the compounds.

B. Biotransformation

1. N-Unsubstituted Carbamates

Early studies on the fate of meprobamate in the animal body by Berger (1954) and by Agranoff *et al.* (1957) showed that about 10% of the orally administered drug was excreted unchanged in the urine of both humans and laboratory animals along with additional amounts of the drug or its metabolic products in the form of a glucuronide. The latter investigators found that a portion of the conjugate was hydrolyzable with β-glucuronidase, and the remainder could be split by chemical hydrolysis to give a meprobamate-like substance.

Walkenstein *et al.* (1958) demonstrated that, unlike urethan, essentially none of the compound labeled in the carbamate position with radioactive carbon was split into radioactive carbon dioxide and concluded that the bulk of the meprobamate, 60% of the ingested dose, was excreted by the dog as 2-hydroxymethyl-2-propyl-1,3-propanediol dicarbamate (XX).

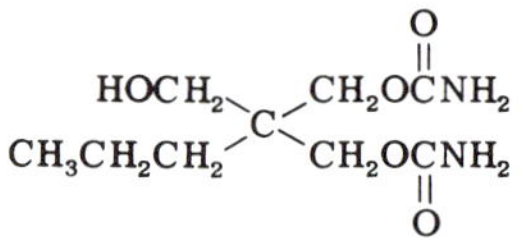

$$(HOCH_2)(CH_3CH_2CH_2)C(CH_2OC(=O)NH_2)_2$$

(XX)

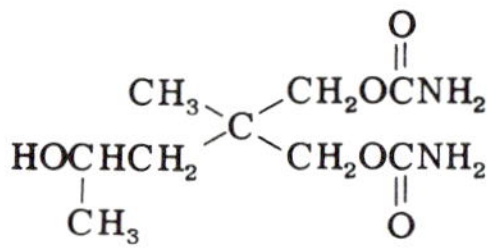

$$(CH_3)(HOCH(CH_3)CH_2)C(CH_2OC(=O)NH_2)_2$$

(XXI)

$$(CH_3)(H_2NC(=O)OCH(CH_3)CH_2)C(CH_2OC(=O)NH_2)_2$$

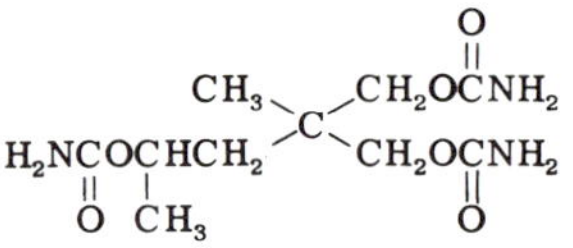

(XXII)

Ludwig *et al.* (1961), in the course of their studies on the metabolism of meprobamate, observed certain discrepancies in the chromatographic behavior of the urinary end product and the synthetic hydroxymethyl derivative. A more extensive investigation by these investigators proved conclusively that the most abundant metabolite of meprobamate was 2-(β-hydroxypropyl)-2-methyl-1,3-propanediol dicarbamate (XXI) instead of the hydroxymethyl compound reported by Walkenstein. This compound (XXI) proved to be a true detoxification product of meprobamate in that it possessed a very high water solubility and in that it was inactive in doses as high as 7 gm/kg when administered intraperitoneally to mice.

Ludwig *et al.* (1969) converted hydroxymeprobamate to the corresponding tricarbamate. Like hydroxymeprobamate, 2-(β-hydroxypropyl)-2-methyl-1,3-propanediol tricarbamate (XXII) dissolves in water in excess of 10% and is essentially devoid of pharmacological activity. The extreme solubility and inactivity of this tricarbamate compound supports the postulate that the 1,3-propanediol *N*-unsubstituted dicarbamates owe their limited water solubility to internal hydrogen binding between the carbamate moieties. The characteristic pharmacological activity exhibited by meprobamate is apparently due in part to the relatively high degree of lipophilicity resulting from this internal hydrogen bonding.

Ludwig *et al.* (1961) also presented evidence that the major conjugated metabolite of meprobamate excreted in human urine was a glucosyluronide of unaltered meprobamate. The identity of this conjugate as the *N*-mono-β-D-glucopyranosiduronic acid of meprobamate (XXIII) and its chemical synthesis have been reported by Tsukamoto *et al.* (1963a,b).

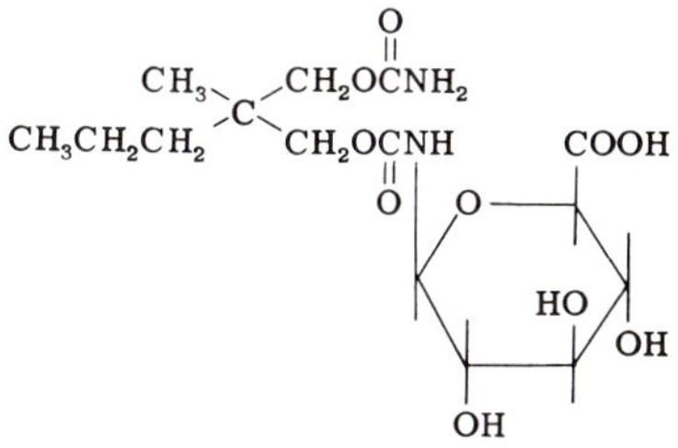

(XXIII)

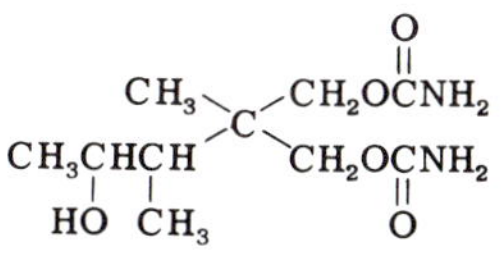

(XXIV)

In addition to their role in elucidating the metabolic fate of meprobamate in the animal body, these findings were of particular interest because they provided the first evidence that a carbamate NH_2 group participates in *N*-glucuronide conjugation. Indication for the occurrence in the urine of experimental animals of other metabolic products of meprobamate, including the keto and carboxylic derivatives, has been presented by Wiser and Seifter (1960) and by Yamamato *et al.* (1962a,b).

Studies carried out by Douglas *et al.* (1962a) revealed that the metabolic transformation of mebutamate leads to similar end products—a hydroxylated derivative, 2-(β-hydroxy-α-methylpropyl)-2-methyl-1,3-propanediol dicarbamate (XXIV), the primary metabolite, and a glucuronide conjugate. Hydroxymebutamate, like hydroxymeprobamate, has an unusually low toxicity and is essentially devoid of other pharmacological properties. Douglas and colleagues observed that the hydroxylated form of mebutamate and unchanged mebutamate are excreted by the dog in a ratio of approximately 30:1 as compared to 4:1 for hydroxymeprobamate and meprobamate. They attribute this difference to a somewhat higher lipid solubility of mebutamate.

2. *N-Substituted Carbamates*

Douglas *et al.* (1962b, 1966) have studied the metabolic fate of carisoprodol and tybamate in laboratory animals. Radiopaper chromatographic investigation of the urine of dogs receiving carisoprodol-^{14}C intravenously revealed that unchanged carisoprodol is excreted to a minor extent, whereas the major urinary products are hydroxycarisoprodol and hydroxymeprobamate. *N*-Dealkylation and alkyl hydroxylation are similarly involved in the metabolism of tybamate. It is noteworthy that each of the four related 1,3-propanediol dicarbamate drug compounds investigated is hydroxylated at the penultimate carbon of their longer alkyl side chain. Table VIII summarizes pharmacokinetic factors of importance to the pharmacological activity of the four carbamate drug compounds and the distribution of the urinary end products resulting from the oral administration of these compounds to dogs.

Douglas *et al.* (1962b) also made a detailed study of the distribution of radioactivity in blood following the intravenous administration of carisoprodol-^{14}C to dogs. The simultaneous *N*-dealkylation and side-chain hydroxylation occurring in the dog and rat results in an interesting pattern of distribution of the various metabolites. Figure 3 shows the relative percentages of carisoprodol, hydroxycarisoprodol, and meprobamate occurring in the blood of dogs following the intravenous administration of carisoprodol. Because of the conversion to the rapidly eliminated hydroxylated derivatives, only minimal concentrations of the dealkylated product, mepro-

TABLE VIII

PHARMACOKINETIC PROPERTIES OF CARBAMATE DRUG COMPOUNDS

Property[a]	Meprobamate	Mebutamate	Carisoprodol	Tybamate
Water solubility (%)	0.3	0.5	0.05	0.05
Oil–water dist. coeff.	0.3	0.4	4.8	>20
Protein binding (%)	0	0	55	80
Plasma $T_{1/2}$, human, p.o. (hr)	10	5	8	3
Urinary excretion, dog, p.o.				
Unchanged (%)	10	2	<1	0–7
Glucuronide (%)	30	60	1–2	1–2
Hydroxylated (%)	60	30–40	40	60
Dealkylated (%)	—	—	15	1–2
Hydroxylated–dealkylated (%)	—	—	40	30

[a] p.o. = Orally.

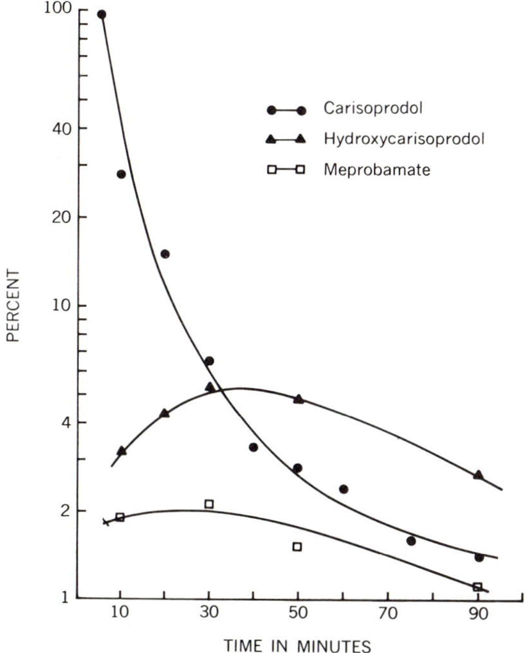

FIG. 3. Distribution of carisoprodol metabolites in blood of dog following intravenous administration of carisoprodol-^{14}C. Percent metabolite based on the initial radioactivity equal to 100%. Radioactivity due to hydroxymeprobamate not included. (From data of Douglas *et al.*, 1962b.)

bamate, are present in the blood of the dog following administration of these *N*-alkyl carbamates. The relatively rare occurrence of fixed drug eruption in humans due to cross-reaction of meprobamate and carisoprodol (Honeycutt and Curtis, 1964; Gore, 1965) may be due to residual blood concentrations of meprobamate resulting from the metabolic dealkylation of carisoprodol.

C. ENZYMATIC INACTIVATION AND DRUG INTERACTION

Many reports have appeared in the literature presenting evidence that the metabolism of meprobamate in laboratory animals is altered by pretreatment with certain chemical compounds and with meprobamate itself. Conney and Burns (1960) first demonstrated that the administration of a number of drugs including phenobarbital, barbital, phenylbutazone, orphenadrine, and aminopyrine shortened the duration of action of meprobamate, and Kato (1960a) has observed a similar effect due to chlorpromazine. Kato (1960b) also demonstrated a lowered tissue concentration and a decreased pharmacological effect of meprobamate following pretreatment with phenobarbital and phenaglycodol.

A comparable induction in rats pretreated with a variety of neurotropic drugs has been reported by Kato and Chiesara (1962) and by Kato and Vassanelli (1962). In these studies, meprobamate was shown to be less potent than phenobarbital in stimulating the metabolism of phenobarbital, when measured by its effect on serum and brain phenobarbital concentrations and by its ability to prolong phenobarbital sleeping time. Meprobamate was also found to be substantially less effective than phenobarbital in accelerating meprobamate metabolism.

Ponomarev and Terekhina (1964) reported that animals pretreated with a number of drugs including phenobarbital exhibited reduced plasma and brain tissue levels of meprobamate due to hepatic microsomal stimulation. Wenzel and Broadie (1966) demonstrated that the administration of nicotine to mice caused an immediate and significant decrease in the duration of ataxia produced by meprobamate. These investigators also found that nicotine administered *in vivo* enhanced *in vitro* metabolism of meprobamate by mouse liver homogenate. Enhanced metabolism of meprobamate in rats after chronic feeding of low dietary levels of dichlorodiphenyltrichloroethane (DDT) has been reported by Datta and Nelson (1968).

Phillips *et al.* (1962) observed that brain and blood concentrations of meprobamate-^{14}C decreased at a more rapid rate in animals made tolerant by pretreatment with meprobamate for 35 days than in nontolerant animals. Also, urinary excretion was more rapid in tolerant animals, and nontolerant rats excreted nearly twice as much unchanged meprobamate as tolerant rats.

Douglas *et al.* (1963) in an investigation of the urinary excretion ratios of meprobamate and hydroxymeprobamate found that human subjects receiving small doses of the drug over a period of at least 30 days excreted a significantly larger proportion of hydroxymeprobamate than did subjects taking a single dose of the drug. In the former group of subjects, the hydroxymeprobamate–meprobamate ratio was 1.8 as compared to 0.9 for the nonchronic drug users. In each case, these values were substantially lower than those found in a similar study utilizing five species of laboratory animals. Most of the animal species voided these compounds in a ratio in excess of 2:1 and in some cases as high as 7:1, and the ratio was essentially independent of the route of administration and prior exposure to the drug. The inability of the rats employed in this study to display evidence of tolerance of the type described by Phillips was probably due to the substantially lower daily dose of meprobamate received by these animals.

The shift observed in the ratio of meprobamate urinary excretion products may be due to stimulation of either the hydroxylation reaction or the glucuronide-forming step. Each produces an inactive water-soluble metabolite, and the stimulation of either reaction would result in an accelerated removal of meprobamate from the bloodstream producing the tolerance observed by Phillips *et al.* (1962), Kato (1960b), and others.

Hollister and Levy (1964) compared meprobamate elimination in acutely dosed, healthy individuals with that of subjects who had received large doses of this drug for prolonged periods. The half-life value of the latter group was considerably higher than that of subjects receiving a single usual dose. This observation does not exclude the possibility of self-induced enhancement of meprobamate metabolism, since the longer half-lives may reflect a dose-dependent absorption and elimination rate.

Enhanced meprobamate metabolism resulting from enzyme induction in humans by administration of low doses of phenobarbital for 10 days could not be readily demonstrated by Held and von Oldershausen (1969). These investigators were unable to find a significant difference in meprobamate blood half-life before and after phenobarbital treatment in 4 subjects, but contrary to the findings of Hollister and Levy (1964), they obtained evidence for enzyme induction in drug-addicted patients. It is apparent that the relatively consistent evidence reported for hepatic microsomal enzyme induction in laboratory animals is not readily reproducible in humans, and further studies are needed to establish the significance of enzyme induction in the drug therapy of patients.

Instances in which the action of meprobamate has been intensified by the enzyme-inhibitory effect of a second drug, or in which meprobamate by the same mechanism enhanced the activity of another drug, have been reported. Kato *et al.* (1962a, 1963) observed that a number of "inducing" drug compounds were capable of inhibiting meprobamate metabolism in rat liver microsomes, and Edelson and Douglas (1967) found that benactyzine inhibited the metabolic transformation of meprobamate in a similar *in vitro* system. Although the results of these studies cannot be directly extrapolated to man, a similar metabolic inhibition in humans could intensify the activity of meprobamate when administered in conjunction with a second drug.

A number of drugs, including meprobamate, have been shown to reduce markedly warfarin half-life in dogs (Hunninghake and Azarnoff, 1968), and meprobamate has been implicated in a similar effect on prothrombin time in humans (Cullen and Catalano, 1967).

Mebutamate is readily oxidized in rat and rabbit microsomes to hydroxymebutamate (Edelson and Douglas, 1968). The enzymatic hydroxylation was found to be stimulated by treatment with phenobarbital, aminopyrine, and tybamate, but pretreatment of the animals with mebutamate itself produced neither a stimulatory nor an inhibitory effect on the *in vitro* metabolism of this compound.

Studies on drug enzyme induction and inhibition of carisoprodol metabolism have also been reported (Kato *et al.*, 1961; Kato and Chiesara, 1962; Kato *et al.*, 1962b, 1963). Kato (1967) has also reported that repeated injections of carisoprodol reduced the duration of paralysis and increased the rate of metabolism of this drug in rats. This observation is comparable to the self-inducing stimulation of metabolism produced by meprobamate in laboratory animals.

IV. Pharmacology of Propanediol Dicarbamates

Because of its unique actions and broad usefulness, meprobamate was the first of the propanediol dicarbamates to be widely studied. Indeed, it became the prototype not only of drugs of similar chemical structure but of antianxiety agents with different chemical structures and pharmacological actions. Since the introduction of meprobamate in 1955, results of over 1200 pharmacological investigations on propanediol carbamates have been published. This review must consequently deal only with the findings of representative experiments.

A. Meprobamate

Early pharmacological investigation demonstrated that the oral administration of small doses of meprobamate to mice produced a state of calm in which the animals appeared to be quiet and relaxed but nonetheless interested in their environment. Somewhat larger doses (100 mg/kg) reduced muscle tone but did not alter respiration. Still larger doses of 150 mg/kg caused greater loss of muscle tone along with ataxia and somnolence. Paralysis of the hind extremities preceded that of the forelimbs. The righting reflex was lost in half of the animals given 300 mg/kg. The effects of very large but sublethal doses were reversible and complete recovery ensued. The lethal dose in mice was estimated to be about 1100 mg/kg. Similar effects were seen in rats. Hostile Rhesus monkeys given 250–400 mg/kg by mouth did not object to handling by humans, tolerated petting, accepted food, and did not show fear. Appetite was not impaired, and the animals retained an interest in their environment. After larger doses, the animals showed some loss of coordination, gradually became paralyzed, and unable to walk (Berger, 1954). These early studies by Berger drew attention to the four most characteristic pharmacological actions of the drug: (*1*) its effects on voluntary muscles, (*2*) its anticonvulsant actions, (*3*) its taming effects in animals, and (*4*) its lack of effect on the autonomic nervous system.

1. Effects on Voluntary Muscles

The skeletal muscle relaxant effects of meprobamate were studied in many animal species and in man using a wide variety of techniques.

a. Effects on Muscle Tone. The administration of meprobamate in doses comparable to those used clinically produces relaxation of the voluntary skeletal muscles in most animal species. Greater doses are required to produce motor deficit and muscle paralysis. In many respects, its actions differ strikingly from those obtained after the administration of other drugs. The extent of muscle relaxation is less intense than that produced by curare and curare-like substances, and respiratory function is not impaired. Meprobamate, unlike barbiturates and other hypnotics, causes no psychomotor excitation and restlessness during the induction period and no signs of tremors, convulsions, or other manifestations of hyperactivity on recovery. Although quantitatively and qualitatively similar to mephenesin, meprobamate is far more effective on oral administration, and its actions are more pronounced and long lasting (Berger, 1966).

b. Effects on Motor Activity. Muscle-relaxing doses of meprobamate do not significantly impair the spontaneous locomotor activity of animals in situations in which the movement of the animal or that of a suspended jiggle cage is counted (Melander, 1959; Caviezel and Baillod, 1958). These doses also do not impair the ability of an animal to remain suspended from a rotating rod (Kinnard and Carr, 1957), to stay on a series of slowly rotating rollers (Dunham and Miya, 1957), to grasp a vertical or inclined screen (Friedman and Ingalls, 1960; Harrison and Albert, 1963; Kondziella, 1964), to climb a smooth, hollow cylinder (Boissier *et al.*, 1960), or to perform similar tasks (Turrian *et al.*, 1957). Even relatively large doses do not significantly reduce the ability of an animal to perform demanding physical tasks, such as swimming with a weighted load under harsh environmental conditions. Indeed, occasionally such performance may be enhanced (Jacob and Michaud, 1960). After the administration of paralyzing doses, exploratory behavior, by which animals become familiar with new or strange environments, is not altered. Such responses may be facilitated in situations in which animals are exposed to relatively strong stimuli (Battig, 1961).

c. Effects on Spinal Reflexes. The amplitude of the monosynaptic patellar reflex is not altered by the administration of relatively large doses of meprobamate (80 mg/kg) to intact animals (Berger, 1954). Likewise, the responses of other simple reflexes, such as the gastrocnemius, are not altered. Equivalent doses markedly depress polysynaptic reflexes such as the flexor (Hendley *et al.*, 1954), extensor (Ngai *et al.*, 1966), and crossed-extensor reflexes (Abdulian *et al.*, 1960). Larger doses are required to abolish higher reflexes such as the linguomandibular (Hendley *et al.*, 1954). Nonetheless, appropriate doses depress monosynaptic spinal reflexes (Wilson, 1958) particularly if given within 1 to 2 hours of barbiturate anesthesia (Del Castillo and Nelson, 1960).

Abdulian *et al.* (1960) found that ataxic doses of meprobamate depressed facilitation and inhibition of the patellar reflex evoked in high spinal cats by contralateral sciatic stimulation. Under these circumstances, meprobamate could be clearly distinguished from mephenesin. Subataxic and ataxic doses of meprobamate shifted the stimulus response curves representative of facilitation and inhibition without altering its slope, whereas mephenesin decreased the slope of the curve itself. The actions of phenobarbital appeared to be less selective. De Salva and Oestler (1960) reported in spinal cats that inhibition and facilitation of patellar reflex responses produced by stimulation of the contralateral sciatic nerve were blocked to a greater extent than inhibition evoked by ipsilateral sciatic stimulation. Wilson and Talbot (1960) demonstrated in spinal cats given cumulative doses of meprobamate that recurrent facilitation was greatly reduced by total doses ranging from 210 to 400 mg/kg. The duration of recurrent inhibition was greatly increased, perhaps as a consequence of the removal of the convergent facilitatory background. Indeed, in experiments in which mixed responses were evoked and conditioning started with an inhibitory phase, meprobamate depressed facilitation, increased the depth of inhibition, and prolonged the interval between onset of inhibition and its reversal to facilitation.

Lynes and Williams (1958) observed in intact cats that meprobamate more readily suppressed facilitation of the patellar reflex evoked by stimulation of reticular sites than that produced by sciatic stimulation. By contrast, mephenesin had a greater effect on sciatic stimulation whereas barbiturates had little differential action. Ngai *et al.* (1966) demonstrated in decerebrate cats that polysynaptic reflex responses were susceptible to depression by meprobamate but became more resistant after spinal cord transection. However, monosynaptic reflexes were hardly affected either in decerebrate or spinal preparations. These results suggest that the site of action of meprobamate and other drugs with similar pharmacological actions may be within supraspinal structures.

2. Anticonvulsant Actions

Although effective against convulsions evoked by a wide variety of stimuli (Berger, 1966), meprobamate is remarkably effective in antagonizing the convulsant effects of pentylenetetrazole. Berger (1954) found that convulsions induced in mice by pentylenetetrazole (120 mg/kg) are prevented by 102 ± 9.5 mg/kg of meprobamate intraperitoneally and that fatalities are completely eliminated by 31 ± 2 mg/kg. By contrast, the median effective doses of mephenesin which protect against convulsions are over 420 mg/kg and against death are 235 ± 25 mg/kg. The effectiveness of meprobamate against these seizures has been subsequently demonstrated by DeSalva and Evans (1960), Maffii and Soncin (1958), Yen *et al.* (1964), and others. Indeed, Weiss and Ewing (1959) observed that intraperitoneal doses of 100 mg/kg were about equally as effective as trimethadione, 400 mg/kg, in antagonizing pentylenetetrazole seizures.

Meprobamate is effective to a somewhat lesser extent in preventing convulsions and death due to strychnine, although in this respect it is somewhat more potent than mephenesin (Berger, 1954). Similarly, meprobamate is also effective in counteracting the spasms accompanying tetanus. Perlstein (1959) found in humans that the intramuscular administration of 400 mg (about 6.5 mg/kg) abolished only the somatically induced spasms such as those induced by loud noises, bright lights, or pin prick. However, spasms produced by proprioceptive or visceral stimuli were not affected by meprobamate so that procedures such as aspirating the trachea, gagging the patient with a tongue depressor, or catheterizing the bladder could provoke seizures.

3. Taming Effect

The observation that the administration of meprobamate reduced hostility in monkeys without causing the animals to lose interest in their surroundings (Berger, 1954) led later investigators to study the actions of the drug on aggressivity and fear and to evaluate its effect on simple forms of learning and conditioning.

a. Effects on Aggressivity and Fear. Meprobamate ameliorates spontaneous or natural aggressivity in most animal species. Doses of 80 to 100 mg/kg, which have no hypnotic effect, reduced fighting among mice prompted by bringing a new animal into an established colony (Oelkers, 1957). Similarly, fighting among rabbits was lessened (Wolf and von Haxthausen, 1960), and the survival of wild hares in captivity was enhanced (Stern and Milin, 1959). Meprobamate reduced the intersexual aggressivity of the praying mantis *Mantis religiosa* (Mercier and Dessaigne, 1964). The fighting behavior of the Siamese fighting fish *Beta splendens* (Walaszek and Abood, 1956) and the guppy *Lebistes reticulatus* was lessened (Oelkers, 1960). Similarly, the hostility of cats produced by human handling was decreased by meprobamate, although there was some loss of sociability as shown by responses such as purring and mewing (Norton and deBeer, 1956). On the other hand, neither the aggressiveness of "killer rats," which attack and kill mice (Karli, 1959) nor the combative behavior of fighting bantam cocks (Hukovic and Stern, 1959) was altered, perhaps because these behavioral responses reflect very complex patterns of learned reactivity.

Meprobamate is also effective in reducing aggressivity evoked in animals by prolonged isolation, painful stimuli, the action of drugs and chemicals, and by surgical lesions of various parts of the brain. For example, aggressivity evoked in mice when these animals were isolated in individual cages for 2 or 3 weeks was abolished by meprobamate, 87 mg/kg, a dose which did not produce neurological deficit, decrease spontaneous activity, or impair the ability of the animals to function normally. By contrast, phenobarbital failed to abolish aggressivity and caused motor agitation (Mantegazzini *et al.*, 1960). Similar observations have been made by Yen *et al.* (1959) and others. Episodes of fighting produced in mice by electroshock to the feet were suppressed by meprobamate (Tedeschi *et al.*, 1959). Similarly, the drug ameliorated aggressive behavior elicited when mice were placed in cages with electrified floors (Randall *et al.*, 1960, 1961). The excitement and agitation induced by the administration of morphine, the injection of mescaline into the cerebral ventricles of cats, and the administration of 3,4-dihydroxyphenylalanine (dopa) were blocked by the administration of meprobamate or pretreatment with it (Silvestrini and Kohn, 1958; Rice and McColl, 1960; Yen *et al.*, 1970). The intraperitoneal administration of 50 to 150 mg/kg reduced by 14 to 88% the "hyperemotionality" produced in rats by surgical ablation of the olfactory bulb, although general activity was reduced to a roughly comparable extent (Kumadaki *et al.*, 1967). Along these lines, sham rage produced by septal forebrain lesions in the rat was offset by the administration of meprobamate (Hunt, 1957; Schallek *et al.*, 1962; Azuma, 1964). The fright or fearlike behavioral and electroencephalographic responses elicited by stimulation of hypothalamic nuclei were inhibited by the intravenous administration of 15 to 30 mg/kg to rabbits (Silvestrini and Kohn, 1958; Bovet *et al.*, 1957) and intraperitoneal doses of 25, 50, and 75 mg/kg to cats, although the largest of these doses produced ataxia (Baxter, 1968).

b. Effects on Conditioning. Although meprobamate does not ordinarily affect autonomic function, it ameliorates the visceral disturbances which are frequently associated with conditioning. Gantt and Newton (1960) observed in dogs that meprobamate, 800–1000 mg, did not diminish the acquisition of a motor-defense response but that it greatly diminished those disturbances in cardiac activity and blood pressure which accompanied conditioning. Similarly, Corson *et al.* (1961) reported that when antidiuretic responses were conditioned in water-loaded dogs by pairing auditory tones with electrical stimulation of the foreleg, diuresis was delayed and electrolytes such as sodium, chloride, and potassium were retained. Administration of meprobamate blocked these conditioned autonomic responses. Treated animals showed prompt diuresis and electrolyte elimination comparable to that of ordinary dogs and these animals continued to make motor-defense responses. Reduction of the autonomic concomitants of conditioning was also demonstrated in humans (Alexander, 1961). These actions may explain, in some instances, how meprobamate facilitates learning in animals and in humans (Berger and Potterfield, 1969).

Meprobamate does not interfere with the acquisition, performance, or extinction of conditioned operant responses reinforced either by negative (punishment) or positive (food) stimuli. Hughes and Kopmann (1960) and Hughes and Rountree (1961) found in rats that meprobamate, 50–100 mg/kg intraperitoneally, did not interfere with lever-pressing responses to avoid electroshock, although it reduced the behavioral responses made in anticipation of punishment. In contrast, phenobarbital (5–10 mg/kg) and ethanol (0.5–1.0 gm/kg) decreased lever-pressing performance and reduced behavioral reactivity. Similarly, Kelleher *et al.* (1961) found in rats that, except at neurotoxic doses, meprobamate did not alter disc-pressing responses to obtain food which was made available only after a fixed number of responses. Phenobarbital consistently produced a small increase in the average number of such responses. When rewards were given at fixed or variable intervals, or were reinforced only after long delays, response rates in control animals were consistently low. The administration of meprobamate increased the rate of responding whereas phenobarbital reduced it.

In more complex conditioned avoidance experiments in which the response was paired to both negative (shock) and positive (food) stimuli, meprobamate reduces avoidance more than approach responses. Geller and Seifter (1960) found that hungry rats given meprobamate, 120 mg/kg intraperitoneally, continued to press a lever to obtain food, despite electroshocks. Pentobarbital (5–15 mg/kg) and phenobarbital (5–10 mg/kg) produced a similar but very transient effect. In contrast, promazine (5–10 mg/kg) and *d*-amphetamine (0.5–2 mg/kg) decreased avoidance responses. Similarly, Ray (1962) showed that 40-mg/kg doses of meprobamate intraperitoneally, which had no significant effect on motor activity, blocked avoidance behavior and increased the latency of avoidance responses, while approach responses were less affected.

Meprobamate counteracts the effects of conditioned suppression, by which operant behavior is eliminated by unavoidable punishment. In relatively simple situations, meprobamate restored to some extent lever-pressing activities to obtain a reward that had been disrupted by unavoidable electroshock (Lauener, 1963). Meprobamate restored positively reinforced lever-pressing behavior in instances in which the activity was suppressed by reinforcement given at regular and variable time intervals (Geller, 1964). In experiments in which feeding behavior and water drinking were suppressed, meprobamate abolished the effects of such aversive conditioning (Naess and Rasmussen, 1958). If cats were given an electric shock whenever they touched a mouse, attack behavior was suppressed by three or more shocks. Small (18-mg/kg) doses of meprobamate restored this intraspecies aggressivity, and the animals attacked the mice despite continued electric shock (Sacra *et al.*, 1957).

In conflict situations in which animals seeking food or water are invariably punished or unsolvable problems are presented, meprobamate attenuates the resulting behavioral disturbances (Jacobsen, 1957; Feldman and Lewis, 1962; Tamura, 1963). It reduced paroxysmal inhibition or "freezing" of behavior which occurs in animals confronted by environmental threats (Davis, 1963). Meprobamate does not impair maze learning and performance in instances in which food and water are used as rewards. Under these circumstances meprobamate facilitated exploratory behavior by reducing fear without impairing activity. The length of time required to attain satisfactory performance was reduced as was the number of instances in which the animals entered blind pathways (Bloch and Silva, 1959; Marriott and Spencer, 1965).

4. Effects on Autonomic Nervous System

Meprobamate and similar drugs do not affect the autonomic nervous system, except after very large doses (Theobald *et al.*, 1965). Meprobamate had almost no effect on responses in isolated smooth muscles such as the intestine, ileum, colon, or seminal vesicles or in the exocrine glands or cardiovascular system caused by various substances such as acetylcholine, physostigmine, pilocarpine, and atropine (Berger, 1954). Cardiac action was not significantly altered. Disturbances in heart rate induced by myocardial infarction, ouabain, and strophanthin were ameliorated in dogs if meprobamate was administered jointly with quinidine (Arora *et al.*,

1962). Large doses decreased extrasystoles in the dog (Royer and Gantt, 1965). In a unique instance, syncope due to heart block was relieved in a human given ordinary clinical doses (Cooper and Davis, 1960). Generally, pulse was not changed except after large doses, and electrocardiographic changes were not observed. Arterial blood pressure was not altered except by near toxic doses and coronary or peripheral blood flow was not changed. Vasopressor responses induced by electrical stimulation of the brainstem, by carotid occlusion, or by the administration of drugs were not significantly reduced (Berger *et al.*, 1961; Kletzkin, 1966). Hypertensive responses to eserine were not changed (Varagic *et al.*, 1964). Similarly, respiration or gastrointestinal activity were not affected (Furuno, 1959; Bornmann, 1961). Except at near toxic doses, kidney function was not altered as demonstrated in animals or humans by renal function studies involving inulin or *p*-aminohippurate (PAH) clearance (Greene, 1963).

5. *Effects on Endocrine and Enzyme Systems*

Meprobamate does not significantly affect overall metabolic processes (Opitz, 1962a,b) and catabolic processes are not influenced. Oxygen consumption was not changed in mice, even after some animals were given thyroid extracts (Falciendo and Minola, 1958). Basal metabolism was not changed except after the administration of large doses (Laporte *et al.*, 1960; Lanza, 1966). Carbohydrate metabolism was generally not altered (Rafelsen, 1959). However, meprobamate caused some hyperglycemia in fasting animals and delayed the onset of insulin convulsions (Glassman *et al.*, 1958). It counteracted the effects of morphine-induced hyperglycemia (De Boer *et al.*, 1959). The administration of meprobamate to rats inhibited the increase in free fatty acids evoked by stress in rats (Khan *et al.*, 1964). It inhibited the formation of aortic plaques in monkeys (Frazier *et al.*, 1964) and slightly reduced the incidence and severity of aortic lesions in these animals possibly because of its ability to counteract stress (Wissler *et al.*, 1962).

Meprobamate does not cause any overall change in the enzyme activity of the brain (Albaum, 1962), and it does not inhibit monoamine oxidase (Bose and Vijayvargiya, 1960). Acetylcholinesterase levels in the dog brain were not altered by this drug (Mehta *et al.*, 1967). Cerebral lactic acid levels were reduced by administration of 40 mg/kg (Mathé and Kassay, 1969). Similarly, in the hypothalamus, but not in the cerebral cortex, there was a slight reduction in brain adenosine triphosphate activity (Decsi and Mehes, 1959). In addition, acetylcholine levels appeared to be increased (Malhotra and Mehta, 1966). These changes may be correlated with the neurophysiological actions of the drug on the limbic system.

Meprobamate does not have any significant effect on most enzyme systems (Koizumi, 1961). Its administration reduced phosphorylase activity in skeletal muscles (Kocsar *et al.*, 1960). Granick (1966) suggested that meprobamate as well as other drugs induced the synthesis of δ-aminolevulinic acid synthetase in chick embryo liver *in vitro* and caused a porphyria-like condition which mimicked the inheritable human disease. Although Racz and Marks (1969) reported that meprobamate had only negligible activity on porphyrin synthesis in mouse liver, porphyria-like states have been reported on very rare occasions in humans (Condaese *et al.*, 1965).

The administration of meprobamate in doses comparable to those used clinically does not alter adrenal–pituitary function. The histological appearance of adrenal tissues was not changed and meprobamate did not compensate for adrenal hypertrophy (Cabrini and Metalli, 1957; Georges *et al.*, 1961). Circadian variations in plasma 17-hydroxycorticosteroid (17-OCHS) levels were not altered (Krieger and Krieger, 1967). Meprobamate did not modify the release of epinephrine from tissues except during insulin shock when it slightly inhibited the increase in corticosteroid content of rat plasma and reduced its eosinophilic effects (Milcu *et al.*, 1958; Kroneberg and Schumann, 1959; Pekkarinen *et al.*, 1963; Weil-Malherbe and Posner, 1963). Along these lines, Makela *et al.* (1959) showed that the administration of large (450 mg/kg) doses to rats by stomach tube inhibited adrenal responses to the stresses of intense light, noise, or prodding with a blunt instrument. Similar observations have been made by others. Meprobamate, unlike chlorpromazine, has not been shown to alter significantly the release of antidiuretic hormones (Ben-David, 1963; Khazan *et al.*, 1963) or prolactin in dogs (Danon, 1963). Reports on the effects of meprobamate on the secretion of intermedin with subsequent dispersion of pigment in melanophores are consistent with an absence of hypophyseal effect (Robinson and Scott, 1960; Scott, 1965; Melnick, 1966).

Thyroid function is not significantly altered by the administration of therapeutic or comparable doses to animals or man (Newman and Fish, 1958; Fischetti and Inselvini, 1959; Molcan *et al.*, 1963), although Friedell (1958) reported that meprobamate significantly reduced elevated levels of iodine uptake in anxious patients. Meprobamate does not affect the estrus cycle in mice even in doses 5 times greater than those used clinically (Döring and Heller, 1960). However, very large doses caused persistent diestrus, particularly when administered for long periods of time (Cranston, 1958; Stegmann and Burger, 1960). Palmieri (1964) did not observe any significant histological changes in the uterus, ovaries, or vaginal mucosa after administration of 77 mg/kg a day for 20 days to mice—a dose equivalent to five human daily therapeutic doses. Indeed, Brar (1969) showed that the chronic oral administration of meprobamate, 180–280 mg/kg, to mice for 30 weeks did not cause changes in the estrus cycle, fertility, duration of gestation, litter size, and viability and development of offspring. There was no evidence of teratogenicity or drug-related abnormalities in the body organs and tissues of the treated animals.

6. *Neurophysiological Actions*

Many extensive investigations have been made of the effect of meprobamate on the electroencephalogram (EEG), both on spontaneous and evoked brain activity. In general, it has been found that ordinary doses have little or no effect on the spontaneous electrical activity of the various brain structures. Responses which are evoked within the limbic system, which is apparently correlated with many emotional processes, are inhibited by meprobamate and other antianxiety tranquilizers as well.

a. Effect on Spontaneous Brain Activity. Meprobamate, in doses of 10 to 20 mg/kg intravenously which decrease muscle tone and exert a marked tranquilizing action in unanesthetized, noncurarized cats or rabbits, produced some synchronization of cerebral electrical activity characterized by high-amplitude, low-frequency slow waves most evident in the thalamus. There were no changes in the spontaneous activity of the midbrain reticular formation, limbic system, respiratory nuclei, or hypothalamus (Berger, 1957; Hendley *et al.*, 1957; Himwich, 1962). The cerebral cortex was not affected, even after the intravenous administration of 40 mg/kg to intact cats (Gangloff, 1959), although with larger doses a slight slowing of cortical activity may occur (Schallek *et al.*, 1962). These observations confirmed studies by Chauchard and Mazoue (1956a,b) and others who showed that comparable doses of meprobamate did not depress the excitability of motor areas of the cerebral cortex. Larger doses (40–80 mg/kg) produced definite increases in slow waves (Magyar, 1960). Even greater doses (100–200 mg/kg) produced further flattening of spontaneous brain wave activity (Longo, 1962).

In humans, the single administration of a 400-mg therapeutic dose of meprobamate does not alter spontaneous brain activity. Indeed, the daily administration of meprobamate up to 1600 mg did not generally change basic electroencephalogram patterns. Alpha rhythms were not altered in frequency and voltage. The average duration and latency of responses were not modified (Glotfelty and Wilson, 1956). Occasionally, barbiturate-like fast-wave activity has been observed, particularly after large doses (Henry and Obrist, 1958). This pattern is characterized by spindling, most pronounced in the parietal area, but it differs from barbiturate spindling which is more general and displayed in the frontal, frontotemporal, or parietal areas (Pfeiffer *et al.*, 1957). Under such circumstances, paroxysmal electroencephalogram changes have been noted after photic stimulation (Bokonjic and Trojaborg, 1960). Even larger doses may evoke such responses more frequently. For example, fast activity was observed in 10 of 12 psychiatric patients given 10 gm daily (Shagass *et al.*, 1959). After the administration of toxic amounts, this increased fast activity persisted even during unconsciousness. Frequencies of less than 6 cps were almost never seen. The electroencephalogram usually returned to its ordinary configuration within 48 hours (Berger, 1963).

b. Effect on Evoked Responses. Meprobamate does not consistently alter the cortical actions of many drugs. For example, responses evoked by *N*,*N*-diethyl-D-lysergamide (LSD-25), ergot alkaloids, dihydroclavine, or dihydroemyloclavine were not altered (Pierre and Cahn, 1957; Yui and Takeo, 1958; Sasaki, 1959; Berger *et al.*, 1964). Yet, meprobamate antagonized the electroencephalographic effects of amphetamine, eserine, hydrocortisone, and other drugs (Silvestrini and Kohn, 1958; Katona *et al.*, 1963). Benactyzine has been shown to potentiate the action of meprobamate in decreasing the duration of limbic seizures produced by electrical stimulation of the fornix (Berger *et al.*, 1967).

Moderately large doses of meprobamate do not greatly alter the overall functioning of the midbrain reticular formation which in part mediates wakefulness and sleep. Gangloff (1959) showed in cats immobilized by gallamine that the intravenous administration of 10 mg/kg inhibited recruiting responses evoked by stimulation of the thalamocortical projections, which constitute the upper part of the activating system. In contrast, the administration of doses up to 80 mg/kg did not alter arousal responses produced by stimulation of the midbrain reticular structures, the other moiety. In cats with midbrain lesions, intravenous 10–20-mg/kg doses increased the threshold for arousal but did not alter the threshold for thalamic recruiting. Bradley and Key (1959) found in *encéphale isolé* preparations that meprobamate (40 mg/kg) neither produced any change in the arousal threshold nor altered cortical activity. Takaori and Ohato (1962) observed that 20-mg/kg intravenous doses had no effect on arousal elicited in high spinal cats by stimulation of the midbrain reticular formation but that larger (50–80-mg/kg) doses shortened the duration of electroencephalographic arousal. Other investigators have made similar observations.

Responses produced by auditory stimulation are not modified by the intravenous administration of 40 mg/kg to cats immobilized by succinylcholine. No significant changes could be observed in responses measured in the medial geniculate nucleus and other specific ascending pathways of the reticular activating system. Consequently, Kletzkin and Swan (1959) concluded that the action of meprobamate cannot be attributed to a selective depression of the reticular activating system.

Subsequent neurophysiological investigation has provided evidence that the tranquilizing effects of meprobamate can be attributed, to a considerable extent, to its effects on the limbic system, an area in which emotional behavior is correlated with the discriminative activities of the cerebral cortex (Kletzkin, 1962). Kletzkin and Berger (1959) showed that the intravenous administration of 20 mg/kg to unanesthetized cats that were immobilized with succinylcholine shortened the duration of afterdischarges evoked by electrical stimulation of the limbic system. Prior to administration of the drug, after discharges from the hippocampus and amygdala persisted for 54 seconds. Ten minutes after administration of the drug, afterdischarges were reduced in duration to only 18 seconds and did not reappear when stimulation was repeated 10 minutes later. Fifty minutes after administration of meprobamate, afterdischarges, although present, were still markedly shorter in duration than before the drug. Responses produced by stimulation of the amygdala seemed to be somewhat more sensitive to the effects of meprobamate than the hippocampus. Activation of the cerebral cortex and hippocampus produced by stimulation of the midbrain reticular formation was not altered. Subsequent studies confirmed these observations (Gogerty *et al.*, 1965; Takagi and Ban, 1960), although some conflicting evidence has been presented (Kobayashi and Ishikawa, 1965).

7. *Toxicity*

The toxicity of meprobamate is relatively low and the ratio between the effective and lethal doses is greater generally than with barbiturates. Data on the acute toxicity of meprobamate in small laboratory animals are summarized in Table IX.

Chronic toxicity studies in dogs showed that animals given 1 gm daily for 60 to 75 days remained in good condition, ate well, and gained weight. Urine analysis and other laboratory tests remained within normal limits. Histopathological examination at autopsy showed no abnormalities of the kidney, stomach, small intestine, liver, bladder, or adrenal glands. The addition of meprobamate (0.5%) to the diet of newly weaned rats for 15 weeks caused no changes in body weight, although somes losses were seen after feeding a diet containing 1 or 2% for this period. Hema-

TABLE IX

ACUTE LETHAL DOSES OF DICARBAMATE COMPOUNDS

Compound	i.p.	i.v.	p.o.
	Mouse, LD_{50} (mg/kg)[a]		
Meprobamate	800 ± 15(a)[b]	482 ± 33(a)	1100 ± 44(a)
	736 ± 53(b)	450 ± 27(b)	1100 ± 176(c)
Mebutamate	460 ± 39(e)	390(f)	550 ± 40(e)
Carisoprodol	1150 ± 84(g)	165(i)	2340 ± 236(h)
	980 ± 78(h)	165 ± 20(h)	3400(j)
Tybamate	540 ± 13(k)	254 ± 13(k)	830 ± 65(k)
	Rat, LD_{50} (mg/kg)[a,b]		
Meprobamate	545 ± 40(a)	—[c]	1600 ± 163(a)
			1522 ± 16(d)
Mebutamate	410 ± 37(e)	300(f)	1400(f)
			1160 ± 73(e)
Carisoprodol	450 ± 61(h)	—[c]	1320 ± 109(h)
			1350 ± 150(g)
Tybamate	465 ± 39(k)	—[c]	1350 ± 150(g)
			1040 ± 94(k)

[a] LD_{50} = lethal dose 50%; i.p. = intraperitoneally; i.v. = intravenously; p.o. = orally.

[b] Key to references.
(a) Berger (1954)
(b) Randall *et al.* (1960)
(c) De Salva *et al.* (1959)
(d) Yeary *et al.* (1966)
(e) Berger *et al.* (1961)
(f) Preti (1961)
(g) Carroll *et al.* (1961)
(h) Berger *et al.* (1959)
(i) O'Dell (1961)
(j) Hofrichter *et al.* (1967)
(k) Berger *et al.* (1964)

[c] Data not available.

tological examination and autopsy of animals consuming 2% meprobamate in their diet for 9 months revealed no statistically significant drug-related changes (Berger, 1954).

Swinyard *et al.* (1957) suggested that tolerance to the anticonvulsant actions of meprobamate occurred in mice. In animals not previously treated with the drug, the oral administration of 300 mg/kg increased the electroshock seizure threshold tenfold. In animals which had been given a total daily dose of 1200 mg/kg for 7 days, then 1800 mg/kg for 10 more days, the same dose of the drug increased the seizure threshold only 2.5-fold. Along these lines, Essig (1958) observed that convulsions occurred in dogs after the abrupt withdrawal of daily doses of 8.0 to 8.6 gm which had been given for 75 to 130 days. Margolin *et al.* (1965) made similar observations in dogs upon the abrupt withdrawal of doses which had been gradually increased over a 6-month period to 570 mg/kg. In these experiments, the doses were at least 25 times greater than those given therapeutically to humans. In dogs made dependent on barbital by prolonged administration, Deneau and Weiss (1968) found that meprobamate, 150 mg/kg, could be substituted for sodium barbital (100 mg/kg) to prevent the occurrence of withdrawal syndromes. Withdrawal symptoms have been observed on rare occasions in humans, most frequently in persons previously dependent on alcohol or barbiturates, who subsequently took large doses of meprobamate for prolonged periods.

B. Mebutamate

Mebutamate has hypotensive actions of a unique and distinctive nature. It differs from other antihypertensive agents in that it probably acts directly on the brainstem medullary vasomotor centers to cause changes in blood pressure and blood flow without reducing cardiac output. It differs sharply from those substances that act on the arteriolar smooth muscles directly and from those that reduce blood volume by increasing the excretion of electrolytes. It also differs from those substances that act on the autonomic nervous system by affecting catecholamines or by interfering with ganglionic transmission (Berger, 1962).

Berger *et al.* (1961) observed that in unanesthetized, normotensive rabbits, the intraperitoneal administration of doses of 18 mg/kg evoked a mild hypotensive effect and 37 mg/kg produced statistically significant reductions of both systolic and diastolic blood pressure. Similarly, mebutamate consistently lowered blood pressure in normotensive rats. The intravenous administration of mebutamate, 20 mg/kg, to 8 dogs anesthetized with sodium pentobarbital reduced mean blood pressure by 36 ± 8.5 mm Hg within 5 minutes. This action persisted for 15 to 45 minutes. Moreover, mebutamate effectively antagonized pressor responses evoked in animals by various mechanisms not only by reducing increased blood pressure but by raising the threshold at which responses could be evoked and by limiting the magnitude of these changes. Even after supramaximal stimulation, vasopressor responses were blocked to a considerable extent. Mebutamate did not appear to have any adverse effect on the heart, blood circulation, or kidney function. The administration of suitable doses of mebutamate produced muscle relaxation and paralysis which sometimes was preceded by excitement. During paralysis, respiration and heart action were not impaired and the pinna and corneal reflexes remained intact. The anticonvulsant action was qualitatively similar to that of meprobamate. Mebutamate did not appear to have a significant effect on autonomic function in general. Early studies suggested that its most characteristic pharmacological actions were (*1*) its effects on blood pressure which are not accompanied by adverse effects on the heart or blood circulation, (*2*) its interneuronal blocking effects, and (*3*) its lack of effect on the autonomic nervous system.

1. Effects on Blood Pressure

Subsequent studies confirmed that mebutamate has a hypotensive effect in normotensive animals (Iwaki *et al.*, 1967; Preti, 1961) and in humans (Baldrighi *et al.*, 1962). Similar responses have been seen in intact anesthetized animals (Rowe *et al.*, 1962; Taccardi *et al.*, 1961), although occasionally barbiturate anesthesia may obscure these effects. Reduction of arterial blood pressure was more pronounced in hypotensive subjects than in normotensives. Generally, the effect was greater as larger doses were given, but the dose–effect relationship may not be strictly linear. The effects of the drug are usually observed within 1 to 2 hours after oral or intraperitoneal administration and persist up to 6 hours (Berger *et al.*, 1961; Morin *et al.*, 1963; Stanton and White, 1965).

Many studies have demonstrated that mebutamate effectively antagonizes pressor responses. Mebutamate reduced by two-thirds the increase in blood pressure elicited by electrical stimulation of the mesencephalon or medulla. Hypertension produced by stimulation of the hypothalamus appeared to be most sensitive to the action of the drug which reduced such pressor effects to about 40% of predrug values. The pressor response evoked by bilateral carotid occlusion in pentobarbital-anesthetized dogs was also reduced by intravenous doses of 10 mg/kg or larger, even after pretreatment with atropine or section of the carotid sinus or glossopharyngeal nerves. The depressor response produced in anesthetized dogs by peripheral vagal stimulation was only slightly reduced after mebutamate, 20 mg/kg, intravenously (Berger *et al.*, 1961). Kayaalp (1966) showed that the pressor response to carotid occlusion was reduced 12–66% of predrug values after the intravenous administration of 10, 20, and 40 mg/kg to anesthetized cats immobilized with gallamine. The pressor responses and bradycardia evoked by endocranial hypertension were reduced by the administration of mebutamate (Baldrighi *et al.*, 1962), and the hypertensive response to stimulation of the right vagus nerve was abolished by 25 to 30 mg/kg (DeCaro *et al.*, 1962). Stanton and White (1965) confirmed earlier observations that mebutamate reduced hypertension elicited in uninephrectomized rats by the acute or chronic administration of Doca. Mebutamate depressed the pressor response evoked by physostigmine and inhibited its action in mobilizing free fatty acids (Westermann and Stock, 1963).

a. Effects on the Heart. Mebutamate does not have a significant effect on the heart. It did not markedly affect the electrocardiogram of dogs or humans with normal heart rhythm (Berger *et al.*, 1964; Mulinos *et al.*, 1961). Mebutamate had a protective action against tachycardia induced in guinea pigs by strophanthin or hypertensin, even when the animals were greatly disturbed by environmental stress (Marino, 1964; Marino *et al.*, 1963). Similarly, mebutamate reduced disturbances in heart rate elicited in dogs by stimulation of the *ruber nucleus* or its neural connections (Carroll *et al.*, 1968). Angiospasm elicited by audiogenic stimulation was ameliorated (Taccola, 1965). Extrasystoles which frequently accompany autonomic conditioning were reduced by large doses (Royer and Gantt, 1965). These cardioprotective actions have been observed in humans (Bosisio and Scaglietti, 1962; Montemartini *et al.*, 1963). Nonetheless, some transient tachycardia was noted after the rapid administration of the compound in propylene glycol solution to anesthetized animals (Elliott, 1969; Rowe *et al.*, 1962). Some changes in the rate and amplitude of contractions of the isolated heart of the guinea pig and the toad *Bufo Marinus* have been reported after perfusion with 500 μg (Kurtz *et al.*, 1965), but no changes were observed in the activity of the isolated heart muscle of the rabbit after perfusion with concentrations of 1:10,000 (Preti, 1961; Taccardi *et al.*, 1961).

b. Effects on Blood Circulation. Mebutamate does not adversely affect circulatory dynamics. The intravenous administration of 20 mg/kg to phenobarbital-anesthetized dogs significantly reduced femoral arterial pressure but did not alter arterial or venous rates of flow in the femoral artery. Coronary blood flow was augmented to a statistically significant extent. Cardiac output was not changed. Pulmonary arterial blood pressure was slightly decreased, but blood flow in the pulmonary artery was not changed. The administration of 20 mg/kg intravenously did not alter blood pressure or flow in the renal artery (Baldrighi *et al.*, 1961; Berger *et al.*, 1961; Rowe *et al.*, 1962; DeCaro *et al.*, 1963). Mebutamate, like meprobamate, has no significant renal effects in laboratory animals or in man. Serum electrolytes were not affected in dogs given mebutamate, 10–50 mg/kg intravenously. A slight reduction in PAH (but not inulin) clearance was reported, but no significant changes were observed in glomerular filtration rate. Neither water and electrolyte excretion was altered nor was diuresis changed (Grisler and Finulli, 1962; Greene, 1963; Bert *et al.*, 1964).

Although it does not appear to have a direct vasodilator effect on peripheral blood vessels, mebutamate effectively lowers vascular resistance in coronary vessels and causes significant reduction in pulmonary vascular resistance. Administration of the compound caused a decrease in total peripheral resistance (Berger *et al.*, 1961; Margolin *et al.*, 1963; Rowe *et al.*, 1962).

2. Effects on Spinal Interneurons

Mebutamate, 20 mg/kg, is as effective as mephenesin in selectively inhibiting polysynaptic reflexes to a greater extent than monosynaptic arcs (Margolin *et al.*, 1963). Unlike some antihypertensive drugs, mebutamate did not significantly alter postural reflexes in animals (Vargas *et al.*, 1965) or in humans (Sibilia and Stoppoloni, 1962). Mebutamate is as effective as carisoprodol in protecting animals from convulsions and death due to pentylenetetrazole, although this action is much less than that of meprobamate. Mebutamate is as effective as meprobamate in protecting against strychnine convulsions, but it is less effective in preventing death due to this convulsant. Mebutamate is about half as effective as meprobamate in preventing extensor tonic electroshock seizures (Berger *et al.*, 1961). Its antitetanic activity is of a magnitude comparable to that of meprobamate (Bhargava and Srivastava, 1965).

3. Effects on the Autonomic Nervous System

Mebutamate appears to have no significant autonomic effects. Unlike sympathetic ganglionic blocking agents, mebutamate did not modify vasopressor effects or vascular actions of epinephrine (Della Bella *et al.*, 1964; Kayaalp, 1966; Lamperi *et al.*, 1962; Preti, 1961; Varagic and Vojvodic, 1962). In contrast to parasympatholytic agents, mebutamate was relatively ineffective in reducing the hypotensive response elicited by stimulation of the vagus nerve (Berger *et al.*, 1961; DeCaro *et al.*, 1962). It did not modify circulatory responses to acetylcholine or to norepinephrine and did not interfere with the synthesis or release of norepinephrine or alter its effects at receptor sites (Preti, 1961; Jori *et al.*, 1964; Kayaalp, 1966).

Spasms of the isolated guinea pig ileum were unaffected by mebutamate in concentrations of 1:15,000, and spasms induced by acetylcholine chloride (0.05 μg/ml) or histamine diphosphate (0.2 μg/ml) were reduced in magnitude by mebutamate 1:10,000 but not affected by this drug in a concentration of 1:20,000. Spasms produced in isolated segments of rat colon by serotonin creatinin sulfate (2.0 μg/ml) were not influenced by mebutamate (1:30,000) (Berger *et al.*, 1961).

4. *Neurophysiological Effects and Site of Action*

Cross-circulation experiments showed that when mebutamate, 20 mg/kg, was injected into the femoral artery of a dog connected only by the intact sciatic nerve to another dog, arterial and venous blood flow significantly increased in an isolated hindlimb of the recipient animal, although none of the drug entered its circulation. This hypotensive action was evident only as long as nerve trunks which connected the isolated perfused limb with the brain were intact. These findings suggested that the primary site of action of mebutamate was the central nervous system (Berger *et al.*, 1961).

Kletzkin (1966) measured the effects of mebutamate on pressor responses produced by stimulating one brainstem vasomotor area and recording the effects in a second region. This drug, like phenobarbital, attenuated pressor responses evoked from the medulla, hypothalamus, and mesencephalon. It enhanced the later phases of the evoked responses and caused trains of slow waves to appear after single shock stimuli. By contrast, phenobarbital suppressed the early phases of such evoked responses. After stimulation was terminated, the spontaneous electrical activity of these areas was altered as shown by decreased frequency and increased amplitude of the electroencephalogram. Neither meprobamate nor reserpine altered the electrophysiological activity of the vasomotor centers. These studies confirm earlier observations which indicate that mebutamate acts primarily on the central nervous system.

Margolin *et al.* (1963) suggested that mebutamate acts on spinal vasomotor centers as well. In trunk-to-limb cross-circulation experiments on dogs with intact vagi, an isolated hindlimb was perfused through the femoral artery and blood was returned to the donor through the femoral vein. Intravenous injection of 20 mg/kg into the trunk of the recipient animal caused a sharp, sustained increase in arterial and venous blood flow in the limb perfused by the donor. A significant decrease in arterial peripheral resistance was observed and blood pressure within the limb was not changed. In head-to-trunk experiments in dogs with intact vagi in which the spinal cord was intact, the vascularly isolated head of the recipient dog was perfused from the common carotid of a donor animal. Intravenous injection of 20 mg/kg into the trunk of the recipient animal caused an almost twofold increase in peripheral limb blood flow in the recipient, and femoral arterial blood pressure and peripheral resistance were significantly decreased. The magnitude of these circulatory changes was reduced when the spinal cord was sectioned in the lumbar region (L_2) but not when the spinal cord was severed at the C_2 level. Conversely, injection of mebutamate, 20 mg/kg, into the perfused head through the carotid arterial flow from the donor did not increase recipient femoral arterial blood flow or change femoral arterial blood pressure or alter peripheral resistance. In the same kind of animal preparations, meprobamate (20 mg/kg) regularly failed to elicit a hypotensive effect. These findings suggested that, as an interneuronal blocking agent, mebutamate has a very selective action on spinal vasomotor pathways and differs from meprobamate which acts on spinal motor tracts. Additional evidence to support this hypothesis was drawn from experiments in which mebutamate was administered intrathecally at levels of the second, third, and fourth lumbar vertebrae. Doses of 1 mg/kg significantly increased peripheral blood flow and reduced blood pressure and peripheral resistance in the femoral artery. The same intrathecal doses of meprobamate or phenobarbital did not produce significant changes. Although intrathecal administration of lidocaine increased limb blood flow, this effect was accompanied by the complete loss of skeletal muscle tone typical of spinal anesthesia. Under these circumstances, the same doses of mebutamate did not cause skeletal muscle relaxation.

Wang and his colleagues (1966) offered some evidence to support these conclusions on the basis of experiments which evaluated the actions of mebutamate in antagonizing pressor responses elicited by brainstem stimulation in head-to-trunk cross-circulation experiments. The vascular and peripheral nerve connections, including the vagi, between the head and neck of the recipients were severed before the animals were perfused from the carotids of donor dogs. As Margolin *et al.* (1963) observed, mebutamate had a hypotensive effect when given to the trunk circulation of the recipient animal but elicited no significant action when administered to the vascularly isolated head. This suggested to these investigators that the site of action was not in the medullary vasomotor center but rather in the spinal cord or more peripheral structures. Moreover, Wang *et al.* (1966) showed that resting splanchnic nerve activity was increased by mebutamate, 20 mg/kg intravenously, in intact cats but decreased in animals in which the cervical vagi and carotid sinus nerves were severed. Indeed, mebutamate inhibited the responses of the urinary bladder to pelvic nerve stimulation and reduced vagal bradycardia by increasing the threshold for vagal slowing. Contrary to the findings of Berger *et al.* (1961) and others, these investigators also reported that the intravenous administration of 20 mg/kg consistently reduced the pressor response to epinephrine, 2–4 μg/kg. Vascular responses to norepinephrine, 1–2 μg/kg, were not changed. On this basis, Wang and his colleagues concluded that mebutamate had substantial actions on the peripheral parts of the sympathetic nervous system.

Elliott (1969), however, concluded that the depressant effects of mebutamate on the sympathetic nervous system were of small magnitude and that its actions were predominantly upon the central nervous system. The action of mebutamate in antagonizing pressor responses evoked from brainstem vasomotor areas was studied in phenobarbital-anesthetized cats in which the vagi were severed. At the same time, the central sympathetic system was stimulated, or epinephrine or norepinephrine was injected intravenously. Nonetheless, the intravenous administration of mebutamate, 20 mg/kg, promptly reduced pressor responses to medullary stimulation by 11 to 36% in animals in which the carotid sinus was intact and by 42 to 74% when the carotid sinus was denervated. Responses to catecholamines administered at the same time pressor responses were evoked were diminished to a slight extent—less than 10 to 15%. No major action on the heart or afferent nervous system could be demonstrated.

5. *Toxicity*

The acute toxicity of mebutamate in mice and rats is summarized in Table IX. Mebutamate incorporated into the diet of rats in concentrations of 0.5 and 1.0% for 28 weeks neither interfered with growth nor produced any abnormal signs or symptoms in these animals. Two percent mebutamate in the diet caused a decreased rate of growth apparently because of reduced food intake. Pathological findings of significance were not evident in animals given 2% mebutamate for 28 weeks. The administration of this drug to dogs at the rate of 100 mg/kg, 5 days a week, for 6 months did not produce any unusual hematology or significant histopathological changes in the organs of these animals (Berger *et al.*, 1961).

C. Carisoprodol

Although carisoprodol resembles mephenesin and meprobamate in some respects, its skeletal muscle relaxant actions are more profound and occur more quickly. In addition, carisoprodol demonstrates unusual analgesic properties. Unlike mephenesin and meprobamate, carisoprodol has no taming effects, and it does not modify conditioned avoidance behavior. Carisoprodol mildly affects the autonomic nervous system, but these actions are transient and do not seem to be clinically significant. These pharmacological effects are correlated with its neurophysiological actions which are substantially different from those of meprobamate and other *N*-unsubstituted propanediol dicarbamates.

Berger *et al.* (1959) observed that in mice, the intraperitoneal administration of carisoprodol in doses of 180 mg/kg produces reversible paralysis of voluntary muscles which persists for nearly 15 minutes in 50 to 70% of the animals. The time interval between intraperitoneal administration of 280 mg/kg to mice and the onset of its paralytic effects is about 6 minutes after carisoprodol but about 33 minutes after meprobamate. The duration of action under these conditions is about 37 minutes for carisoprodol as compared to about 91 minutes for meprobamate. In mice, immediately prior to the onset of flaccid paralysis, there may be some signs of excitement. During paralysis, at minimal effective doses, tremors and twitching are absent, and there is no evidence of impairment of respiration or heart beat. The animals respond to painful stimulation by withdrawing or turning the body. Even during complete paralysis, the leg responds promptly to sciatic nerve stimulation, indicating that the peripheral nerve, interneuronal junction, and muscle itself are not significantly affected. The righting reflex is abolished. The corneal reflex is blocked in half of the animals by the administration of 310 mg/kg, but larger doses are required to suppress the pinna reflex. The administration of intraperitoneal doses larger than 1 gm/kg in mice produces death from respiratory paralysis. The heart continues to beat for a few minutes after respiration ceases. Similar responses occur in other animals, except that excitement may not be observed before the onset of paralysis.

Carisoprodol is remarkably effective in abolishing decerebrate rigidity. As little as 3 mg/kg given intravenously is sufficient to abolish completely spasticity in cats due to decerebration. It appears that carisoprodol is about 8 times more potent in this respect than mephenesin or meprobamate, since 24-mg/kg doses of these drugs are required to achieve a comparable effect. In addition to its unusual muscle relaxant properties, carisoprodol has a striking effect on pain produced by injection of silver nitrate into the joints of rats, although it shows no analgesic action when evaluated by commonly used pharmacological tests for analgesia, such as the hot plate test or procedures involving withdrawal from a painful stimulus as a measure of analgesic activity. The early pharmacological studies suggested that the most characteristic actions of carisoprodol were (*1*) its effects on voluntary muscles and (*2*) its analgesic action (Berger *et al.*, 1959).

1. Effects on Voluntary Muscles

The effects of carisoprodol on skeletal muscle have been appraised by many investigators, using techniques similar to those employed for the evaluation of meprobamate, in mice (Frommel *et al.*, 1960b), rats (Matthews *et al.*, 1963), rabbits (Del Castillo and Nelson, 1963), dogs (Cahn and Herold, 1967), and in humans by electromyography and other objective tests (Campbell and Green, 1965; Hofrichter *et al.*, 1967; Levine *et al.*, 1960).

a. Effects on Muscle Tone. Diamantis and Kletzkin (1966) showed that in rabbits with normal skeletal muscle tone, carisoprodol is twice as active as tybamate or mephenesin, 8 times more active than meprobamate, and 20 times as active as methocarbamol in terms of the ratios between mean paralyzing and lethal doses. Other investigators have reported similar findings. Carisoprodol produces loss of the righting reflex in rats after doses which are about one-fourth of the oral lethal dose. Mephenesin abolishes the righting reflex only after administration of three-fourths or more of the mean lethal dose (Carroll *et al.*, 1961). Similarly, Del Castillo and Nelson (1960) and others confirmed the earlier observations of Berger *et al.* (1959) that carisoprodol effectively abolishes decerebrate rigidity. The tonic component of the mechanically elicited stretch reflex is depressed to a greater extent than the phasic response. Some observers, however, disagree about the relative potencies of carisoprodol, mephenesin, and meprobamate in abolishing decerebrate rigidity (Chin and Smith, 1962).

b. Effects on Motor Activity. The intravenous administration of 5 to 10 mg/kg to unrestrained intact animals did not significantly alter spontaneous motor activity, although occasionally small doses produced excitement (Berger *et al.*, 1959, 1960; O'Dell, 1961). The administration of carisoprodol seemed less likely than mephenesin or meprobamate to impair the ability of rats to hang on a vertical or inclined plane (Stille, 1962; Hofrichter *et al.*, 1967). Relatively large doses (of about 260 mg/kg in mice or 305 mg/kg in rats) which also cause sedation, hypnosis, and a loss of the righting reflex significantly altered motor performance (Hoffmeister, 1964).

c. Effects on Spinal Reflexes. Carisoprodol has a slight but definite effect on reflex excitability. Doses of 5 to 10 mg/kg blocked the potentiation of spinal reflexes produced in decerebrate cats by the action of physostigmine (eserine), 0.1–0.2 mg/kg. Pretreatment with atropine blocked the antagonistic action of carisoprodol on physostigmine-enhanced reflexes (Del Castillo and Nelson, 1963). Like meprobamate, carisoprodol depressed in intact animals polysynaptic reflexes more profoundly than monosynaptic arcs (Berger *et al.*, 1959, 1960; Inoki *et al.*, 1961). Larger doses were required to abolish the more complex linguomandibular reflex (Carroll *et al.*, 1961), although O'Dell (1961) reported that, in pentobarbital-anesthetized dogs, carisoprodol, 20–30 mg/kg, given intravenously caused a dose-related increase in the flexor and linguomandibular reflexes. Fukuda *et al.* (1968) observed in young chicks that the depressant effects of carisoprodol on polysynaptic crossed extensor reflexes were about twice as great in intact as in spinal animals and suggested that this demonstrated that carisoprodol acted principally on supraspinal levels. Support for this mode of action was provided by Del Castillo and Nelson (1960) who found that even large injections (70 mg/kg) did not alter inhibition of the patellar reflex in cat preparations, decerebrated by intercollicular sectioning, in which either facilitatory or inhibitory sites of the brainstem were stimulated at supramaximal intensity. However, 10-mg/kg doses markedly depressed facilitation of this arc and 15–20 mg/kg completely blocked the patellar reflex for 120 minutes or longer. Similarly, carisoprodol, 3 mg/kg, suppressed the enhancement of reflex activity evidenced by the prolonged increase in the amplitude of spinal reflexes after facilitatory stimuli. In contrast, mephenesin depressed both facilitation and inhibition in decerebrate preparations. Subsequent studies (Del Castillo and Nelson, 1963) showed that when both facilitatory and inhibitory sites in the brainstem were stimulated at submaximal intensity, inhibition of the patellar reflex was augmented by doses of carisoprodol as small as 1–2 mg/kg. Reductions of 25 to 40% in the amplitude of the knee jerk were completely inhibited by 10 to 15 mg/kg, probably because of the profound depression of facilitation. Neither mephenesin nor meprobamate was capable of augmenting such spinal inhibition. When facilitatory and inhibitory stimulation were alternated, carisoprodol tended to augment inhibition, although 20 mg/kg was required to reduce muscle tension evoked in nonactivated preparations by stretching the soleus or gastrocnemius muscles. Jurna (1965) found that facilitation evoked in intercollicular decerebrate cats by stimulation of the brainstem was markedly depressed by intravenous doses of 5 mg/kg. Doses twice as large were required to depress facilitation elicited at spinal levels by stimulation of ipsilateral cutaneous nerves. Carisoprodol, 5 mg/kg, reduced the frequency of discharge of muscle spindles caused by reticular stimulation, but 10 mg/kg was required to produce this effect after stimulation of ipsilateral cutaneous nerves, indicating that carisoprodol depresses facilitation in the gamma motoneurons. Facilitatory responses in the alpha motoneurons are depressed as well. Doses of 5 mg/kg inhibited potentiation of the monosynaptic reflex response by 60% and depressed activation of single motoneurons evoked by stretching the gastrocnemius muscle.

The ability of carisoprodol to depress the exaggerated muscle tone which is associated with spasticity has also been demonstrated in humans. Goodgold *et al.* (1959) demonstrated by electromyography that the oral administration of carisoprodol reduced abnormal monosynaptic (H) reflex activity elicited by electrical stimulation in humans with upper neuron motor diseases but not in persons without neuromuscular disease. Similarly,

Campbell and Green (1965) observed that carisoprodol decreased the anterior horn excitability after H-wave activity in persons with cerebral palsy and tended to normalize these responses. Likewise, the oral administration of carisoprodol, 700–1200 mg, reduced the exaggerated quadriceps potentials typical of some spastic states in humans (Peterson and Wise, 1961).

d. Anticonvulsant Actions. Carisoprodol is a less potent anticonvulsant than meprobamate or mephenesin. It is a weak strychnine antagonist. Even extremely large doses are ineffective in preventing convulsions or death, although carisoprodol modifies the characteristics of the seizures and prolongs survival time. Pretreatment of mice with carisoprodol, 250 mg/kg by mouth, did not prevent convulsions or death in 80% of the animals.

Carisoprodol protected animals against the convulsive and lethal effects of pentylenetetrazole, although in this respect it was only about one-half as effective as meprobamate (Berger *et al.*, 1959, 1960; Carroll *et al.*, 1961; Yamamoto *et al.*, 1963; Duchene-Marullaz *et al.*, 1965). Carisoprodol is less effective than meprobamate in antagonizing electroshock seizures (Hofrichter *et al.*, 1967) but is as effective as meprobamate in antagonizing audiogenic seizures. Unlike meprobamate, it shortened the survival time of mice to which scorpion venom was administered (Greenberg and Ingalls, 1963).

2. *Analgesic Actions*

Many studies have demonstrated that carisoprodol possesses some analgesic activity in animals (Cahn and Herold, 1967; Carpi, 1960; Frommel *et al.*, 1960a,b) and in man (Lynn and Eysenck, 1963; Margolin, 1960). In some experiments, it appeared to be more potent that acetylsalicylic acid, and its effects were more long lasting.

Berger *et al.* (1959) showed that carisoprodol reduced pain and other behavioral responses evoked by the manipulation of the joints of animals injected with silver nitrate. Although it was considerably less potent, it seemed to resemble morphine, pethidine, and codeine since it reduced pain without substantially reducing edema. Subsequent studies indicated that carisoprodol could be distinguished from aspirin and substances such as indomethacin and phenylbutazone which have potent anti-inflammatory properties (Margolin, 1964).

Margolin (1960) demonstrated in man that carisoprodol was effective in raising threshold to pain evoked by electrical stimulation in the dental pulp. Oral doses of 350 mg produced a statistically significant long-lasting increase in pain threshold, whereas meprobamate and placebo were without effect. Aspirin, 1200 mg, produced comparable but shorter-lasting effects. Although similar findings were reported by some investigators (Frommel *et al.*, 1960a; Holliday and Dille, 1960; Lynn and Eysenck, 1963), others were not able to replicate these findings in animals or humans (O'Dell, 1961; Lasagna *et al.*, 1962).

Carisoprodol does not modify withdrawal responses to painful stimulation evoked by heat. Indeed, under these circumstances, experimental animals reacted even more quickly after the administration of 50 or 100 mg/kg. It did not modify the writhing movements of the abdomen, trunk, and limbs induced in mice by phenylquinone, even after administration of doses that abolished the righting reflex (Berger *et al.*, 1959, 1960; Dandiya and Menon, 1963; Hoffmeister and Wirth, 1963; O'Dell, 1960, 1961). Carisoprodol has relatively slight antipyretic action; it is about one-half as effective as aspirin in reducing the fever produced in rabbits by pyrogens such as typhoid–paratyphoid vaccine (Berger *et al.*, 1959) or yeast (Buch, 1960). Although carisoprodol is as effective as phenylbutazone in reducing edema produced in mice by serotonin, it is only half as effective against that evoked by formalin and dextran (Buch, 1960). Carisoprodol does not affect the dermal spreading action of hyaluronidase or inhibit granuloma tissue formation. It does not change the number of circulating eosinophiles or alter Schwartzman reactivity (Berger *et al.*, 1959).

3. Taming Effect

Carisoprodol has no taming effect. Intraperitoneal doses of 235 mg/kg do not abolish fighting behavior produced in mice by 21 days of isolation (DaVanzo *et al.*, 1966). Oral doses of 100 to 200 mg/kg do not affect conditioned suppression in rats (Lauener, 1963). Carisoprodol, 10–20 mg/kg, in rabbits produces a transitory enhancement of paroxysmal inhibition, a "fearlike" behavioral state, whereas meprobamate antagonizes this acute emotional response (Davis, 1963). Its effect on imprinting is more profound than that of meprobamate, which suggests that muscle tension is deeply involved in the imprinting process. The optimal periods for this simple form of reactivity are prolonged by carisoprodol which does not affect learning of a simple color discrimination task (Hess, 1960).

4. Autonomic Effects

Carisoprodol, 20 mg/kg, given intravenously to dogs or cats anesthetized with pentobarbital sodium causes a transient lowering of blood pressure of about 20 mm Hg or less. The blood pressure returns to its original level within 5 minutes. In 6 dogs, cardiac slowing and fall of blood pressure produced by stimulation of the peripheral stump of the cut vagus nerve was inhibited by 20 to 90% after administration of carisoprodol, 20 mg/kg. The same dose of carisoprodol in 4 dogs reduced by 20 to 60% the fall in blood pressure induced by administration of acetylcholine (25 μg/kg). The drug does not affect the pressor effect of epinephrine and reduces only slightly (by 10 to 35%) the amplitude of contraction of the nictitating membrane produced by stimulation of the preganglionic nerve. The carotid sinus pressor reflex in dogs is not affected (Berger *et al.*, 1959).

Carisoprodol does not greatly alter contractions of the isolated guinea pig ileum. It does not significantly alter spasms evoked by acetylcholine, histamine, or serotonin. Although somewhat more effective than meprobamate, carisoprodol is a relatively weak antispasmodic agent compared to atropine or diphenhydramine (Berger *et al.*, 1959; Dandiya and Hemnani, 1964; DiMaggio, 1966). Salivary secretion produced in mice by intracerebral injection of acetylcholine is not significantly reduced by carisoprodol given in amounts as large as 620 mg/kg. Carisoprodol does not alter body temperature, basal metabolism, intestinal motility, or respiration, except after near-toxic doses (Berger *et al.*, 1959; Diamantis and Kletzkin, 1966; Lanza and Goude, 1967).

5. *Neurophysiological Actions*

Meprobamate and carisoprodol differ in almost every respect in their neurophysiological actions. Whereas meprobamate neither modifies the spontaneous EEG nor alters cortical or hippocampal activation, carisoprodol depresses these patterns. The ability to attenuate limbic seizures so characteristic of meprobamate is not shared by carisoprodol. These differences have been observed with respect to spontaneous and evoked patterns of electrical activity in cats (Berger *et al.*, 1959, 1960; Kletzkin, 1960, 1962), rabbits (Del Castillo and Nelson, 1960; Longo, 1960), and in man (Fraser *et al.*, 1961; Manzini, 1960).

a. Spontaneous Activity. Unlike meprobamate, which does not affect spontaneous EEG activity, intravenous administration of 5 to 10 mg/kg of carisoprodol to unanesthetized cats or rabbits produced a marked decrease in the frequency and increase in the amplitude of cortical and subcortical electrical activity. Although these patterns were typical of sleep, behavior changes were not evident. Spindling in the frontal leads characteristic of the action of barbiturates was seldom seen. Larger doses caused progressive slowing of frequency and further increase of amplitude. After 40 to 60 mg/kg, irregular high-voltage, very low-frequency waves were interspersed with periods of isoelectricity. Still larger doses caused further reductions of activity and longer periods of electrical silence (Berger *et al.*, 1959, 1960; Kletzkin, 1960, 1962). Similar changes were observed in rabbits (Del Castillo and Nelson, 1960; Longo, 1960). The oral administration to humans of 2 gm for 3 days (Manzini, 1960) or 4.8 gm for 18 to 54 days (Fraser *et al.*, 1961) had no significant effect on spontaneous electrical brain wave activity.

b. Evoked Responses. The actions of carisoprodol on the spontaneous and evoked EEG suggested that the site of its muscle relaxant and analgesic actions is the midbrain reticular formation. In sharp contrast to meprobamate, carisoprodol did not shorten the duration of evoked limbic seizures, even after intravenous administration of 40 mg/kg, which may explain its lack of tranquilizing action. Carisoprodol, 10 mg/kg, depressed activation evoked in unanesthetized cats by stimulation of the midbrain reticular formation, diffuse thalamic system, hypothalamus, and by peripheral nerve stimulation in intact cats immobilized with gallamine or succinylcholine. Carisoprodol, 10–20 mg/kg, enhanced recruiting responses evoked by low-frequency stimulation of the diffuse thalamic nuclei (Berger *et al.*, 1959, 1960; Kletzkin, 1962; Margolin, 1960). These actions sharply contrasted with the effect of meprobamate on the EEG, and in some respects these effects resembled those of morphine and atropine. Longo (1960) made similar observations in unanesthetized noncurarized rabbits and observed that there was a parallelism between the myorelaxant effects of carisoprodol and its EEG action in blocking reticular activation, which further suggested that its site of action in the neuraxis is more rostral than the spinal cord.

These neurophysiological observations supported the conclusions of Del Castillo and Nelson (1960, 1963) and others (Jurna, 1965) that carisoprodol has a direct action on the midbrain reticular formation. Apparently, carisoprodol augments inhibition of the excitatory processes mediated by the brainstem by selectively depressing facilitatory responses. It does not significantly interfere with the transmission of nonfacilitated responses. Its actions on spinal structures are of secondary consequence. Larger doses are required to block facilitation evoked by ipsilateral cutaneous stimulation than stimulation evoked from facilitatory sites in the midbrain.

6. *Toxicity*

Carisoprodol appears to have about the same toxicity as meprobamate. The mean lethal doses of this drug in mice and rats are shown in Table IX. The incorporation of 0.5 and 1% of the drug into the diet of rats for 1 year did not alter food intake or body weight. Animals receiving 2% of the drug in their diet had a lower food intake and lower weight gain for the first few weeks of the study, but eventually these values matched those of the controls. No evidence of drug-induced changes was found on macroscopic and microscopic examination of the various organs of animals which received diets containing 0.5 and 1% of the drug for 1 year. The liver and kidneys of the animals receiving the 2% diet were somwehat enlarged but appeared normal in texture and color. No drug-related pathological changes were observed on histological examination of these organs. The administration of 50 mg/kg twice daily, 5 days a week, for 6 months did not cause any changes in the appearance, behavior, or neurological status of 3 Beagle puppies. Changes connected with administration of the drug were not detected on postmortem examination (Berger *et al.*, 1959).

Fraser *et al.* (1961) observed that the administration of daily doses of 3000 to 4800 mg did not suppress abstinence syndromes in humans dependent on morphine. Similarly, the chronic administration of doses of up to 4800 mg for 18 to 54 days to individuals with a history of drug dependence suggested that physical dependence to carisoprodol does not occur. However, Deneau and Weiss (1968) found that carisoprodol, 200 mg/kg, could be substituted for sodium barbital (100 mg/kg) to prevent the recurrence of withdrawal syndromes in dogs made dependent on barbital by prolonged administration. Yet, no instances of dependence on carisoprodol in humans have been reported.

D. Tybamate

Tybamate has pharmacological activities typical in some respects to other propanediol dicarbamates. Suitable doses relax skeletal muscles and produce taming in animals without causing neurological deficit or sensory impairment. These effects correlate with its neurophysiological actions which are similar to meprobamate and unlike mebutamate and carisoprodol. Yet tybamate also has pharmacological actions suggestive of antipsychotic drugs such as chlorpromazine. It markedly reduces pressor responses to serotonin and antagonizes the effects of the hallucinogen LSD-25 on the spontaneous EEG. Like chlorpromazine, tybamate blocks conditioned avoidance responses in rats at doses which do not affect unconditioned escape responses.

Berger *et al.* (1964) observed in mice that tybamate produced profound muscle relaxation which became greater with increasing doses in intact and decerebrate animals. As with meprobamate and other interneuronal blocking agents, tybamate blocked polysynaptic arcs such as the flexor reflex in doses which did not affect monosynaptic reflexes. The onset of action was rapid and the effect persisted for 1 to 3 hours. Tybamate was less effective than meprobamate in antagonizing convulsions and preventing fatalities due to the administration of pentylenetetrazole. It was as effective as meprobamate in antagonizing convulsions and death produced by strychnine and in eliminating the occurrence of the tonic extensor phase of maximal electroshock seizures in mice. Intraperitoneal doses of 50 to 100 mg/kg produced a long-lasting and profound taming effect in extremely aggressive cats which remained alert but became calm and tractable and tolerated handling for 4 to 5 hours. The same doses of meprobamate had similar but less long-lasting effects. These behavioral effects appeared to be related to the action of tybamate in suppressing limbic seizures in laboratory animals. Although many of the actions of this compound on the EEG resembled those of meprobamate, small doses of tybamate, which by themselves had no effect on the EEG, completely abolished activation produced by LSD-25. These studies demonstrated that the most significant pharmacological actions of tybamate were (*1*) its effects on voluntary muscles, (*2*) its effects on aggressivity in animals, and (*3*) its lack of significant effects on the autonomic nervous system. Although some of these actions resemble those of meprobamate and other propanediol dicarbamates, tybamate has some pharmacological actions characteristic of drugs which are clinically effective in the treatment of neuroses and psychoses.

1. Effects on Voluntary Muscles

Tybamate is a more potent muscle relaxant than meprobamate in abolishing the righting reflex in intact animals. The oral administration of about 235 mg/kg to mice produced flaccid paralysis of the skeletal muscles but did not alter respiratory and other vital functions. The lethal dose was about 830 mg/kg, and the safety ratio between paralyzing and lethal doses was greater than that of meprobamate. Similar muscle relaxant effects were seen in rats and dogs. The intravenous administration of 10 mg/kg to cats decerebrated at an intercollicular level abolished decerebrate rigidity. The characteristic high-voltage, high-frequency potentials of the electromyogram of animals in this spastic state were normalized. For meprobamate and carisoprodol to produce similar relaxation of decerebrate rigidity, 24 and 3 mg/kg, respectively, were required. Indeed, Diamantis and Kletzkin (1966) confirmed that tybamate was a more potent muscle relaxant than meprobamate or mephenesin in producing head drop in rabbits and in reducing decerebrate rigidity in cats, particularly in terms of its safety.

Tsui-Chin Tseng and his colleagues (1970) attributed these muscle-relaxant effects to its actions at spinal levels. In midcollicularly decerebrated cats in which the spinal cord was intact, tybamate, 10–20 mg/kg intravenously, abolished the polysynaptic contralateral extensor reflex evoked by stimulation of the sciatic nerve, but ipsilateral arcs were more resistant to the action of the drug. No changes in the activity of the contralateral reflexes occurred when the spinal cord was severed at high cervical levels (C_1) and the drug was administered during the time that the extensor reflexes were depressed, although ipsilateral responses often were augmented markedly. A similar action occurred when tybamate was administered to these decerebrate preparations only after spinal transection. Doses of 5 to 20 mg/kg promptly reduced exaggerated responses of the monosynaptic patellar reflex. Tybamate had a greater effect on polysynaptic reflexes such as the contralateral crossed extensor reflex than on the ipsilateral crossed extensor reflex, in which there is a substantial monosynaptic component. The monosynaptic patellar reflex was not affected under these circumstances. In cats in which the cervical spine was severed at C_1 and jerks were elicited by sciatic nerve stimulation, administration of 5 to 20 mg/kg intravenously depressed both facilitation and inhibition. These investigators interpreted these results as demonstrating that tybamate can act independently of higher brain centers to produce an effect on spinal reflexes. Indeed, these actions are in marked contrast to the effects of meprobamate and carisoprodol on reticulospinal or spinal inhibition and facilitation. Moreover, further experiments showed that the administration of 2 to 5 mg/kg to cats decerebrated by midcollicular section slightly diminished the spontaneous activity of mesencephalic neurons recorded extracellularly with microelectrodes. Augmented neuronal activity elicited in these nerve cells by stimulation of the sciatic nerve was not affected. The same doses markedly reduced polysynaptic crossed extensor responses. These investigators concluded that tybamate has a more profound effect on inhibitory pathways than on those concerned with facilitation and attributed this action chiefly, but not entirely, to its effect at spinal levels.

2. Effects on Aggressivity in Animals

Tybamate reduces hostility in animals. Valzelli *et al.* (1967) showed that the intraperitoneal administration of 10 to 40 mg/kg completely abolished or markedly reduced aggressivity produced by prolonged isolation in male Swiss albino mice. The administration of these doses did not cause neuromuscular impairment, and the effect of the drug lasted for 4 to 6 hours. By contrast, the administration of meprobamate, 10 to 20 mg/kg, caused less reduction in aggresiveness and this action persisted for 1 to 2 hours. Although the administration of 40-mg/kg doses of tybamate ameliorated aggressive behavior almost completely for 1 to 2 hours, signs of overt neuromuscular impairment were evident. Geller (1966) demonstrated that the administration of 200 mg/kg orally blocked avoidance behavior in rats; escape behavior was not changed. In this respect, tybamate was like chlorpromazine and unlike meprobamate, chlordiazepoxide, diazepam, or pentobarbital which blocked avoidance behavior only in doses that also blocked escape. However, tybamate resembled meprobamate and other antianxiety agents in that the administration of 200 mg/kg attenuated punishment discrimination. The attenuation was less than that produced by meprobamate and was accompanied by a reduction of the overall response rate.

3. *Effects on the Autonomic Nervous System*

Tybamate, like mebutamate, has some effects on the autonomic nervous system, but the magnitude of these actions is slight. Rapid intravenous injection of tybamate, 20 mg/kg, to anesthetized normotensive dogs reduced arterial blood pressure for 20 to 30 minutes. No significant hypotensive action could be demonstrated in unanesthetized rabbits. The carotid sinus pressor response, induced by the occlusion of the common carotid arteries, and the pressor effect of central vagal stimulation were diminished by 60 to 70% after the administration of tybamate, 20 mg/kg. The pressor response to electric stimulation of hypothalamic, mesencephalic, or medullary vasomotor centers was reduced by 30 mg/kg tybamate intravenously. Vasopressor responses to epinephrine (2 μg/kg) and acetylcholine (20 μg/kg) were not significantly altered by tybamate, 20 mg/kg intravenously. Pressor responses to serotonin (100 μg/kg) were markedly reduced, and in this respect, tybamate appeared to be about one-half as potent as chlorpromazine, whereas meprobamate showed no such activity. Cardiac arrest elicited by electric stimulation of the peripheral end of the vagus was prevented in 5 of 10 dogs by tybamate, 20 mg/kg (Berger *et al.*, 1964).

In cats, contractions of the nictitating membrane produced by preganglionic stimulation of the isolated superior cervical ganglion were reduced by 25% after administration of tybamate, 20 mg/kg. It did not possess marked antispasmodic action when evaluated on the isolated guinea pig ileum. Contractions of the ileum produced by acetylcholine or histamine were not antagonized by the drug. To prevent serotonin-induced contractions, tybamate in a concentration of 17 μg/ml was required. Tybamate possessed no analgesic action when evaluated in mice on the hot plate and was ineffective in protecting dogs from apomorphine-induced emesis (Berger *et al.*, 1964)—an observation which was later confirmed by Falutz *et al.* (1966).

4. Effects on the Central Nervous System

In anesthetized immobilized cats, the intravenous administration of 10 mg/kg produced no effect on the spontaneous electrical activity of the cortex. Doses of 20 mg/kg caused a decrease of high-frequency components and a moderate increase in the amplitude of slow waves with the occasional appearance of spindling. The effects of 40 mg/kg were more pronounced. Tybamate was less potent than meprobamate in reducing the threshold for recruiting after low-frequency stimulation of the diffuse thalamic system, and doses of 40 mg/kg only had slight depressant effects. Tybamate doses of 20 to 40 mg/kg caused a slight depression of cortical activation consequent to stimulation of the mesencephalic reticular formation and elevated the threshold for such activation. These same doses sharply reduced the duration of hippocampal seizures induced by electrical stimulation of the fornix. The long-lasting activation of the EEG produced by the administration of LSD-25 (10 μg) to rabbits was completely abolished by tybamate, 5 to 10 mg/kg intravenously, doses that by themselves had no effect on the EEG. Apparently, tybamate possesses some pharmacological actions characteristic of both antianxiety and antipsychotic tranquilizing agents, and this combination of pharmacological activities indicates that it belongs to a class of substances intermediate between these drugs (Berger *et al.*, 1964; Kletzkin, 1964).

5. Toxicity

The toxicity of tybamate, like that of other propanediol carbamates, is low (see Table IX). The addition of 0.5, 1.0, and 2.0% of this drug to the diet of newly weaned rats for 18 months produced no significant changes, except for some lowering of body weight gain in females on the 2% drug diet. Examination of the blood showed that hemoglobin, erythrocytes, and leukocyte differential values remained within normal limits. At autopsy, no signs of drug-induced alterations were found, except for some liver enlargement in animals receiving 2% tybamate in their diet. The livers of these dogs grossly appeared normal in color and texture, and histological examination showed no abnormal findings which would suggest that the enlargement of the liver was due to its role in tybamate detoxification. No gross or histological changes were observed in dogs given 150, 250, 350, and 550 mg/kg orally, 5 days a week, for 4 months. In dogs treated with 50, 150, and 300 mg/kg a day for 18 months, administration of the highest dose caused pronounced weight loss. This was probably due to the inability of these animals to take sufficient nourishment since they were seriously depressed and ataxic for the greater part of the day. Pathological alterations were not found. Sulfobromophthalein and blood urea nitrogen values were normal, but serum transaminase and alkaline phosphatase concentrations were elevated. Hematological and urine tests remained within normal limits. The oral administration of 50, 150, and 450 mg/kg, 5 days a week, for 26 consecutive weeks to Rhesus monkeys caused no changes which could be attributed to the drug (Berger *et al.*, 1964).

Margolin *et al.* (1965) observed that, unlike meprobamate, there was no evidence of abstinence upon abrupt withdrawal in dogs given doses up to 570 mg/kg of tybamate daily for 6 months.

E. Comparison of Activities

There are some striking similarities in the pharmacological actions of meprobamate, mebutamate, carisoprodol, and tybamate. All of these substances act primarily on the central parts of the nervous system and have little effect on sympathetic, parasympathetic, or peripheral components.

Except in animals under behavioral stress, these compounds do not significantly affect the autonomic nervous system. Even though mebutamate and carisoprodol may have greater activity in this respect than meprobamate or tybamate, the propanediol dicarbamates do not substantially alter visceral function. Respiration, heart action, gastrointestinal motility, and excretion are not altered. The activity of smooth muscles is not changed. These substances do not substantially affect the exocrine or endocrine glands nor influence overall metabolic processes. In situations of stress, meprobamate, and perhaps mebutamate and tybamate, mitigate disturbances in autonomic reactivity which frequently accompany these reactions.

All of these propanediol dicarbamates have skeletal muscle-relaxant effects which can be attributed to the inhibition of interneuronal conductivity within the spinal cord. The mechanism by which these effects occur has not yet been elucidated but it appears that these actions are mediated at supraspinal levels. This action seems to depend on the number of neurons interposed between sensory and motor segments of the spinal reflexes. Consequently, these substances depress polysynaptic arcs more profoundly than monosynaptic ones. Indeed, investigations of the actions of these drugs in antagonizing convulsions produced by pentylenetetrazole and strychnine support this hypothesis, although there does not seem to be any correlation between muscle-relaxant and anticonvulsant activities.

Despite these similarities, there are marked differences in the phar-

TABLE X

COMPARISON OF PHARMACOLOGICAL AND NEUROPHYSIOLOGICAL ACTIVITIES OF PROPANEDIOL DICARBAMATES

Effects[a]	Meprobamate	Mebutamate	Carisoprodol	Tybamate
Autonomic nervous system	0	++	+	0
Blood pressure	0	++	0	0
Skeletal muscle tone	++	+	++++	+++
Convulsions evoked by pentylenetetrazole	+++	+	+	++
Convulsions evoked by strychnine	++	++	+	+++
Taming	++	*	0	+++
Basal ganglia	0	*	+	0
Cortical and hippocampal activation	0	*	+	++
Recruiting	+	*	+	0
Limbic seizures	+	*	0	+
Spontaneous cortical activation	0	*	++	+
Neurohormones	*	*	*	+

[a] + Represents magnitude of particular actions; 0 no effect; * data not available.

macological actions of these compounds. The biological activities of these propanediol dicarbamates are compared in Table X which also enumerates the effects of these drugs on the EEG. Both meprobamate and tybamate possess a number of pharmacological properties in common: a taming action along with the ability to shorten the duration of afterdischarges evoked by electrical stimulation of the fornix or other parts of the limbic system. Yet tybamate, unlike meprobamate, can counteract the EEG activation produced by the hallucinogen LSD-25. Moreover, it counteracts the pressor response produced by serotonin, an action like that displayed by LSD. Carisoprodol has no taming effect and even the administration of paralyzing doses does not attenuate limbic seizures. With the exception of mebutamate, none of these drugs significantly affect blood pressure.

V. Clinical Uses

Meprobamate has been widely used in the treatment of anxiety states and in other conditions in which anxiety and tension are associated with irritability and hyperemotionalism. It also has been successfully employed in the treatment of musculoskeletal disorders and in certain neurological diseases such as petit mal epilepsy and tetanus. Several reviews evaluated its efficacy in these disorders (Berger, 1968; Ban, 1969). Serious adverse effects have been rarely encountered after the ingestion of therapeutic doses, but occasionally reports have been made of idiosyncratic reactions characterized by allergic symptoms. In a relatively few instances, dependence has been observed in persons taking excessive amounts of this drug for prolonged periods of time. Most of these individuals have been dependent previously on substances such as alcohol or barbiturates.

Tybamate appears to be potentially useful in the treatment of more severe psychiatric disturbances, particularly in patients with marked somatic complaints. Although a number of carefully controlled clinical trials have demonstrated its superiority in these situations to antianxiety agents such as meprobamate and chlordiazepoxide, its exact place in psychiatric therapy remains to be established. Carisoprodol has been successfully employed for the symptomatic management of muscle spasm in a variety of inflammatory, traumatic, and degenerative disorders. Mebutamate has had some use in the treatment of certain types of hypertension.

This review of the actions of propanediol dicarbamate compounds demonstrates that it is difficult to predict biological activity on the basis of chemical structure. Pharmacologically active substances may affect many interrelated physiological functions in different ways or to varying extents. Consequently, the testing and evaluation of drugs remains pragmatic. Strain and species differences, particularly those existing between animals and man, make this task difficult. Yet the careful evaluation of compounds with seemingly similar structures or activities will help provide the knowledge necessary for the discovery of new and more effective remedies.

Acknowledgment

The authors gratefully acknowledge the contributions and helpful suggestions made by Frank M. Berger.

References

Abdulian, D. H., Martin, W. R., and Unna, K. R. (1960). *Arch. Int. Pharmacodyn. Ther.* **128,** 169.

Agranoff, B. W., Bradley, R. M., and Axelrod, J. (1957). *Proc. Soc. Exp. Biol. Med.* **96,** 261.

Aitchison, J. D. (1960). *Brit. Med. J.* **ii,** 387.

Albaum, H. G. (1962). *Acta Neurol. Scand.* **38,** 68.

Alexander, L. (1961). *In* "Neuro-Psychopharmacology" (E. Rothlin, ed.), Vol. II, pp. 93–123. Elsevier, Amsterdam.

Arora, R. B., Somani, P., and Lal, A. (1962). *Indian J. Med. Res.* **50,** 720.

Azuma, N. (1964). *Nippon Yakurigaku Zasshi* **60,** 259.

Baldrighi, V., Baldrighi, G., DeCaro, L. G., Jr., Ferrari, V., Montemartini, C., and Tronconi, L. (1961). *Arch Ital. Sci. Farmacol.* **11,** 225.

Baldrighi, V., DeCaro, L. G., Jr., Ferrari, V., Montemartini, C., Tronconi, L., and Baldrighi, G. (1962). *Minerva Cardioangiol.* **10,** 558.

Ban, T. A. (1969). "Psychopharmacology," pp. 313–325. Williams & Wilkins, Baltimore, Maryland.

Battig, K. (1961). *J. Physiol.* (*Paris*) **53,** 266.

Baxter, B. L. (1968) *Int. J. Neuropharmacol.* **7,** 47.

Ben-David, M. (1963). *Bull. Res Counc. Isr., Sect. E* **10,** 236.

Berger, F. M. (1949). *Proc. Soc. Exp. Biol. Med.* **71,** 270.

Berger, F. M. (1952a). *J. Pharmacol. Exp. Ther.* **104,** 468.

Berger, F. M. (1952b). *J. Pharmacol. Exp. Ther.* **104,** 229.

Berger, F. M. (1954). *J. Pharmacol. Exp. Ther.* **112,** 413.

Berger, F. M. (1957). *Ann. N.Y. Acad. Sci.* **67,** 685.

Berger, F. M. (1962). *N.Y. State J. Med.* **62,** 1580.

Berger, F. M. (1963). *Clin. Pharmacol. Ther.* **4,** 209.

Berger, F. M. (1966). *In* "Methods in Drug Evaluation" (P. Mantegazza and F. Piccinini, eds.), pp. 218–233. North-Holland Publ., Amsterdam.

Berger, F. M. (1968). *In* "Psychopharmacology (A Review of Progress 1957–1967)" (D. H. Efron, ed.), pp. 139–152. U.S. Govt. Printing Office, Washington, D.C.

Berger, F. M., and Bradley, W. (1946). *Brit. J. Pharmacol.* **1,** 265.

Berger, F. M., and Ludwig, B. J. (1950). *J. Pharmacol. Exp. Ther.* **100,** 27.

Berger, F. M., and Ludwig, B. J. (1960) Unpublished observations.

Berger, F. M., and Potterfield, J. (1969). *In* "Drugs and Youth" (J. R. Wittenborn, H. Brill, J. P. Smith, and S. A. Wittenborn, eds.), pp. 37–43. Thomas, Springfield, Illinois.

Berger, F. M., Hendley, C. D., Ludwig, B. J., and Lynes, T. E. (1956). *J. Pharmacol. Exp. Ther.* **116,** 337.

Berger, F. M., Kletzkin, M., Ludwig, B. J., Margolin, S., and Powell, L. S. (1959). *J. Pharmacol. Exp. Ther.* **127,** 66.

Berger, F. M., Kletzkin, M., Ludwig, B. J., and Margolin, S. (1960). *Ann. N.Y. Acad. Sci.* **86,** 90.

Berger, F. M., Douglas, J. F., Kletzkin, M., Ludwig, B. J., and Margolin, S. (1961). *J. Pharmacol. Exp. Ther.* **134,** 356.

Berger, F. M., Kletzkin, M., and Margolin, S. (1964). *Med. Exp.* **10,** 327.

Berger, F. M., Kletzkin M., and Margolin, S. (1967). *In* "Anti-depressant Drugs" (S. Garattini and M. N. G. Dukes, eds.), pp. 241–246. Excerpta Med. Found., Amsterdam.

Bert, G., Anfossi, F., Anselmino, A., Gagna, C., Mathis, I., Ruschena, A., and Miheli, B. (1964). *Minerva Cardioangiol.* **12,** 499.

Bhargava, K. P., and Srivastava, R. K. (1965). *Brit. J. Pharmacol.* **25, 74.**

Bloch, S., and Silva, A. (1959). *J. Comp. Physiol.* **52,** 550.

Boissier, J. R., Tardy, J., and Diverres, J. -C. (1960). *Med. Exp.* **3,** 81.

Bokonjic, N., and Trojaborg, W. (1960). *Electroencephalogr. Clin. Neurophysiol.* **12, 177.**

Bornmann, G. (1961). *Arzneim.-Forsch.* **11,** 89.

Bose, B. C., and Vijayvargiya, R. (1960). *J. Pharm. Pharmacol.* **12,** 99.

Bosisio, P., and Scaglietti, C. (1962). *Minerva Med.* **53,** 1101.

Bovet, D., Longo, V. G., and Silvestrini, B. (1957). *In* "Psychotropic Drugs" (S. Garattini and V. Ghetti, eds.), pp. 193–206. Elsevier, Amsterdam.
Boyd, L. J., Huppert, V. F., Mulinos, M. G., and Hammer, H. (1959). *Amer. J. Cardiol.* **3,** 229.
Bradley, P. B., and Key, B. J. (1959). *Brit. J. Pharmacol.* **14,** 340.
Brar, B. S. (1969). *Arch. Int. Pharmacodyn. Ther.* **177,** 416.
Buch, O. (1960). *Naunyn-Schmiedebergs Arch. Exp. Pathol. Pharmakol.* **238,** 92.
Cabrini, G., and Metalli, P. (1957). *Boll. Soc. Med.-Chir. Pavia* **71,** 1527.
Cahn, J., and Herold, M. (1967). *In* "Anti-Depressant Drugs" (S. Garattini and M. N. G. Dukes, eds.), pp. 116–120. Excerpta Med. Found., New York.
Campbell, E. D. R., and Green, E. A. (1965). *Ann. Phys. Med.* **8,** 4.
Carpi, C. (1960). *Farmaco, Ed. Prat.* **15,** 311.
Carroll, M. N., Jr., Luten, W. R., and Southward, R. W. (1961). *Arch. Int. Pharmacodyn. Ther.* **130,** 280.
Carroll, M. N., Jr., Lyon, A. F., Golinko, R. J., Dunst, M., Rene, H. F., Jr., and Ford, D. H. (1968). *Arch. Int. Pharmacodyn. Ther.* **171,** 462.
Caujolle, F., de Boislambert, P., de Gout, R., and Gout-Tarbouriech, Y. (1960). *Therapie* **15,** 791.
Caviezel, R., and Baillod, A. (1958). *Pharm. Acta Helv.* **33,** 469.
Chambon, M. (1959). *Therapie* **14,** 771.
Charkes, N. D. (1958). *Arch. Intern. Med.* **102,** 584.
Chauchard, P., and Mazoue, H. (1956a). *C. R. Soc. Biol.* **150,** 679.
Chauchard, P., and Mazoue, H. (1956b). *C. R. Acad. Sci.* **243,** 89.
Chiesara, E., and Conti, F. (1964). *Boll. Soc. Ital. Biol. Sper.* **40,** 825.
Chin, J. H., and Smith, C. M. (1962). *J. Pharmacol. Exp. Ther.* **136,** 276.
Condaese, A., Radelscu, E., Jelezov, M., and Iosif, I. (1965). *Viata Med.* **12,** 973.
Conney, A. H., and Burns, J. J. (1960). *Ann. N.Y. Acad. Sci.* **86,** 167.
Cooper, J., and Davis, W. A. (1960). *J. Med. Soc. N.J.* **57,** 20.
Corson, S. A., O'Leary Corson, E., Dykman, R. A., Peters, J. E., Reese, W. G., and Seager, L. D. (1961). *Biochem. Pharmacol.* **8,** 174.
Cranston, E. M. (1958). *Proc. Soc. Exp. Biol. Med.* **98,** 320.
Cullen, S. J., and Catalano, P. M. (1967). *J. Amer. Med. Ass.* **199,** 582.
Dandiya, P. C., and Hemnani, K. L. (1964). *Indian J. Physiol. Pharmacol.* **8,** 161.
Dandiya, P. C., and Menon, M. K. (1963). *Arch. Int. Pharmacodyn. Ther.* **141,** 223.
Danon, A. (1963). *Bull. Res. Counc. Isr., Sect. E* **10,** 236.
Datta, P. R., and Nelson, M. J. (1968). *Toxicol. Appl. Pharmacol.* **13,** 346.
DaVanzo, J. P., Daugherty, M., Ruckart, R., and Kang, L. (1966). *Psychopharmacologia* **9,** 210.
Davis, W. M. (1963). *Arch. Int. Pharmacodyn. Ther.* **142,** 349.
De Boer, B., Engelstaat, O., and Gray, D. (1959). *Fed. Proc. Fed. Amer. Soc. Exp. Biol.* **18,** 382.
DeCaro, L. G., Baldrighi, V., Minelli, R., Baldrighi, G., and Buniva, G. (1962). *Arch. Ital. Sci. Farmacol.* **12,** 160.
DeCaro, L. G., Baldrighi, V., Baldrighi, G., and Tronconi, L. (1963). *Atti Soc. Ital. Cardiol.* **2,** 267.
Decsi, L. and Mehes, J. (1959). *Arch. Int. Pharmacodyn. Ther.* **119,** 294.
del Castillo, J., and Nelson, T. E., Jr. (1960). *Ann. N.Y. Acad. Sci.* **86,** 108.
del Castillo, J., and Nelson, T. E., Jr. (1963). *Arch. Int. Pharmacodyn. Ther.* **142,** 572.
Delga, J., Laboure, J. and Olive, G. (1962). *Sem. Hop.* **38,** 270.
Della Bella, D., Gandini, A., and Preti, M. (1964). *Brit. J. Pharmacol.* **23,** 540

Deneau, G. A., and Weiss, S. (1968). *Pharmakopsychiat. Neuro-Psychopharmakol.* **1,** 269.

De Salva, J. D., and Oestler, Y. T. (1960). *Arch. Int. Pharmacodyn. Ther.* **124,** 255.

De Salva, S. J., and Evans, R. (1960). *Toxicol. Appl. Pharmacol.* **2,** 397.

De Salva, S. J., Clements, G. R., and Ercoli, N. (1959). *J. Pharmacol. Exp. Ther.* **126,** 318.

Diamantis, W., and Kletzkin, M. (1966). *Int. J. Neuropharmacol.* **5,** 305.

DiMaggio, G. (1966). *Biochim. Biol. Sper.* **5,** 111.

Döring, G. K., and Heller, A. (1960). *Arch. Gynaekol.* **194,** 138.

Douglas, J. F. (1962). Unpublished observations.

Douglas, J. F., Ludwig, B. J., Ginsberg, T., and Berger, F. M. (1962a). *J. Pharmacol. Exp. Ther.* **136,** 5.

Douglas, J. F., Ludwig, B. J., and Schlosser, A. (1962b). *J. Pharmacol. Exp. Ther.* **138,** 21.

Douglas, J. F., Ludwig, B. J. and Smith, N. (1963). *Proc. Soc. Exp. Biol. Med.* **112,** 436.

Douglas, J. F., Bradshaw, W. H., Ludwig, B. J., and Powers, D. (1964). *Biochem. Pharmacol.* **13,** 537.

Douglas, J. F., Ludwig, B. J., Schlosser, A., and Edelson, J. (1966). *Biochem. Pharmacol.* **15,** 2087.

Duchene-Marullaz, P., Tercinet, A., Lakatos, C., and Vacher, J. (1965). *Therapie* **20,** 737.

Dunham, N. W., and Miya, T. S. (1957). *J. Amer. Pharm. Ass., Sci. Ed.* **46,** 208.

Dunsmore, R. A., Dunsmore, L. D., Bickford, A. F., and Goldman, A. (1957). *Amer. J. Med. Sci.* **233,** 280.

Edelson, J., and Douglas, J. F. (1967). *Biochem. Pharmacol.* **16,** 2050.

Edelson, J., and Douglas, J. F. (1968). *Arch. Int. Pharmacodyn. Ther.* **173,** 182.

Elliott, R. C. (1969). *Int. J. Neuropharmacol.* **8,** 117.

Emmerson, J. L., Miya, T. S., and Yim, G. K. W. (1960). *J. Pharmacol. Exp. Ther.* **129,** 89.

Essig, C. F. (1958). *AMA Arch. Neurol. Psychiat.* **80,** 414.

Ewaldsson, B. (1963). *Arch. Int. Pharmacodyn. Ther.* **142,** 163.

Falciendo, P., and Minola, G. C. (1958). *Arch. Sci. Med.* **106,** 312.

Falutz, S. E., Chenier, L. P., and McColl, J. D. (1966). *Rev. Can. Biol.* **25,** 225.

Feldman, R. S., and Lewis, E. (1962). *J. Neuropsychiat.* **3,** S27.

Ferrari, G., and Casagrande, C. (1963). *Farmaco, Ed. Sci.* **18,** 780.

Fessenden, R. J., and Coon, M. D. (1965). *J. Med. Chem.* **8,** 604.

Fischetti, B., and Inselvini, M. (1959). *Arch. Ital. Sci. Farmacol.* **9,** 159.

Fraser, H. F., Essig, C. F., and Wolbach, A. B., Jr. (1961). *Bull. Narcotics* **13,** 1.

Frazier, L. E., Mann, A. N., Rasmussen, R. A., Hughes, R. H., and Wissler, R. W. (1964). *Circulation Suppl.* **3,** 9.

Friedell, M. T. (1958). *J. Amer. Med. Ass.* **167,** 983.

Friedman, S. L., and Ingalls, J. W. (1960). *Quart. J. Stud. Alc.* **21,** 217.

Frommel, E. Fleury, C., and Schmidt-Ginzkey, J. (1960a). *Helv. Physiol. Pharmacol. Acta* **18,** 109.

Frommel, E., Fleury, C., and Schmidt-Ginzkey, J. (1960b). *Ann. N.Y. Acad. Sci.* **86,** 162.

Fukuda, H., Watanabe, K., Kudo, Y., and Ohshima, T. (1968). *Yakugaku Zasshi* **88,** 1338.

Furuno, K. (1959). *Igaku Kenkyu* **29,** 3653.

Gangloff, H. (1959). *J. Pharmacol. Exp. Ther.* **126,** 30.

Gantt, W. H., and Newton, E. O. (1960). *Pharmacologist* **2**, 63.
Geller, I. (1964). *Arch. Int. Pharmacodyn. Ther.* **149**, 243.
Geller, I. (1966). *J. Psychopharmacol.* **1**, 48.
Geller, I., and Seifter, J. (1960). *Fed. Proc. Fed. Amer. Soc. Exp. Biol.* **19**, 20.
Georges, G., Herold, M., and Gautier, E. (1961). *Agressologie* **2**, 605.
Glassman, J. M., Hudyma, G. M., and Seifter, J. (1958). Meeting of the American Society of Pharmacology and Experimental Therapeutics, Ann Arbor, Michigan.
Glotfelty, J. S., and Wilson, W. P. (1956). *N.C. Med. J.* **17**, 401.
Gogerty, J. H., Houlihan, W., Dzamba, F., Takesue, E. I., and Trapold, J. H. (1965). *Fed. Proc. Fed. Amer. Soc. Exp. Biol.* **24**, 134.
Goodgold, J., Hohmann, T., and Tajima, T. (1959). *In* "The Pharmacology and Clinical Usefulness of Carisoprodol" (J. G. Miller, ed.), pp. 66–76. Wayne State Univ. Press, Detroit, Michigan.
Gore, H. C., Jr. (1965). *Arch. Dermatol.* **91**, 627.
Granick, S. (1966). *J. Biol. Chem.* **241**, 1359.
Greenberg, L., and Ingalls, J. W. (1963). *J. Pharm. Sci.* **52**, 159.
Greene, F. E. (1963). *Proc. Soc. Exp. Biol. Med.* **114**, 165.
Grisler, R., and Finulli, M. (1962). *Riforma Med.* **76**, 817.
Harrison, D. L., and Albert, J. R. (1963). *Pharmacologist* **5**, 254.
Held, H., and von Oldershausen, F. (1969). *Klin. Wochenschr.* **47**, 78.
Hendley, C. D., Lynes, T. E., and Berger, F. M. (1954). *Proc. Soc. Exp. Biol. Med.* **87**, 608.
Hendley, C. D., Lynes, T. E., and Berger, F. M. (1957). *In* "Tranquilizing Drugs" (H. E. Himwich, ed.), pp. 35–46. Amer. Ass. Advan. Sci., Washington, D. C.
Henry, C. E., and Obrist, W. D. (1958). *J. Nerv. Ment. Dis.* **126**, 268.
Hess, E. H. (1960). *In* "Drugs and Behavior" (L. Uhr and J. G. Miller, eds.), pp. 268–271. Wiley, New York.
Himwich, H. E. (1962). *J. Neuropsychiat.* **2**, 279.
Hoffman, A. J., and Ludwig, B. J. (1959). *J. Amer. Pharm. Ass., Sci. Ed.* **48**, 740.
Hoffmeister, F. (1964). *Arch. Int. Pharmacodyn. Ther.* **148**, 382.
Hoffmeister, F., and Wirth, W. (1963). *Med. Chem. Abhandl. Med. Chem. Forschungsstaetten Farbenfabriken Bayer* **7**, 99.
Hofrichter, G., Roesch, A., Roesch, E., and Schenk, G. (1967). *Arzneim.-Forsch.* **17**, 242.
Holliday, A. R., and Dille, J. M. (1960). *Ann. N.Y. Acad. Sci.* **86**, 147.
Hollister, L. E., and Levy, G. (1964). *Chemotherapia* **9**, 20.
Honeycutt, W. M., and Curtis, A. C. (1964). *J. Amer. Med. Ass.* **180**, 691.
Hughes, F. W., and Kopmann, E. (1960). *Arch. Int. Pharmacodyn. Ther.* **126**, 1958.
Hughes, F. W., and Rountree, C. B. (1961). *Arch. Int. Pharmacodyn. Ther.* **133**, 418.
Hukovic, S., and Stern, P. (1959). *Atti Soc. Lomb. Sci. Med. Biol.* **14**, 80.
Hunninghake, D. B., and Azarnoff, D. L. (1968). *Arch. Intern. Med.* **121**, 349.
Hunt, H. F. (1957). *Ann. N.Y. Acad. Sci.* **67**, 712.
Inoki, R., Otori, K., and Komura, I. (1961). *Nippon Yakurigaku Zasshi* **57**, 280.
Iwaki, R., Kudo, Y., Ishihi, J., and Irikura, T. (1967). *Nippon Yakurigaku Zasshi* **63**, 472.
Jacob, J., and Michaud, G. (1960). *Med. Exp.* **2**, 323.
Jacobsen, E. (1957). *In* "Psychotropic Drugs" (S. Garattini and V. Ghetti, eds.), pp. 119–124. Elsevier, Amsterdam.
Jori, A., Mortari, A., Sioli, G., and Valzelli, L. (1964). *Boll. Soc. Ital. Biol. Sper.* **40**, 1421.

Jurna, I. (1965). *Int. J. Neuropharmacol.* **4,** 245.
Karli, P. (1959). *J. Physiol.* (*Paris*) **51,** 497.
Kato, R. (1960a). *Experientia* **16,** 427.
Kato, R. (1960b). *Med. Exp.* **3,** 95.
Kato, R. (1967). *Pathol. Biol.* **15,** 158.
Kato, R., and Chiesara, E. (1962). *Brit. J. Pharmacol.* **18,** 29.
Kato, R., and Vassanelli, P. (1962). *Biochem. Pharmacol.* **11,** 779.
Kato, R., Chiesara, E., and Frontino, G. (1961). *Jap. J. Pharmacol.* **11,** 31.
Kato, R., Vassanelli, P., and Chiesara, E. (1962a). *Experientia* **18,** 453.
Kato, R., Vassanelli, P., Frontino, G., and Bolego, A. (1962b). *Med. Exp.* **6,** 149.
Kato, R., Chiesara, E., and Vassanelli, P. (1963). *Biochem. Pharmacol.* **12,** 357.
Katona, F., Tomka, I., and Obal, F. (1963). *Acta Physiol.* **22,** 29.
Kayaalp, S. O. (1966). *Arch. Int. Pharmacodyn. Ther.* **162,** 69.
Kelleher, R. T., Fry, W., Deegan, J., and Cook, L. (1961). *J. Pharmacol. Exp. Ther.* **133,** 271.
Khan, A. U., Forney, R. B., and Hughes, F. W. (1964). *Arch. Int. Pharmacodyn. Ther.* **151,** 466.
Khazan, N., Ben-David, M., and Sulman, F. G. (1963). *Proc. Soc. Exp. Biol. Med.* **112,** 490.
Kinnard, W. J., Jr., and Carr, C. J. (1957). *J. Pharmacol. Exp. Ther.* **121,** 354.
Kletzkin, M. (1960). *Fed. Proc. Fed. Amer. Soc. Exp. Biol.* **19,** 270.
Kletzkin, M. (1962). *Ann. N.Y. Acad. Sci.* **96,** 263.
Kletzkin, M. (1964). *Fed. Proc. Fed. Amer. Soc. Exp. Biol.* **23,** 197.
Kletzkin, M. (1966). *Arch. Int. Pharmacodyn. Ther.* **164,** 71.
Kletzkin, M., and Berger, F. M. (1959). *Proc. Soc. Exp. Biol. Med.* **100,** 681.
Kletzkin, M., and Swan, K. (1959). *J. Pharmacol. Exp. Ther.* **125,** 35.
Kobayashi, T., and Ishikawa, T. (1965). *In* "Neuro-Psychopharmacology" (D. Bente and P. B. Bradley, eds.), Vol. IV, pp. 320–326. Elsevier, New York.
Kocsar, L., Veress, O., and Kajtor, F. (1960). *Ideggyogy. Szemle* **13,** 90.
Koizumi, H. (1961). *Naika Hokan* **8,** 167.
Kondziella, W. (1964). *Arch. Int. Pharmacodyn. Ther.* **152,** 277.
Krieger, D. T., and Krieger, H. P. (1967). *Neuroendocrinology* **2,** 232.
Kroneberg, G., and Schumann, H. J. (1959). *Arzneim.-Forsch.* **9,** 442.
Kumadaki, N., Hitomi, M., and Kumada, S. (1967). *Jap. J. Pharmacol.* **17,** 659.
Kurtz, G. S., Santos, Y. V., dos Bueno, J. R., and Sollero, L. (1965). *Hospital* (*Rio de Janeiro*) **67,** 71.
Lamperi, S., Caponnetto, S., and Iannetti, M. (1962). 23rd Congress of the Italian Society of Cardiology, Lido, Venice.
Lanza, M. (1966). *C. R. Soc. Biol.* **159,** 1998.
Lanza, M., and Goude, F. (1967). *C. R. Soc. Biol.* **161,** 640.
Laporte, J., Valdecasas, F. G., and Salva, J. A. (1960). *Rev. Espan. Fisiol.* **16,** 147.
Lasagna, L., Tetreault, L., and Fallis, N. E. (1962). *Fed. Proc. Fed. Amer. Soc. Exp. Biol.* **21,** 326.
Lauener, H. (1963). *Psychopharmacologia* **4,** 311.
Leaffer, M. A., Skinner, W. A., and Ludwig, B. J. (1965). *J. Med. Chem.* **8,** 208.
Levine, I. M., Jossmann, P. B., Yood, B., DeAngelis, V., and Friend, D. (1960). *Ann. N.Y. Acad. Sci.* **86,** 208.
Longo, V. G. (1960). *Ann. N. Y. Acad. Sci.* **86,** 143.
Longo, V. G. (1962). *In* "Rabbit Brain Research" (V. G. Longo, ed.), Vol. 2, pp. 91–102. Elsevier, New York.

Ludwig, B. J., and Piech, E. C. (1951). *J. Amer. Chem. Soc.* **73,** 5779.
Ludwig, B. J., Douglas, J. F., Powell, L. S., Meyer, M., and Berger, F. M. (1961). *J. Med. Pharm. Chem.* **3,** 53.
Ludwig, B. J., Stiefel, F. J., Powell, L. S., and Diamond, J. (1964). *J. Med. Chem.* **7,** 174.
Ludwig, B. J., Powell, L. S., and Berger, F. M. (1969). *J. Med. Chem.* **12,** 462.
Lynes, T. E., and Williams, H. L. (1958). *J. Pharmacol. Exp. Ther.* **122,** 46A.
Lynn, R., and Eysenck, H. J. (1963). *In* "Experiments with Drugs" (H. Eysenck, ed.), pp. 324–328. Macmillan (Pergamon), New York.
McGregor, L. (1928). *Arch. Pathol.* **5,** 630.
Maddock, R. K., Jr., and Bloomer, H. A. (1967). *J. Amer. Med. Ass.* **201,** 999.
Maffii, G., and Soncin, E. (1958). *Brit. J. Pharmacol.* **13,** 357.
Magyar, I. (1960). *Electroencephalogr. Clin. Neurophysiol.* **12,** 222.
Makela, S., Naatanen, E., and Rinne, U. K. (1959). *Acta Endocrinol.* **32,** 1.
Malhotra, C. L., and Mehta, V. L. (1966). *Brit. J. Pharmacol.* **27,** 440.
Mantegazzini, P., Fabbri, S., and Magni, C. (1960). *Arch. Ital. Sci. Farmacol.* **10,** 347.
Manzini, B. (1960). *Minerva Med.* **51,** 2007.
Margolin, S. (1960). *Proc. Soc. Exp. Biol. Med.* **105,** 531.
Margolin, S. (1964). *In* "Non-Steroidal Anti-Inflammatory Drugs" (S. Garattini and M. N. G. Dukes, eds.), pp. 214–217. Excerpta Med. Found., Amsterdam.
Margolin, S., Plekss, O. J., and Fedor, E. J. (1963). *J. Pharmacol. Exp. Ther.* **140,** 170.
Margolin, S., Plekss, O. J., and Berger, F. M. (1965). *Pharmacologist* **7,** 143.
Marino, A. (1964). *Nature (London)* **203,** 1289.
Marino, A., Parise, A., and Galdi, R. (1963). *Arch. Int. Pharmacodyn. Ther.* **145,** 276.
Marriott, A. S., and Spencer, P. S. J. (1965). *Brit. J. Pharmacol.* **25,** 432.
Mathé, V., and Kassay, G. (1969). *Arzneim.-Forsch.* **19,** 419.
Matthews, R. J., DaVanzo, J. P., Collins, R. J., and Vander Brook, M. J. (1963). *Arch. Int. Pharmacodyn. Ther.* **143,** 574.
Mehta, V. L., Kalrah, N. S., and Malhotra, C. L. (1967). *Indian J. Physiol. Pharmacol.* **11,** 159.
Melander, B. (1959). *J. Med. Pharm. Chem.* **1,** 443.
Melnick, B. E. (1966). *Dokl. Akad. Nauk SSSR* **166,** 253.
Mercier, J., and Dessaigne, S. (1964). *C. R. Soc. Biol.* **158,** 1535.
Milcu, M., Holban, R., Sahleanu, V., Iancu, L., and Dragomirescu, M. (1958). *Rev. Fiziol. Norm. Patol.* **4,** 500.
Molcan, J., Dufkova, A., and Janotka, M. (1963). *Activ. Nerv. Super.* **5,** 190.
Montemartini, C., Tronconi, L., Baldrighi, G., and Massoni, G. (1963). *Atti Soc. Ital. Cardiol.* **2,** 265.
Morin, Y., Turmel, L., Grantham, H., and Fortier, J. (1963). *Can. Med. Ass. J.* **89,** 980.
Mulinos, M. G., Saltefors, S., Boyd, L. J., and Cronk, G. A. (1961). *Fed. Proc. Fed. Amer. Soc. Exp. Biol.* **20,** 113.
Naess, K., and Rasmussen, E. W. (1958). *Acta Pharmacol. Toxicol.* **15,** 99.
Newman, S., and Fish, V. J. (1958). *J. Clin. Endocrinol. Metab.* **18,** 1296.
Ngai, S. H., Tseng, D. T. C., and Wang, S. C. (1966). *J. Pharmacol. Exp. Ther.* **153,** 344.
Norton, S., and deBeer, E. J. (1956). *Ann. N.Y. Acad. Sci.* **65,** 249.
O'Dell, T. B. (1960). *Ann. N.Y. Acad. Sci.* **86,** 191.
O'Dell, T. B. (1961). *Arch. Int. Pharmacodyn. Ther.* **134,** 154.
Oelkers, H. A. (1957). *Aerztl. Forsch.* **11,** 530.
Oelkers, H. A. (1960). *Arzneim.-Forsch.* **10,** 392.
Opitz, K. (1962a). *Arzneim.-Forsch.* **12,** 525

Opitz, K. (1962b). *Arzneim.-Forsch.* **12,** 618.
Pallos, F. (1963). *Promotionsarb. Zurich* No. 3370, **77** pp.
Palmieri, A. (1964). *Arch. Ostet. Ginecol.* **69,** 552.
Pekkarinen, A., Luostarinen, L., and Tala, E. (1963). *Biochem. Pharmacol.* **12,** 54.
Perlstein, M. A. (1959). *J. Amer. Med. Ass.* **170,** 1902.
Peterson, C. R., and Wise, C. S. (1961). *Arch. Phys. Med. Rehabil.* **42,** 566.
Pfeiffer, C. C., Riopelli, A. J., Smith, R. P., Jenney, E. H., and Williams, H. L. (1957). *Ann. N.Y. Acad. Sci.* **67,** 734.
Phillips, B. M., Miya, T. S., and Yim, G. K. W. (1962). *J. Pharmacol. Exp. Ther.* **135,** 223.
Pierre, R., and Cahn, J. (1957). *In* "Psychotropic Drugs" (S. Garattini and V. Ghetti, eds.), pp. 286–289. Elsevier, Amsterdam.
Ponomarev, G. A., and Terekhina, A. I. (1964). *Farmakol. Toksikol.* (*Moscow*) **27,** 432.
Preti, M. (1961). *Arch. Ital. Sci. Farmacol.* **11,** 216.
Racz, W. J., and Marks, G. S. (1969). *Biochem. Pharmacol.* **18,** 2009.
Rafelsen, O. J. (1959). *Acta Psychiat. Neurol. Scand.* **136,** 73.
Randall, L. O., Schallek, W., Heise, G. A., Keith, E. F., and Bagdon, R. E. (1960). *J. Pharmacol. Exp. Ther.* **129,** 163.
Randall, L. O., Heise, G. A., Schallek, W., Bagdon, R. E., Banziger, R., Boris, A., Moe, R. A., and Abrams, W. B. (1961). *Curr. Ther. Res. Clin. Exp.* **3,** 405.
Ray, O. S. (1962). *American Psychologist* **17,** 398.
Rice, W. B., and McColl, J. D. (1960). *Arch. Int. Pharmacodyn. Ther.* **128,** 249.
Riley, R. F., and Berger, F. M. (1949). *Arch. Biochem. Biophys.* **20,** 159.
Robinson, M. A., and Scott, G. T. (1960). *Biochem. Biophys. Res. Commun.* **2,** 19.
Rowe, G. C., Castillo, C. A., Afonso, S., Leicht, T. R., Kyle, J. C., Lugo, J. E., and Crumpton, C. W. (1962). *Amer. J. Med. Sci.* **243,** 496.
Royer, F. L., and Gantt, W. H. (1965). *Fed. Proc. Fed. Amer. Soc. Exp. Biol.* **24,** 329.
Sacra, P., Rice, W. B., and McColl, J. D. (1957). *Can. J. Biochem. Physiol.* **35,** 1151.
Sasaki, S. (1959). *Nippon Yakurigaku Zasshi* **55,** 570.
Schallek, W., Kuehn, A., and Jew, N. (1962). *Ann. N.Y. Acad. Sci.* **96,** 303.
Scott, G. T. (1965). *Limnol. Oceanogr.* **10,** Suppl., R230.
Shagass, C., Azima, H., and Sangowicz, J. (1959). *Electroencephalogr. Clin. Neurophysiol.* **11,** 275.
Shane, A. M., and Hirsch, S. (1956). *Can. Med. Ass. J.* **74,** 908.
Sibilia, D., and Stoppoloni, A. (1962). *Minerva Med.* **53,** 1123.
Silvestrini, B., and Kohn, R. (1958). *Rend. Ist. Super. Sanita* (*Ital. Ed.*) **21,** 328.
Stanton, H. C., and White, J. B., Jr. (1965). *Arch. Int. Pharmacodyn. Ther.* **154,** 351.
Stegmann, H., and Burger, R. (1960). *Arch. Gynaekol.* **192,** 420.
Stern, P., and Milin, R. (1959). *Proc. Soc. Exp. Biol. Med.* **101,** 298.
Stewart, R. O., Gudmunsen, C., Dervinis, A., Glassman, J. M., and Seifter, J. (1962). *Pharmacologist* **4,** 183.
Stille, G. (1962). *Arzneim.-Forsch.* **12,** 340.
Swinyard, E. A., Chin, L., and Fingl, E. (1957). *Science* **125,** 739.
Taccardi, B., Maccari, M., and Valli, A. (1961). *Arch. Ital. Sci. Farmacol.* **11,** 207.
Taccola, A. (1965). *Boll. Soc. Ital. Biol. Sper.* **41,** 428.
Takagi, H., and Ban, T. (1960). *Jap. J. Pharmacol.* **10,** 7.
Takaori, S., and Ohato, K. (1961). Cited by Domino, E. F. (1962). *Annu. Rev. Pharmacol.* **2,** 215.
Tamura, M. (1963). *Jap. J. Pharmacol.* **13,** 133.
Tedeschi, D. H., Tedeschi, R. E., and Fellows, E. J. (1959). *J. Pharmacol. Exp. Ther.* **126,** 223.

Theobald, W., Buch, O., and Kunz, H. A. (1965). *Arzneim.-Forsch.* **15,** 117.
Tseng,Tsui-Chin, Przybyla, A. C., Shung Tsing Chen, and Wang, S. C. (1970). *Int. J. Neuropharmacol.* **9,** 211.
Tsukamoto, H., Yoshimura, H., and Tatsumi, K. (1963a). *Chem. Pharm. Bull.* **11,** 421.
Tsukamoto, H., Yoshimura, H., and Tatsumi, K. (1963b). *Life Sci.* **6,** 382.
Turrian, H., Doebelin, R., and Gross, F. (1957). *Helv. Physiol. Pharmacol. Acta* **15,** C39.
Valzelli, L., Giacalone, E., and Garattini, S. (1967). *Eur. J. Pharmacol.* **2,** 144.
van der Kleijn, E. (1969a). *Arch. Int. Pharmacodyn. Ther.* **178,** 457.
van der Kleijn, E. (1969b). "Pharmacokinetics of Ataractic Drugs," pp. 33–58. St. Catherine Press, Bruges.
Varagić, V., and Vojvodić, N. (1962). *Brit. J. Pharmacol.* **19,** 451.
Varagić, V., Krstić, M., and Mihajlović, L. (1964). *Int. J. Neuropharmacol.* **3,** 273.
Vargas, R., Carrillo, R., and Pardo, E. G. (1965). *Gac. Med. (Caracas)* **95,** 621.
Walaszek, E. J., and Abood, L. G. (1956). *Science* **124,** 440.
Walkenstein, S. S., Knebel, C. M., MacMullen, J. A., and Seifter, J. (1958). *J. Pharmacol. Exp. Ther.* **123,** 254.
Wang, H. H., Markee, S., Kahn, N., Mills, E., and Wang, S. C. (1966). *J. Pharmacol. Exp. Ther.* **151,** 285.
Wasson, B. K., and Parker, J. M. (1959). U.S. Patent No. 2,901,501.
Weil-Malherbe, H., and Posner, H. S. (1963). *J. Pharmacol. Exp. Ther.* **140,** 93.
Weiss, B., and Ewing, C. G. T. (1959). *Amer. J. Pharm.* **131,** 307.
Wenzel, D. G., and Broadie, L. L. (1966). *Toxicol. Appl. Pharmacol.* **8,** 455.
Westermann, E., and Stock, K. (1963). *Naunyn-Schmiedebergs Arch. Exp. Pathol. Pharmakol.* **245,** 102.
Wilson, V. J. (1958). *J. Gen. Physiol.* **42,** 29.
Wilson, V. J., and Talbot, W. H. (1960). *J. Gen. Physiol.* **43,** 495.
Wiser, R., and Seifter, J. (1960). *Fed. Proc. Fed. Amer. Soc. Exp. Biol.* **19,** 390.
Wissler, R. W., Hughes R. H., Frazier, L. E., and Rasmussen, R. A. (1962). *Circulation* **26,** 673.
Witkin, L. B., deStevens, G., O'Keefe, E., Spitaletta, P., Wilson, D., and Jablonski, J. (1962). *Pharmacologist* **4,** 167.
Wolf, A., and von Haxthausen, E. F. (1960). *Arzneim.-Forsch.* **10,** 50.
Yamamoto, A., Yoshimura, H., and Tsukamoto, H. (1962a). *Chem. Pharm. Bull.* **10,** 522.
Yamamoto, A., Yoshimura, H., and Tsukamoto, H. (1962b). *Chem. Pharm. Bull.* **10,** 540.
Yamamoto, I., Inoki, R., Kurogochi, Y., and Nishio, H. (1960). *Nara Igaku Zasshi* **11,** 49.
Yamamoto, I., Inoki, R., and Otori, K. (1963). *Nippon Yakurigaku Zasshi* **59,** 242.
Yeary, R. A., Benish, R. A., and Finkelstein, M. (1966). *J. Pediat.* **69,** 663.
Yen, H. C. Y., Stanger, R. L., and Millman, N. (1959). *Arch. Int. Pharmacodyn. Ther.* **123,** 179.
Yen, H. C. Y., Sigg, E. B., and Warner, C. L. (1964) *Int. J. Neuropharmacol.* **2,** 337.
Yen, H. C. Y., Katz, M. H., and Krop, S. (1970). *Toxicol. Appl.Pharmacol.* **17,** 597.
Yui, T., and Takeo, Y. (1958). *Jap. J. Pharmacol.* **7,** 162.

Drug Effects and Learning and Memory Processes

WALTER B. ESSMAN

Departments of Psychology and Biochemistry
Queens College of the City University of New York
Flushing, New York

I. Introduction

Pharmacological agents, one effect of which may suggest the modification of learning and/or memory processes, present a difficult issue to consider. It appears that one aspect of this issue is whether such an effect—facilitation or disruption—is a unique property of the drug molecule, perhaps shared by others of such a molecular family, or whether the effect is, perhaps, better dealt with in terms of a central nervous system event to which such an agent bears the proper time, locus, and site of action, as well as the event being one that is properly accorded a meaningful relationship to the cognitive processes which are drug-altered. The latter consideration—one of central mechanisms correlated with learning and memory processes—is often, of necessity, dealt with beyond the scope of traditional pharmacology, especially in those instances where concern with molecular substrates or models, cellular interactions, or subcellular sites of change necessitate cross-disciplinary investigative tools. The end point toward which such theory may be directed, around which such tools (pharmacological, as well as other) are employed, and for which questions or hypotheses of drug effect are generated is ultimately a behavioral event for which "learning" or "memory" processes are inferred. Such a behavioral change eventuating in a criterion response, the maintenance of a behavior in a response repertoire, or a predicted motor pattern or effect following stimulation or stimulus specific cuing has traditionally been that which drug effects have been titrated against and from which theories of central action of a wide segment of the pharmacopaeia have sprung, as well as theories about mechanisms related to the central processes of learning and memory. The rules for drug effects and behavioral change are neither simple nor are they or have they been guidelines for psychopharmacological research. Certainly there are other behavioral events, states, and processes which may be contributory to learning or memory, but not of necessity a critical component of either system; these are usually the behavioral conditions most obviously affected by drugs but not necessarily isolated from their disruptive or facilitatory effects posed for learning or memory. Performance, motivation, sensory capacity, etc., although they are all components of learning and memory capacity and capability, are not ideally bound to the same processes. This consideration raises the relevant question as to what is disrupted or facilitated by drug action—response capability, sensory input, response capacity, behavior storage, retrieval, etc.?

It would appear that the relevant literature in this area suggests two possible alternatives toward a possible solution of this problem; one approach has been essentially phemenological, i.e., to catalog which drugs affect which specific response—sometimes with the added consideration of dose, route of administration, and time course provided. A second approach has invited investigation of specific pharmacological agents on the basis of their established or presumed mode, site, or consequence of central action and, then, to deal with one or more of such central events as correlates of facilitated or impaired learning or memory.

It becomes rapidly obvious that psychoactive drugs, including those for which clinical therapeutic indications are the basis for use, as well as others for which such indications may be quite secondary, can exert facilitatory, disruptive, or no effect upon learning and/or memory, depending not only upon the drug but also upon the behavioral indices used to define the processes as well as the effects. The majority of the reveiws dealing with drug effects upon learning/or memory have been technique-oriented in their approach; i.e., learning or memory have been considered as definable within the context of a specific class of responses and for several parameters of the method through which the response is altered—such as aversive stimulation used to provide escape, condition avoidance, or assume fear (Brady, 1956a,b; Riley and Spinks, 1958; Dews and Morse, 1961; Cook and Kelleher, 1963; Golob and Brady, 1965). In considering which technique yields measures that are more reliable indices of learning memory or which are more valid indices of how drugs affect such processes, one is, indeed, faced with a dilemma. In animal investigation, aversive control of behaviors such as escape, avoidance, motility, and activity, have probably been used with the greatest frequency in drug studies, but it would seem that other than strictly behavioral properties of drugs thus investigated would become an issue of some concern as well; i.e., analgesic effects, motor effects, state-specificity, etc.

Related to the foregoing general considerations is a relevant issue of acute versus chronic effects of agents that modify either learning or memory; these two effects may be quite different, but, unfortunately, the comparison has only been infrequently made and the chronic effects of drugs upon learning or memory has been given regrettably little attention.

The relationship between drug dose, central levels thereof, and the rate of accumulation and loss would appear to be fundamental to the time course over which some behavioral training procedure potentially provides for a "learned response" and a "memory" of the acquired behavior. Yet, if the foregoing relationship were applied in every study concerned with drug effect and learning or memory, then one would very rapidly discover the disturbing fact that either such a relationship could not always be meaningfully demonstrated or that the distinction between disruption and facilitation could possibly apply for the same agent depending upon differences in dose, uptake, disposition, time course, etc.

Disruption of learning or memory by drugs appears to have been a more popular subject of experimental investigation, either by intent or accident, probably because behavioral disruption appears more easily demonstrable than facilitation. It can be inferred from behaviors such as prolonged response time, increased response errors, and absence of response. These responses, however, bear a striking similarity to those which might characterize behavioral toxicity from drug action. It would appear, therefore, that some more meaningful resolution of this difficulty could derive from a methodological distinction between process disruption and toxicity (these could be confused even with isotonic sodium chloride solution given in sufficient volume, systemically), or from a process-oriented definition of drug action). This basic argument is directed at the rationale underlying drug–learning/memory studies; if such rationale is based upon the use of behavioral methods, from which processes are inferred, to study the central action of a drug or drugs (behaviors as tools for pharmacology), then behavioral disruption might provide little more than screening information or indications for effective dosage; such might be the case if disruption of avoidance conditioning is interpreted as a behavioral analogy for an effective antianxiety index. The problem here again has been that such indications—generalized to either cautionary or therapeutic positions—have been largely derived from studies of acute dosage in experimental animals. It would appear that an experimental animal, an experimental behavioral method, and, more than usual, a single drug dose, constitute sufficient components of a model system for drug evaluation in impaired learning or memory, or in other behavioral processes. The other direction that research in this general area has taken is to utilize either the drug or an implied or established central effect resulting from drug action as a means of defining basic mechanisms underlying such behavioral processes as learning or memory (drugs as tools for behavioral investigation). One definite problem posed by this approach is the fact that the "process' is always an intervening variable and that the behavior based upon that process is operationally defined. Such a relationship allows for considerable "mechanism speculation" of which drug action may be but one of several possibilities. Also, very frequently, the specificity of one compound to a given central mechanism may be relatively similar to that of another drug (with dose, onset, and time course taken into account) and, yet, the nature of the behavioral effect (facilitatory or disruptive) may be entirely different. Such disturbing discrepancies are usually dealt with by reference to the complex nature of molecular interactions at the cellular level or in terms of side effects.

The interaction of behavior and drugs, insofar as changes in drug distribution, metabolism, and reciprocating behavioral effects are concerned has been very sparingly dealt with in the specific context of learning and memory. This concern has been applied mainly in toxicity studies, where initial observations regarding differences in toxicity were described as a function of differential housing (Gunn and Gurd, 1940). This issue has been treated more recently with regard to a variety of behaviors related to aggression (see Garattini and Sigg, 1969), where several behavioral paradigms certainly related to the processes of learning and memory seem relevant to the behavioral contributions of differential housing. In Section VIII of this chapter this issue will be specifically considered with regard to potentially facilitative drug action, although clear indication has been given (Essman, 1970a) that differentially housed mice acquire conditioned avoidance behavior at different rates and show clear differences in their susceptibility to amnesic events.

With the issue of facilitation of learning and/or memory by drugs there also arises the problem of rationale. Drugs which presumably facilitate do so by reducing response times, decreasing or eliminating response errors, increasing the rate at which a criterion of task performance is reached, reduce the effects of agents or events which disrupt such behaviors, etc. In order to investigate such drug effects, it seems as if one aspect of the underlying rationale must involve hypotheses regarding the mechanisms that are facilitated and the central event or process initiated, changed, or inhibited through drug action. The same problems confronting the interpretation of results from studies in which drugs impair learning or memory apply to those results wherein these processes are apparently facilitated by drug action. Unfortunately, there appear to be relatively few behavioral paradigms wherein both facilitation and disruption can be demonstrated with different drugs and where the basis for such an effect resides in either a common behavioral mechanism or obverse central effects of the drugs studied. In a rather unexplained fashion the impairment–facilitation dichotomy has been generally paralleled by a central nervous system sedative–depressive–stimulant dichotomy, where the nature of the resultant depression or stimulation (structural, physiological, or metabolic) may, in fact, constitute a methodological barrier to emerging guiding principles in such research.

It would appear that, generally, disruption or facilitation of learning or memory processes suggest in some direct or indirect manner that such processes are correlated with specified central events altered by drug action. It will not be our purpose to weigh the relative merits or limitations of such correlated central events whether they be electrical potential changes, biochemical changes, immunological responses, etc. It will rather be our purpose to consider some of those pharmacological agents, the central action of which may confer some degree of direction in one or more aspects of learning and memory processes. What qualifies one agent for consideration above another or one class of drug to the exclusion of another has largely been based upon (*1*) predefined limitations in the scope and depth of this reveiw, (*2*) the extent to which our own research in this general area is relevant to one aspect of the drug–learning/memory issue, and (*3*) our decision to omit from this writing related reviews and research reported elsewhere (Essman, 1971a,b,c).

A final point perhaps deserves some comment at this juncture, since no attempt will be made to deal with it later; that is, what pharmacological considerations are appropriate or relevant for inclusion. Specifically there are two areas that have been singled out for omission, but mention is made of their possible relevance to the general area. One area concerns the use of cerebral protein-synthesis inhibitors, essentially as tools for the study of learning ability or memory storage. These studies have been reviewed (Agranoff, 1969) but provide little in the way of useful additional information regarding the mechanism, locus, or cellular site at which such inhibition is accomplished by the drug, nor is relevant attention given to the qualitative nature of the inhibited protein synthesis. The latter consideration, in particular, would appear to constitute not only a relevant answer to a pharmacological question but also provide some much-needed insight into the relevant role of protein synthesis for the fixation and storage of acquired information. The second omitted area concerns the highly controversial and often popularly publicized issue of intraanimal information transfer via ingestion or injection of tissue extracts from "experience-endowed donors." Some of the more recent progress in this area has been summarized in several volumes (Byrne, 1970; Ungar, 1970; Adám, 1970) and further review and summary appears redundant. It might be appropriate to indicate that such investigations, which have suffered the pains of nonreplicability, criticism on neurobiological feasibility, and inherent variability of results, may find some more satisfactory resolution were the "extracts" with their presumed "information"-carrying ability treated methodologically as any sound pharmacological agent; in such a case, it might be appropriate first to raise relevant questions such as effective dose, administration time, route differences, and chronicity of treatment.

Since both the areas mentioned above have invoked, either by mechanism or hypothesis, the possible role of macromolecular events as substrates for learning or memory, which, in turn, has influenced the selection of drugs studied in experiments dealing with learning and memory, this may be an appropriate issue with which to proceed.

II. Learning and Memory Processes: Effects of Drugs on Macromolecular Substrates

Pharmacological studies in which the use of macromolecules or specific compounds capable of altering their synthesis, storage, or degradation have been derived, probably to a large extent, from theory regarding their central role in cognitive events; such theory has suggested that macromolecular concentration, structure, locus, or interaction in brain cells may constitute regulatory processes for or provide substrates of the input, storage, and retrieval of information. The focus of such hypotheses has often been ribonucleic acid (RNA) and its role in protein synthesis. An early view favoring the import of this molecule in brain processes (Hydén, 1959) was that changes in the ionic equilibrium of the cell cytoplasm, brought about by frequency-modulated inputs to the central nervous system, affected the stability of a nitrogenous base at a site on the RNA molecule. Base modification, conferring altered molecular structure, and newly synthesized RNA-dependent proteins can then interact with molecules of complementary structure; after an appropriate time course such an interaction could provide for transmitter molecule release. Although this proposal was elegant and remnants thereof may still be appropriate and feasible, it fails to resolve the difficulty in dealing with an RNA molecule, ostensibly nuclear, and the release of quanta of transmitter molecules, presumably synaptic. The mechanism for such cellular and molecular information transduction appears a weak foundation upon which to build hypotheses about macromolecules as drugs. The pharmacological modification of learning or memory, where these are considered in terms of macromolecular substrates upon which the drugs act, creates the further problem in relating the time course of macromolecular change to the time course of behavioral effect. Such relationships have, unfortunately, been rarely demonstrated, infrequently investigated, and seldom considered.

A related theoretical position that developed on a parallel chronological course (Katz and Halstead, 1960) maintained that a theoretical model for learning and memory could be based upon a nucleoprotein-constituted lattice, representing the memory trace; this was viewed in terms of the regional specificity of experience-specific nucleoproteins. If one could accept such theory as a sufficient basis for pharmacological investigation of presumably protein-dependent learning and memory, then one property of such specific agents might reside in their ability to interact with these proteins or in the subcellular machinery through which they are synthesized. This would, unfortunately, necessitate involved further investigation that extends considerably beyond the more general issues of learning or memory. In another regard the issue under consideration raises questions with regard to drugs that do have very specific, well-defined effects upon and interactions with macromolecules—effects, which one might predict from available macromolecular theory to alter learning or memory—if the former were, indeed, substrates of the latter. This expectation does not always find empirical support; for example, the behaviorally disruptive effects of puromycin (Davis, 1968) presumably relevant to its inhibition of protein synthesis (Flexner and Flexner, 1968) are considerably greater than those produced by acetoxycyclohexamide (Barondes and

Cohen, 1968) at the same level of inhibited synthesis (Flexner and Flexner, 1966). Similarly, the effects of the former upon cortical electrical activity during peak inhibition of protein synthesis are dramatic, virtually complete depression of the electroencephalogram (EEG); whereas, the latter compound at comparable levels of inhibition, produces only slight voltage changes. It seems apparent that inhibition of gross macromolecular events in the central nervous system constitutes a weak basis for relating such events to cognitive processes. It is even more relevant to consider the mechanism, site, and time course over which the synthesis of specific cerebral proteins are modified, and from such evidence then test the generality of the relationship. It may be again appropriate to emphasize that because a pharmacological agent results in the modification of brain protein synthesis does not immediately qualify such an agent as a candidate for behavioral investigation, nor does it permit the assumption that the change in rate of protein synthesis will be temporally, morphologically, or functionally consistent with a parallel directional alteration in the rate at which any learning or memory process occurs. A case in point may be illustrative.

We gave ethidium bromide to mice, over a wide dose range, sufficient, with central localization, to result in graded inhibition of cerebral microsomal protein synthesis. This compound also modifies the charging reaction of transfer RNA (tRNA) and presumably acts by intercalating with tRNA, distorting the secondary structure of the molecule. Such treatment at periods of peak, cerebral, microsomal protein-synthesis inhibition did alter the ability of mice to (*1*) acquire a single choice spatial response in a maze, with response times during acquisition comparable to those of saline-injected controls; (*2*) reduce successfully, to a final errorless criterion, the incidence of errors committed during four spaced training trials; (*3*) reverse the acquired maze response; (*4*) show a high incidence of 1-trial passive-avoidance conditioning; (*5*) show complete and long-term retention of the conditioned avoidance response; and (*6*) show effective criterion acquisition of escape behavior and conditioned active avoidance behavior in a one-way shuttle box. The possibility that these observations may be unique because of the mode and/or site of central action of the drug is obviated by further data concerned with cerebral protein-synthesis inhibition brought about as a result of 5-fluorouracil treatment in mice. At doses sufficient to produce significant inhibition, presumably as a consequence of the compound being incorporated into tRNA, those conditions for the assessment of learning and memory, as mentioned above, were similarly unaffected. The suggestion could easily follow that microsomal protein synthesis may not be related to either the disruption or facilitation of events coincident with the learning or memory process. However, this alternative can be set aside in view of our findings that one very consistent and reliable event for the time-dependent disruption of the memory consolidation process, electroconvulsive shock (ECS), also results in a time-related, regional inhibition of protein synthesis in brain, which, on the basis of *in vitro* studies is maximally accounted for by the microsomes. There is, of course a question as to the relationship between the altered synthesis at a given site, and the amnesic properties of ECS; this relationship could well derive from any one or combination of central consequences which also follow ECS, such as RNA decrements (Mihailović *et al.*, 1958; Essman, 1965), altered levels of brain biogenic amines (Garattini and Valzelli, 1957; Essman, 1967a), decrease in brain acetylcholine levels (Richter and Crossland, 1949; Essman, 1971d), and modification of the electrical activity measured over several different regions of the brain (Fink and Green, 1958; Aird *et al.*, 1956). The relationship between ECS as an amnesic agent and the interaction of its amnesic effect with drugs has been considered on a macromolecular level (Essman, 1965) as well as in terms of psychoactive drug screening (Weissman, 1967). This issue will again be treated in a later section of the present discussion. It might be appropriate to anticipate that issue with a comment regarding the interaction of amnesic agents or events and drugs that change the course of such an amnesia. Should macromolecular events or changes, indeed, constitute, at least in part, substrates for the processes of learning or memory, then amnesia induction could be expected to alter the course of such molecular events, and drugs interacting with amnesic agents would either potentiate the alteration or attenuate it, depending upon either the augmentation or reduction of the amnesia. At least on pharmacological grounds, the central effect should bear some relationship to the molecular event if either are considered relevant to cognitive processes.

In view of considerable speculation regarding the role of RNA in learning and memory, a directly emerging result has been to test the hypothesis that these processes can be directly affected by RNA treatment.

III. Ribonucleic Acid

The hypothesis that learning or memory processes can be affected or modified by treatment with exogenous RNA is subject to several criticisms on both theoretical as well as methodological grounds. A first question concerns the issue of the fate of systemically administered RNA and the possibility of its central deposition as an intact molecule, or its central effect. In this regard it would appear (Roll *et al.*, 1949; Sved, 1965) that systemic administration of RNA is ultimately resolved centrally by entry of only very few molecules; it would, therefore, be suggested that any effects of RNA upon learning or memory might depend upon only few molecules in the brain to accomplish such effects, only a portion of the molecule being necessary, or that any effects may be accounted for by peripheral consequences of either the RNA molecule, its nitrogenous bases, or intermediates in the metabolism of these bases.

In general, most studies in which RNA treatment has resulted in a positive behavioral result have indicated that this result favors the view that learning or memory has been facilitated. It would appear that with RNA treatment, the potentially weak stimulant effect upon processes such as attention, motivation, and performance must be weighed against any possible learning or memory effect (or at least considered methodologically). The facilitative properties of yeast RNA were initially reported as a consequence of both oral and intravenous administration (Cameron and Solyom, 1961); improved retention and enhanced interest and alertness were noted when the drug was given to a geriatric population over a 3-month period. In a population of senile and senescnet patients given a lower yeast RNA dosage, orally, no improvement as previously reported was observed (Kral *et al.*, 1967). The two studies are difficult to compare, since the former, a double-blind investigation indicated significantly improved memory function at an ED_{50} of about 540 gm (a summated dosage of 700 gm over 3 months occurred); pre- and posttreatment tests of memory were used in the latter study, where senile (senile dementia, artereosclerotic brain disease, or amnestic syndrome) patients were compared with senescent (free of psychiatric or neurological signs) patients. In this latter study, 7 days of treatment (42 gm of RNA versus placebo) did not provide for statistically significant improvement in memory scores. The generally improved memory scores on the posttreatment memory tests might be accounted for by a task-specific "practice effect" or, perhaps, by a more generally task-derived performance skill. The improved performance or retention tests by persons with diffuse memory disorders by yeast RNA treatment could also be accounted for by the possibility of antifatigue effects or other factors by which attention could be sustained. Another consideration applies to whether chronic RNA treatment in a clinical population tested on memory tasks reflects the same aspect of the memory process as might characterize a population free of apparent memory pathology; this consideration gives rise to the further question of what phase of the memory process as might characterize a population free of apparent memory pathology; this consideration gives rise to the further question of what phase of the memory process in man is assessed by a task such as the Wechsler Memory Scale (WMS) as utilized in the foregoing study. Registration, storage, or retrieval of stimuli can be reflected differently, both between individuals as well as within subject populations, so that recognition, recall, or relearning when improved can fall to any combination of these inferred events.

There are, perhaps, somewhat fewer but no less complex problems of interpretation of results associated with animal studies in which RNA has been given. The chronic administration of yeast-derived RNA to rats (160 mg/kg/day for 53 successive days) led to an increase in the rate at which such animals acquired a conditioned avoidance pole-climbing response, and led to a prolongation of maintence of this response in the repertoire ("retention") (Cook *et al.*, 1963). In a partial replication of this study, the systemic treatment of rats with yeast RNA was shown to enhance acquisition of the avoidance behavior; however, the drug treatment had no apparent effect upon a spatial or temporal discrimination based upon shock reinforcement (Corson and Enesco, 1966). The possibly facilitative effect of yeast RNA, at least insofar as pole-climbing avoidance conditioning was concerned, was further considered in view of the possible contribution that the age of the animal might make to such findings (Solyom *et al.*, 1967). Ribonucleic acid treatment, independent of age (young vs. old rats treated with RNA or saline), led to an increased rate of acquisition of bar-pressing behavior for continuous reinforcement, variable interval reinforcement, and conditioned emotional responding. Old rats were more prominently affected by RNA treatment during the continuous reinforcement phase, where their acquisition was greater than that of the young RNA-treated rats; the latter, however showed a greater RNA-induced effect, as reflected in better rates of variable-interval reinforcement responding, conditioned emotional response acquisition, and in the rate at which this response was extinguished. Measures of locomotor activity (activity wheel) and of heart rate were both reduced as a consequence of RNA treatment in both the young and old rats. These data are offered in support of the premise that locomotor excitation or autonomic activity are not necessarily correlaries of or contributors to the observed behavioral effect of yeast RNA. A somewhat contrasting view may be derived from data (Brown, 1966) showing that rats chronically treated with yeast RNA (160 mg/kg, i.p.) for 30 days and trained to bar-press for food reinforcement (100 reinforcements per session) showed twice the rate of bar-pressing than that of controls. This finding may offer a stronger argument for a yeast RNA-induced stimulatory effect inasmuch as increased bar-pressing for food reinforcement is probably a better reflection of task-specific (bar-pressing) activity level than is activity wheel performance, which is physically removed from, motivationally independent of, and operationally different from the task. Especially appropriate to the latter study is the issue of appetitive behavior as affected by yeast RNA, and in the case of the former study the issue of "equivalence" of the negative reinforcement in the age × drug interaction remains also in question.

The earlier findings of yeast RNA treatment leading to enhancement of learning and memory in rats have been replicated and extended (Cook, 1964; Cook and Davidson, 1968). Continuous injection of yeast RNA (160 mg/kg/day for 53 days, i.p.) led to acquisition to 100% criterion level for conditioned pole-jumping to the onset of a buzzer conditioned stimulus (CS) by 10 trials; rats treated over the same period with saline required 36 trials to achieve the same 100% criterion of pole-jumping. When pretraining drug treatment duration was reduced to 28 or 30 days, more rapid acquisition rates were still observed, in addition to a prolonged rate of extinction for the pole-climbing response. Control animals had reached a 100% level of criterion nonresponse to the CS onset (extinction) by 24 trials, whereas among the drug-treated rats 20% criterion responding was still observed after 41 trials. The process of extinction may be viewed in at least two ways in interpreting the results—a prolonged rate of active avoidance behavior following UCS cessation could reflect either prolonged memory or a reduced rate by which the adaptive behavior reflected in new learning is acquired. That is, does extinction reflect retention of original learning or acquisition of a new response? If the former possibility were applicable, it would appear that the facilitated memory, reflected in prolonged extinction of the avoidance behavior, is dependent upon RNA effects upon learning. The differences in acquisition rate brought about by pretraining RNA treatment, when eliminated through RNA injections for 2 weeks after rats were trained to criterion, still resulted in slower rates of extinction among the RNA-treated rats. It is, therefore, apparent that the slowed extinction rate relates more directly to the drug effect than to the acquired response, but other alternatives for RNA effect may reside in CS responsivity (the drug could increase reactivity to the buzzer), reaction time may be distorted by the drug, or sensory threshold could be altered. If the effective time interval during active avoidance acquisition and drug treatment for the "incubation" of a "fear" response is taken into account, then possible time differences arising out of autonomic side effects could also be utilized in accounting for such results.

The apparent facilitation, by injection of yeast RNA, of pole-climbing avoidance acquisition and prolongation of extinction has been further corroborated (Cook and Davidson, 1968); administration of the drug, either for 53 (160 mg/kg/day) or 34 days (170 mg/kg/day) brought about those results previously observed in treated rats, whereas comparable drug doses (160 mg/kg/day) given from 3 to 56 days resulted in enhancement of acquisition and prolongation of extinction of simultaneous or delayed conditioned responses by rats. The extension of the number of trials required for yeast RNA-treated rats to extinguish these responses was shown to be independent of drug-induced acquisition differences. Treatment with RNA, at the same dose levels over the same duration failed to modify the rate at which rats lever-pressed, when maintained on a schedule of continuous shock avoidance, and yet acquisition of a discrimination response maintained by food reinforcement was enhanced by such treatment. The effects of yeast RNA upon the motivational states upon which negative or positive stimuli serve to reinforce behavior have not been clearly distinguished, nor have they necessarily been eliminated as possible contributions to the observed effects; i.e., if RNA treatment effects a reduced pain threshold, and shock is most easily avoided by the pole-climbing, and hunger or appetite are increased by the drug, sufficiently to accelerate behaviors that are food-reinforced, then relatively parsimoneous principles could obtain to explain the findings. A central theory would have difficulties with these results, as it would with further findings that yeast deoxyribonucleic acid (DNA; 500 mg/kg/day) or guanylic acid (300 mg/kg/day) given to rats for 3 weeks, also enhanced conditioned pole-climbing avoidance conditioning and prolonged the rate at which this response was extinguished. Prolonged retention was again inferred from the prolonged extinction trials. Again, there does not appear to be any simple readily available explanation for such findings nor any indication as to the extent to which nucleic acid treatment is indicated as a requisite for apparent enhancement. The possibility that specific nucleotides, their degredation products, or concomitant metabolic or physiological consequences thereof could account for such effects is questionable. Why this effect is specific for the pole-climbing avoidance is also an interesting point. Whereas other investigators have clearly confirmed the more rapid acquisition and prolonged extinction of this behavior as a consequence of RNA treatment (Corson and Enesco, 1966; Wagner *et al.*, 1966), comparable doses failed to exert effects upon shock-reinforced spatial or temporal discrimination tasks and upon maze response discriminations by rats for food reward, The possible motivational role of RNA treatment as well as the possibility of a task-specific dose dependency may be feasible alternatives that remain to be investigated. Further studies have also indicated either responses or task situations where yeast RNA treatment was without effect—acquisition and retention of a maze-discrimination response based upon water reinforcement and shock-based acquisition of a Miller-Mowrer-type conditioned response were not altered by RNA treatment (Boissier *et al.*, 1966). Acquisition, by mice, of a Y-maze was not modified by treatment with yeast RNA (Barondes and Cohen, 1966).

Some preliminary indication that the central effects of RNA may be quite different from the consequences of its peripheral disposition, as well as follow a different time course of action that could not occur following systemic administration, is that a conditioned response established in rabbits, although unaffected by direct implanted cannuala delivery to cortical motor or visual areas of either saline or serum albumin, was reversibly inhibited by RNA delivered to these areas (17.7 to 20%, respectively). A more marked degree of inhibition of conditioned responses (80%) occurred after RNA was delivered to the hippocampus (Voronin *et al.*, 1968). Although this study does not indicate adequate dosage, drug diffusion area in brain, nor altered tissue levels following intracranial administration, it might suggest that macromolecular intervention can affect emission of a behavior without the necessity of attending to the issues of acquisition or memory processes; particularly implicated is the probability that regional electrolyte changes following RNA invasion of the extracellular milieu may likely depress cell functions. In any case, there appears to be a marked discrepancy between the estimated number of intact RNA molecules that can penetrate into the brain following systemic administration and the number of such molecules that were introduced directly into the brain in the foregoing study. A careful dose–response study for both routes of administration would appear indicated.

In view of the possibility that RNA treatment might alter, acutely, the course over which memory trace fixation would occur, if there were, indeed, a functional tie of the drug to the latter process, an experiment was designed to weigh the potential effect of the drug against the memory-disruptive effects of posttraining ECS. Yeast RNA was given to mice (50 to 100 mg/kg, i.p.) 60 minutes prior to training for a 1-trial passive avoidance response, within 10 seconds of training a single ECS was administered, which under control conditions led to a retrograde amnesia (absence of a conditioned passive-avoidance response among 90% of the mice, when tested 24 hours after training). The RNA-treated mice showed approximately 85% incidence of amnesia when tested, indicating that there was no indication of drug-mediated acceleration of memory fixation or ECS–amnesia antagonism, at least at those doses and times at which RNA was given (Essman, 1970b).

Several agents which result in altered levels of RNA have also been suggested as candidates for learning or memory modifiers. As we have indicated earlier, the relationship between macromolecular theory and macromolecular synthesis or concentration change is not always consistent or prevailing. Inhibition of brain RNA synthesis by 8-azaguanine did not affect the retention of a well-learned water-maze response in rats but did prevent the learning of a new maze (Dingman and Sporn, 1961). Apparent RNA degredation with ribonuclease, present in pond water where head and tail sections of conditioned planaria were allowed to regenerate led to an absence of conditioned response retention in the regenerated tail section, whereas the regenerated head section was not affected; i.e., retention was shown (Corning and John, 1961). Ribonucleic acid inhibition of 8-azaguanine caused a slowing of conditioned discrimination responses made by rats for food reinforcement (25 mg/kg) on a fixed interval schedule (Jewett *et al.*, 1965), but no really clear indication of a learning deficit could be derived from these results.

In a series of studies comparing inhibitors and stimulators of RNA and protein synthesis in rats, several findings of interest emerged (Dergachey, 1970). Actinomycin D, administered in moderate, multiple doses to rats, prolonged the transition of memory from fixation to permanent storage and prevented the consolidation of the memory trace, suggesting that the stage of the memory process affected is temporally linked to the drug effect upon RNA or protein synthesis. Memory consolidation by rats, as well as mild memory disturbance in children were improved by treatment with such presumed stimulants to nucleic acid and protein synthesis as folic acid, vitamin B_{12}, and orotic acid. Although the latter is incorporated into RNA, and folate and cyanocobalamin are possibly related to RNA synthesis by coenzymic linkage providing for formation of purines in one case and condensation with ribose in the other, the hypothesis would still appear to be too thin to support the weight of the implied mechanism or the causal relationship between macromolecular synthesis and cognitive change. A similar venture in the same direction has suggested a correlation between the level of functional activity of the central nervous system and an overall increase in RNA metabolism (DiCarlo *et al.*, 1970); this relationship has sought support with amphetamine sulfate as the origin of such increased level and learning as the end point. Mice given amphetamine sulfate (15 mg/kg., i.p.) showed an increase of 7.12% in total RNA within 2 hours of treatment, and an increase of 52.4% in the specific activity of total RNA. Central nervous system stimulants, including the amphetamines, have been employed in many studies of learning or memory, some with an implied tie to macromolecular theory and others that have been simply empirically based. Since some central nervous system stimulants and several analeptic drugs have been related to the general theme under consideration, but in addition bring into focus the issue of synaptic processes, by way of synthesis, storage, and release effects which such compounds additionally relate to in terms of their effects upon putative transmitter molecules, it might be appropriate to consider this issue.

IV. Amphetamines

The effects of amphetamines in the central nervous system have been extensively studied, and are well summarized (see Costa and Garattini, 1970) to the point where varieties of electrophysiological and biochemical effects may serve as a basis for a number of positions to be taken concerning learning or memory processes. Both cortical and subcortical EEG activation have been noted after amphetamine treatment, and facilitation of synaptic transmission (Luco *et al.*, 1949), both mono- and polysynaptically, has supported the more general excitatory effects observed, such as righting, postural changes, and modified recovery among animals with brain lesions. Possible depressant properties of this compound have also been suggested (Marrazzi, 1953; Longo and Silvestrini, 1957). In relation to brain biogenic amines, the amphetamines have traditionally been believed to effect norepinephrine release from nerve terminals; this release and consequent depletion of catecholamines by 6 to 8 hours following drug treatment—persisting for 24 hours, or more—beyond the limits of drug retention by the tissue, present several evaluative problems. It would initially suggest a triphasic sequence of changes produced by amphetamines, to which behavioral effects might well be related. An initial phase of catecholamine release and ensuing cellular excitation, followed by degredation, removal, and reconstitution of adequate stores—differences in excitation or depression of central events might well depend upon the time course of the drug effect as well as on when a particular learning or memory task was introduced.

On the basis of an extensive review of the effects of amphetamines upon operant behavior in animals (Stein, 1964), it is immediately apparent that because of the drug's hypothalamic effects in areas mediating hunger and/or thirst, assessment of any behavior maintained under either motivational state creates a difficult problem. A paradoxical effect, suggesting a still more complex interaction emerges from the results that rats induced to drink water based upon thirst showed depressed drinking as a consequence of amphetamine treatment, but when drinking mediated escape from shock, amphetamine produced increased drinking. When reinforcements other than food or water have been used to maintain behaviors, there has been a generally increased response after amphetamine. The distinction between psychomotor excitation, elevated performance level, or reduced fatigue effects appear to constitute the major interpretative considerations that apply to amphetamine-induced changes in learning and memory. Performance of responses initiated by shock avoidance has generally been indicated as being increased by the amphetamines, and even where electrical stimulation to the brain has been utilized as positive reinforcement, amphetamine has facilitated such behaviors as well. It has been largely based upon such evidence that the suggestion that amphetamine lowers reward thresholds has emerged (Stein, 1964).

The relatively poor performance shown by rats in a discriminatory escape–avoidance situation was improved by diamphetamine (3 mg/kg) without the drug exerting any effects upon lever-pressing during periods of nonavoidance. Diamphetamines also affected responses to exteroceptive stimuli that were not previously associated with the shock. These findings were interpreted as a drug-induced disruption of central nervous system-mediated freezing patterns (Hearst and Whalen, 1963). Further indication of possibly facilitative effects of the amphetamines have emerged in cases where the temporal discrimination involved in the shift of interresponse times to avoid shock was improved (Verhave, 1961), the response rate was increased, and the number of punishing shocks decreased in acquisition of a temporal schedule of operant responding (Sidley and Schoenfeld, 1963) and in facilitation of avoidance response acquisition by rats (Kelemen and Bovet, 1961a). The escape latency in rats where amphetamine led to an increased rate of avoidance learning was not affected (Gatti and Bovet, 1963), and in hamsters the drug has been reported to increase the rate of discrimination learning (Rensch and Rahmann, 1960; Rahmann, 1961). In contrast, no differences in the number of conditioned avoidance responses made by rats in a shuttle box were observed after treatment with diamphetamine (2 mg/kg, i.p.), where gross activity, as measured by intertrial hurdle-crossing, was increased without enhanced performance in this situation (Powell *et al.*, 1965). In a learning task wherein the approach, shock escape, and shock avoidance responses of rats were assessed after response equalization, methamphetamine led to increased running speed (Barry and Miller, 1965). The equivalence of task performance upon which the drug effect is evaluated may perhaps obscure inherent relationships between individual differences among animals and response to the drug; for example, rats that showed criterion "poor performance" when trained in a shuttle box (20 trials/10 sessions) were then given *d*-amphetamine prior to 5 sessions—after 300 to 400 trials. The optimal dose range within which improvement of performance was observed was 0.125–2.00 mg/kg, i.p. (Rech, 1966). The dose dependency of an amphetamine effect may be reflected in the enhanced fixed-interval response rates produced by low doses and the reduction or reversal of this effect at higher doses (Bignami and Gatti, 1969). When amphetamine (2 mg/kg) was given to rats on 4 operant trials, spaced 1 week apart, intermittently reinforced behavior was depressed and food-motivated discrimination was retarded. Recovery of the operant rate and nonimproved discrimination on later nondrug trials suggested that discrimination learning was retarded by the drug, rather than repressing it as a consequence of the operant rate effect (Cole, 1968). A greater difficulty in the acquisition of avoidance responding was observed in rats tested on the thirty-sixth day after 35 days of daily methamphetamine hydrochloride treatment [6 mg/kg, subcutaneously]; the drug-treated animals showed slower extinction and also responded in a dull and fearful manner (Moriguchi, 1963). Because of the possibility, mentioned earlier, that the amphetamines may serve to provide facilitation of learning that is actually an antifatigue property of the drug, mice were trained to respond to light onset in a shuttle-box avoidance task during a 2000-trial session; immediately following this session, amphetamine (1.5 mg/kg) was administered and a 100-trial session was given. Whereas the best performance (criterion responses during the 2000 trials was 24, amphetamine-treated mice reached a level of 70 out of the 100 additional trials (Oliverio, 1967). The implication of adrenergic mechanisms in this effect was suggested by data showing that the potentiating effect of amphetamine was antagonized when the mice were pretreated, 2 hours before drug injection, with α-methyltryosine (10–30 mg/kg). This implication, however, is rather poorly supported in the absence of any evidence indicating that the exceedingly low dose of a tyrosine hydroxylase inhibitor in fact leads to reduced brain catecholamine levels in mice, especially by 2 hours after treatment. It has been our observation that in mice a 100-mg/kg dose is required to bring about a peak catecholamine depletion (approx. 56%) by 4 hours following i.p. injection (Essman, 1970a).

Several studies have considered the effects of amphetamine administered in combination or mixture with another compound, or used as a presumed drug antagonist. This rationale, at least insofar as learning and memory are concerned, seems to rest upon either a presumed potentiation effect, or maximizing the cognitive while reducing the psychomotor stimulant effect of amphetamine. A combination of amphetamine sulfate (0.75 mg/kg) and amylobarbitone sodium (15 mg/kg) led to a dose-specific increase in rat exploratory behavior that could not be accounted for by either of the constituents of this combination alone (Rushton and Steinberg, 1963). The acquisition of a lever-pressing response, for water reinforcement, by rats was also enhanced by this drug combination (Bösser *et al.*, 1970). In further studies with this drug combination, water-deprived rats, trained to an errorless criterion to a left–right discrimination position in a T-maze for water reinforcement, learned more rapidly than saline-treated controls; these rats did not differ from others given amphetamine (0.75 mg/kg), alone, except that during the initial trials fewer errors were made. Rats given amylobarbitone (15 mg/kg), alone, showed significantly impaired maze acquisition. When reversal training of an acquired maze response was given under either saline, individual drug, or drug combination, reduced interference with the original learning (fewer trials or impaired response retention) resulted when the reversal training was given under amylobarbitone. The mixture appeared to provide intermediate effects, which suggested impaired retention following drug withdrawal; this was not observed with amphetamine alone (Porsolt *et al.*, 1970). The implication that mutual antagonism or reversal of a learning deficit by amphetamine can occur appears to be an issue that requires considerably more study; the duration of drug treatment and dose appear important considerations in this regard. When rats, chronically treated with sodium barbitone, were tested in a multiple T-maze, their running time, food intake, and body weights were increased as compared with untreated rats; this effect was not antagonized by amphetamine treatment (Leonard, 1969). In a discriminated avoidance task, rats treated with 0.5 to 2.0 mg/kg of amphetamine given following 1.0 or 2.0 mg/kg of chlorpromazine, showed a significant enhancement of acquisition. The difference between the effects of amphetamine alone and those of the drug combination appeared to reside in the rate at which conditioned responding increased over total response rate, particularly for the latter animals at the lower chlorpromazine pretreatment dose (Del Rio, 1970).

Conclusions regarding the effect of amphetamines upon memory, particularly in animal studies, have not been clearly offered. There appears to be several facets of the techniques utilized in either task acquisition or stimulus-contingent response problems where memory could be assumed as operative or within which a criterion for its operation could be applied; this has infrequently been the case. The observation that *d*-amphetamine, given to mice prior to training for passive avoidance, resulted in a deficit, tested 24 hours later, has been used not only to invoke an untested adrenergic mechanism of drug action and learning, but also as possible evidence for a memory deficit (Bohdanecky and Jarvik, 1967). In a 1-trial active-avoidance task, mice treated with amphetamine sulfate (5 mg/kg) prior to training showed a reduced incidence of active avoidance retention 24 hours later as compared with saline-treated controls (Essman, 1970b). Since foot shock threshold is not apparently modified by such drug treatment, and precluding any possible drug–foot shock interaction on the central level, one might expect passive avoidance behavior (freezing response) to be enhanced, particularly if the adrenergic effect and augmented arousal favor memory consolidation of a nonmotile emotional response. With more specific regard to memory consolidation, the disruptive effects brought about by treatment with cyclohexamide were antagonized in mice treated with amphetamine (Barondes and Cohen, 1968); this finding may bear possible relevance to previously mentioned correlates of cellular excitation and metabolic activity, or perhaps even pose a role for amphetamine in protein synthesis or as an antagonist of its inhibitors. In a related context, when memory consolidation was disrupted with ECS (which inhibits microsomal and synaptosomal protein synthesis) given to mice within 10 seconds following single-trial passive avoidance training, pretraining amphetamine (5 mg/kg), posttraining treatment, or post-ECS administration did not appreciably reduce the high incidence (~90%) of retrograde amnesia determined on a testing trial given 24 hours later (Essman, 1966, and unpublished observations). The posttraining administration of amphetamine to rats has been observed to facilitate the acquisition of one-way conditioned avoidance responding in a shuttle box and also to facilitate both discriminated avoidance responding and reversal of the discriminated avoidance response; as the training–drug treatment interval was increased, the magnitude of the amphetamine-induced facilitation was reduced, whereas the magnitude of the drug effect was greater in older animals (Doty and Doty, 1966).

The enhancement of performance by the amphetamines in man has been critically reviewed (Weiss and Laties, 1962), and it was suggested that reduced reaction time, improved hand-steadiness and coordination, and counteraction of motor performance decrements produced by alcohol could be attributed to the drug effect. Reduced work-performance decrements and restoration of performance levels lowered by fatigue also appear to be drug-related. It is apparent that inasmuch as the amphetamines lead to improved performance on arithmetic and complex verbal tasks, it is difficult to extract this effect and separate it from the drug's action on learning. Some studies (Franks and Trouton, 1958) have indicated that the rate of human conditioning is accelerated by diamphetamine. In a similar regard, facilitative effects were observed after 10 days of *d*-amphetamine treatment, as reflected in tests of abstract reasoning, free association, sentence completion, addition, writing speed, etc. (Nash, 1962). Statistically significant increases in the solution of arithmetic problems following only a single 10-mg dose of diamphetamine was also noted; in this regard, the drug-treated subjects made fewer errors than placebo-treated controls, and the characteristic performance decrement among fatigued subjects was prevented by drug treatment. Administration of *d*-amphetamine 2 hours prior to an experimental session decreased disjunctive reaction time (Evans and Jewett, 1962). Where sleep deprivation was used to induce moderate fatigue, performance error was decreased in highly motivated, drug-treated subjects given addition and subtraction tasks (Holliday, 1965). In a double-blind study with a saline-placebo, methamphetamine (15 mg/68 kg) was given i.v., and running memory span for strings of digits from 8 to 20 items in length was measured; in testing both item/second and 4/items/second, and calling for the reproduction of the last five items in the correct sequence, the drug produced differences (Talland and Quarton, 1965). In a drug–placebo comparison the effects of *d*-amphetamine were assessed on the acquisition and persistence of paired-associate learning and upon delayed recall. There was a significant increase in the acquisition of "low-competetive" lasts, but during recall the drug had no effect (Hurst *et al.*, 1969).

The amphetamines, as sympathomimetic amines, exert multiple effects, both central and peripheral, which might bear upon more fundamental mechanisms with which learning and memory processes are involved. The striking contrast between the animal and human studies with these drugs is the absence, in the latter area, of motivating conditions requiring avoidance or escape from painful stimulation, whereas among the animal studies the interaction of drug with arousal states specific to the behavioral task might constitute a source of question regarding any potential facilitatory effect of the amphetamines. Still at issue is the apparent antifatigue property of amphetamines that clearly emerges in either repetetive tasks, multiple trials, or sustained task intervals, where performance appears improved, as compared to controls. It appears that an important consideration in such studies would be the methodological separation of motor learning from cognitive learning and a predrug or drug-independent assessment of the relative contribution of each to a given task where both are involved in an ultimate critierion definition of learning or memory. In the case of how varieties of such processes are modified by the amphetamines, then, a distinction between differential drug effects upon system-specific and task-related learning could prove to be extremely useful in specifying the route by which a presumed effect is mediated.

Analeptic agents, the central nervous system stimulatory effect of which may well involve a number of putative transmitter molecules in the central nervous system and which offer some promise insofar as more direct approaches to biochemical mechanisms through which learning and memory processes may be altered, have found some degree of support as presumed facilitators of such processes. Among these drugs are strychnine, pentylenetetrazol, and picrotoxin. Indirect stimulants of a related nature, such as nicotine and caffeine have also been implicated.

V. Strychnine

The apparent action of this central nervous system stimulant upon spinal cord synapses—presumably to block inhibitory substances at the sites, that mediate such transmission—and the effect of the analeptic in depressing postsynaptic inhibitory impulses and *in vitro* cholinesterase inhibition (Nachmansohn, 1938), all appear to be weak as a framework, within which subconvulsive doses of this compound, could be considered to facilitate learning and memory. This latter observation probably originated with the report that rats showed improved maze acquisition ability following treatment with strychnine sulfate (Lashley, 1917); the apparent rationale of such a drug–behavior relationship appears to reside in assumptions regarding either the status of brain excitability at the time of learning or presumed neural events activated by stimuli accompanying the learning experience. A vast majority of studies involving this compound have been essentially phenomenological and descriptive, rather than based upon a drug–central nervous system relationship; as such, the concept of a facilitatory effect of strychnine upon learning or memory processes has referred to behavioral rather than process facilitation. With the implied hypothesis that differences in inbred strains of rats, selected for maze learning ability, may also be affected differently by high and low doses of strychnine sulfate—based upon endogenous cholinergic differences (?)—no significant differences in errors emerged when rats were treated with either 0.33 or 1.00 mg/kg, i.p., of strychnine sulfate (McGaugh, 1961). These animals, trained in a 14-unit alley maze, were in some instances facilitated by low doses, and in other instances adversely affected by high doses. In this study the potential interaction between an appetitive task and the drug effect, exerted when given 10 minutes prior to the onset of training trials, presents a possible methodological hazard to the interpretation of the results. Although the possible locomotor effects of such treatment could contribute to a partial account of the behavioral effect, this effect appears obviated in view of the failure of several subconvulsive doses to affect locomotion (Dews, 1953). In subsequent studies of the presumed facilitatory effect of strychnine upon learning and memory, the previously implied cholinergic hypothesis (McGaugh, 1961) has been discarded in favor of a drug-induced facilitation upon temporally labile phases of the memory fixation process—a phase which corresponds generally to that hypothesized over 70 years ago (Müller and Pilzecker, 1900) and described as the consolidation–perseveration hypothesis. In more recent studies, the hypothesis has been omitted and consolidation of memory is taken to be an event. Reviews of the strychnine–consolidation relationships have been made (McGaugh and Petrinovich, 1965; McGaugh, 1966, 1968), and again the effect of strychnine upon this brief phase of the memory process has not been linked to any molecular or electrical event in the brain. Although such attempts have occasionally been made, i.e., the observation that a 27% increase in whole-brain RNA followed six daily i.p. injections of strychnine (Carlini and Carlini, 1965), such molecular correlates fail to explain the behavioral results.

When strychnine sulfate (0.1 to 0.3 mg/kg) was given to rats tested for escape behavior, more rapid escape and the automatization thereof was improved (Keleman and Bovet, 1961a,b). A compound similar in structure to strychnine, 5,7-diphenyl-1,3-diazemantan-6-OL (1757 I.S.) was also shown (0.6–1.2 mg/kg) to promote more rapid escape behavior. This latter compund (1 mg/kg) was given to rats of "maze-bright" and "maze-dull" derived sublines 10 minutes prior to maze training trials; A first generation cross of these sublines (S_3 and F_1) showed the greatest degree of facilitated maze acquisition when the training trials were massed over time (McGaugh *et al.*, 1961). In a simultaneous discrimination learning task, rats from maze-dull and maze-bright sublines were given strychnine sulfate (0.33 mg/kg) or saline 6 minutes pretrial; although no significant differences between sublines appeared as a function of drug treatment, the strychnine-treated rats, in general, showed superior performance. Whereas control animals required an average of 81.5 trials to reach criterion performance (40.5 median), the drug-treated animals reached criterion by 30.5 trials (13.0 median). Weight differences or a differential response to shock could not account for the behavioral differences (McGaugh and Thomson, 1962). In further studies (McGaugh *et al.*, 1962), maze-aptitude and sex differences were considered where strychnine sulfate was administered (1.0 mg/kg) either 6 minutes before or 1, 15, 30, or 90 minutes after each training trial. Superior performance was shown, generally, among those rats treated either before or 15 minutes after training, and the greatest degree of variance was observed between the performance scores of sublines when the received strychnine 30 minutes after each trial. The lowest mean trials to reach criterion among the S_3 (maze-dull) rats occurred when they were treated either before or within 15 minutes after each training trials, whereas the lowest S_1 (maze-bright) means to criterion were observed when drug treatment was given at 1, 15, or 30 minutes after each trial. In a successive visual discrimination problem, strychnine sulfate-treated rats (1.0 mg/kg) learned faster than either saline or nontreated controls (Petrinovich, 1963). The observation was made (Walsh, 1947) that strychine can accelerate visual acuity; thus, if the nature of the available visual cues were altered or visual cues could be more extensively utilized by an animal, either in maze learning or discrimination learning, then a drug effect could be more properly assigned to a sensory process rather than a cognitive event. The potential contribution of the drug to visual acuity in animals, however, remains to be investigated. Although earlier studies have suggested rather specific time limits within which low doses of this analeptic agent serve to improve learning, female rats, given strychnine sulfate (1.25 mg/kg) either 24 or 72 hours before training in a Hebb-Williams maze, showed improved preformance (Cooper and Krass, 1963), even when tested 7 days later. A single strychnine injection given 72 hours prior to maze testing also led to a reduced number of errors. Evidence, such as that cited, for persisting performance effects of strychnine points to a methodological flaw in studies where the drug is given prior to or during training and results of such a paradigm are interpreted in terms of memory processes. This objection is met, in part, where the drug has been given following training, based upon the assumption that the drug effect is linked to the "perseverative neural activity" that persists for a brief interval of time following an experience. Such posttrial treatment also meets the objectives of possible sensory, sensorimotor, or motivational effects of the drug during learning. Strychnine sulfate (1.0 mg/kg, i.p. was given to female rats, either 2 days prior to training, immediately following training, or 2 days prior to 5 retention trials given following 2 training trials; the training consisted of a maze problem wherein a correct choice was reinforced with water (Greenough and McGaugh, 1965). The data, unfortunately, failed to support a memory-specific rather than a generalized performance effect of the drug, since the incidence of maze errors did not differ for either the 2 training trials or the 5 criterion trials as a function of treatment conditions.

The administration of strychnine sulfate either 1 or 60 minutes after each trial of a 14-unit water maze, beginning after the ninth day of training, led to facilitated acquisition for both maze-bright and maze-dull rats; the latter showed a facilitative effect when the drug was given at either 1 or 60 minutes after each trial, but the former was facilitated only at the 1-minute posttrial interval. These results have been viewed in favor of a required acetylcholine–cholinesterase ratio in the brain, operating at a maximum for efficient learning (Ross, 1964). The basis upon which facilitation of learning by strychnine rests would appear to constitute an important consideration in the evaluation of studies in this area. For example, rats given strychnine sulfate (1.0 mg/kg) after each daily trial in a maze, required fewer trials to reach a criterion of 3 out of 4 correct responses; there were, however, no significant differences in maze errors or response times as a consequence of drug treatment (Loutit, 1965).

Negative or dubious effects of strychnine upon instrumental avoidance conditioning in rats have been reported (Bovet and Gatti, 1965), whereas the presumed facilitation has been indicated as dose- and time-specific. One might ask further whether it is not also task-specific. In mice, trained on an avoidance learning task, 0.3 mg/kg of strychnine sulfate given immediately after each training session facilitated avoidance acquisition; longer delays in drug administration (60 minutes) or higher doses (0.6 mg/kg) did not provide for a facilitative effect (Bovet *et al.*, 1966). It is rather surprising that an avoidance task for mice imposes limits upon treatment time and drug dosage that apparently were not critical parameters in other rodents or in other tasks. For example, rats given strychnine sulfate (1.0 mg/kg) after the first 2 trials of an alternation task for which 3 trials/day were given, showed significantly better performance when long interval delays were imposed (Petrinovich *et al.*, 1965). This phenomenon appeared independent of strain differences, yet strain differences have been subsequently invoked to deal with failure to find strychnine as facilitative. This suggestion was based upon the view that "sensitivity" to strychnine is strain-dependent (Petrinovich, 1967). Food-deprived rats given 0.125 mg/kg of strychnine sulfate made fewer maze errors for wet-mash reinforcement than either saline-treated controls or rats given the drug in doses ranging from 0.25 to 1.75 mg/kg. Although these data support the possibility that a facilitative effect may occur at lower doses, they hardly provide support for strain-related dose effects nor do they effectively resolve the problem of presumed facilitation reported for higher doses of the drug. If this study is offered as an excuse for failure to obtain facilitation of learning at higher doses of strychnine, then it hardly justifies any success in learning facilitation at such higher doses as well. The task-related specificity of a facilitative effect of this drug has been indicated (Coker and Abbott, 1967), and imposition of sensory stimulation (blinking light and intermittent auditory stimuli) upon a posttraining strychnine treatment (0.6 mg/kg., i.p.) impaired learning (Calhoun, 1966). These observations raise questions regarding certain basic assumptions of strychnine action; whereas the prevailing view has held that the drug, at those doses given, leads to increased activation, an opposite view has also been presented. Although reduced home cage activity results from strychnine treatment (Calhoun, 1965), it is not likely that this may bear upon its performance effects during learning. The hypothesis ascribing learning effects to dose-dependent relationships might have difficulty in explaining the finding that rats, trained to lever-press to avoid shock signalled by a buzzer, showed significant enhancement (lower response latency and more avoidance responses) when given 1.0 mg/kg of strychnine sulfate, but at a lower dose (0.5 mg/kg) there was no difference from saline-treated controls (Gibby *et al.*, 1965). These observation were made for Wistar strain rats; hooded rats given either 0.75 or 1.0 mg/kg strychnine sulfate did not show facilitated maze learning (Prien *et al.*, 1963). The question of strain difference remains to be systematically explored with regard to dose differences and task specificity before any more general conclusions can be derived from such studies.

Arguments for a central effect of strychnine upon neural processes associated with learning, rather than a performance effect have been offered. Food- and water-deprived rats, trained in a Y-maze for food reward, were given 3 massed trials/day, followed by strychnine injection (0.33 mg/ kg); drug-treated rats showed fewer errors and required fewer trials than saline-treated controls, with little performance effect of the drug (Krivanek and Hunt, 1967). It is of interest to note that facilitative effects appear dependent upon the intertrial interval or number of trials in relation to drug treatment. With pretrial strychnine treatment, rats given massed trials to acquire a maze response showed facilitation (fewer trials and errors to criterion), but under distributed training trials no drug effect occurred (Livecchi and Dusewicz, 1969). Posttrial administration of strychine (0.2 LD_{50}) to rats given either massed 5/day or distributed 1/day trials in a 12-choice elevated T-maze for food reinforcement was without significant effect for either condition (Dusewicz and Livecchi, 1969).

The effects of strychnine treatment have been considered in at least one classical conditioning study (Cholewiak *et al.*, 1968). Response acquisition of a classically conditioned nictitating membrane in rabbits was facilitated by a presession injection of strychnine; the effect, however, was attributed to performance factors because pretreated animals showed a higher level of conditioned responses following unpaird CS–unconditioned stimulus (UCS) presentations. In the case of postsession strychnine injection, conditioning of the nictitating membrane response was appreciably depressed.

One proposed action of strychnine upon a memory process has been its presumed effect upon the temporally labile phase of memory fixation that follows closely and persists briefly beyond an experience; this hypothesized "memory consolidation" period has been assigned a rate factor and one action of strychnine is apparently to accelerate the rate at which the trace is consolidated (McGaugh, 1966, 1968; McGaugh and Petrinovich, 1965). Evidence in support of this suggestion derives from findings of postexperimental drug treatment, i.e., treatment during the consolidation period leads to facilitation as measured in a subsequent retention test. It is still more surprising to find the same basic rationale applied in a paradigm wherein passive avoidance training in mice, followed by ECS given at 8, 18, or 60 seconds after training, results in reduced retrograde amnesia when strychnine sulfate was given immediately after the ECS at 18 or 60 seconds posttraining, or even by 3 hours after ECS (McGaugh, 1968). In studies reported previous to these, the potential interaction of a posttraining, amnesia-producing ECS and ECS–amnesia attenuator, strychnine, have been considered; in mice, trained in a single-trial avoidance situation, strychnine sulfate (0.16 or 0.33 mg/kg), given 10 minutes before the training trial, was effective, at the latter dose, in attenuating the amnesic effect of ECS given 15 seconds after training, and effective, at both doses, in attenuating the amnesic effect of ECS given 30 seconds after training (Bivens and Ray, 1966). It is difficult to assess the potential interaction of pretraining drug and the conditioning shock or the electroshock; if the threshold to the former were decreased with the centrally arousing effects of strychnine, one might simply be titrating stronger aversive stimulation against ECS, the outcome of which might predictably be a reduced efficacy of the latter. Shoud the central effect of strychnine reduce the seizure activity that leads to ECS-induced amnesia, then the amnesia-inducing potency of the ECS might be predictably reduced. Both of these alternatives to a strychnine-induced memory facilitation require testing before the former hypothesis becomes clearly supported. In rats trained to suppress lever-pressing the injection of strychnine sulfate (1.0 mg/kg) 20 minutes prior to ECS led to some, but not any convincing incidence of attenuated retrograde amnesia (Weissman, 1967). Titration of strychnine dosage against ECS magnitude (superthreshold current) has not been systematically done, nor have chronic treatments been independently considered. It does become apparent that variables such as species, strain, drug dose, treatment times, and testing times can individually or interactively contribute to the success or failure of this analeptic in facilitating learning or memory, impairing such inferred processes, or having no effect discernible from that of saline. The potential role of this analeptic as an antifatigue agent bears some consideration, especially in view of the reported facilitative success of acute doses in those learning situations wherein response measures are derived from experimental paradigms that may maximize fatigue factors, i.e., massed training trials for maze acquisition, increased number of discriminative choices in maze training, or differences in "fatiguability" determining the maze brightness or maze dullness of rats, etc. Several of the foregoing considerations apply, as well, to the contributions of other stimulants and analeptics to learning and memory.

VI. Pentylenetetrazol

The rather general range, from the brainstem to the cerebral cortex, over which pentylenetetrazol (PTZ) acts has complicated the localization of its central site(s) of action when the compound has been administered in both convulsive and subconvulsive doses. The latter has found some favor in treatment of semile attentional and social disorders (Goodhart and Helenore, 1963) and also in memory disorders in geriatric patients with arteriosclerosis or associated chronic brain syndrome (Wolff, 1962).

In animal studies concerned with the application of PTZ toward learning and memory processes, considerable support for subconvulsive doses of this analeptic as a mediator of enhancement of such processes has been provided. It should be pointed out, however, that this agent, given in convulsive doses in close temporal proximity with a single-trial conditioning experience (suppression of bar-pressing for water reinforcement by shock presented through the drinking tube), produces a profound degree of retrograde amnesia in rats (Pearlman *et al.*, 1961); this PTZ-induced amnesia was observed even when the training–PTZ interval was as long as 8 hours, but it appears quite likely that rather than constituting a retroactive effect upon the training experience, this treatment produced a proactive effect upon the testing session. Since recurrent seizures can be easily triggered by interoceptive or peripheral sensory stimuli following recovery from the initial postictal depression following PTZ injection, it is quite possible that such seizure sequalae may explain the long-lasting effect. The temporal gradient for PTZ-induced retrograde amnesia appears more extensive than that for ECS, and the same possible rationale mentioned above may also apply. It is clear that just as the occurrence or nonoccurrence of a PTZ-induced convulsion is not a determinant of whether such postraining treatment produces retrograde amnesia, dose considerations for this compound do not simply entail the principle that subconvulsive doses serve to facilitate learning or memory. It has been shown that the retrograde amnesia, produced in mice for a passive avoidance response by posttraining PTZ injection (60 mg/kg), was not affected when the PTZ-induced convulsion was abolished by pretreatment with lidocaine (Essman, 1968a). In a related series of experiments, it was further pointed out that a PTZ-induced amnesia in mice could not be simply accounted for by a PTZ-induced brain RNA decrement; this relationship was obviated by evidence indicating that PTZ, in the absence of an overt convulsion, does not lead to appreciable changes in whole-brain RNA level. Further evidence for the disruptive effect of PTZ upon learning in the rat has been provided in a study of operant conditioning (lever-pressing for water reward) where continuous reinforecment for responding was followed by a mixed schedule (FR 30, FI 5) of reinforcement (Kahan, 1966); following 35–80 training sessions, rats were given from 10 to 40 mg/kg of PTZ over a period of 5 to 7 weeks. At 10 mg/kg, a slight depression in the initial response rate was observed; at 20 mg/kg, a significant depression in response rate during the first 2 mixed schedule periods was noted; no significant effect resulted from the 30-mg/kg dose, and complete disruption, for over 1 hour, of the response schedules followed the 40-mg/kg treatment. The return to pretreatment baselines of these response levels following drug treatment offers considerable support for the view that a presumed disruptive effect of PTZ may be performance-related within a time interval for which the drug is maximally active. Since this experiment did not actually consider response acquisition or retention, the transient disruption of ratio performance and acquired timing behavior in the rat by PTZ may well correspond to a period of postictal depression following seizure (but not overt convulsive) activity. Whether such activity is varied in duration, magnitude or locus as a function of drug dose remains to be considered.

An early report of the presumed facilitatory effect of PTZ (Loken, 1940, 1941) indicated that the retention and relearning of a single-alternation alley maze by rats was improved when these animals had been given PTZ. Other maze studies of a comparable vintage (Bunch and Mueller, 1941; Heron and Carlson, 1941) did not find differences between PTZ- and saline-treated rats (daily injections of progressively increased dosage and acute sc treatment, respectively) in acquisition (trials and times) or error incidence, respectively. In the case where PTZ was used to elicit convulsions, it has been reported that this state is sufficient to restore experimentally extinguished, conditioned responses (Gellhorn, 1943), but this phenomenon appears contingent upon the convulsion rather than the agent utilized to bring it about.

It has been reported that mice treated with PTZ (1–30 mg/kg) either 30 minutes before or immediately after a 1-trial passive avoidance, training experience show facilitated learning and improved memory (Irwin and Benuazizi, 1966). Using an escape latency to hurdle-crossing after the onset of foot shock, the maximum facilitative effect was observed at a dose of 3 mg/kg. With a pretraining treatment of 10 to 20 mg/kg, rats demonstrated a drug-related enhancement of several discrimination tasks; similarly, drug-treated mice trained to a black–white discrimination in a T-maze showed an enhanced ability to learn simultaneous and successive discriminations, although response speed was reduced (Hunt and Krivanek, 1966). Among two strains of mice, posttrial PTZ treatment facilitated Lashley III alley maze acquisition (McGaugh, 1966). For C57 BL/6 strain mice the greatest initial maze error decrement occurred with 10 mg/kg of PTZ, whereas when BALB/C strain mice were given 5 mg/kg of PTZ, these mice with a lower overall initial error score, showed a greater maze error decrement. In studies using foot shock in avoidance training and posttrial PTZ injection, no apparent effect was noted (Bovet *et al.*, 1966), and the replicability of the memory enhancing properties of this agent, as considered for passive avoidance behavior, has also been negative (Pearl and McKean, 1967).

An interesting hypothesis has been proposed to account for earlier findings and generate further experiments; that is, that because PTZ decreased maze running speed, it provided the animal with more maze time and a greater duration of exposure to relevant cues (Krivanek and Hunt, 1967). For rats given PTZ (20 mg/kg) immediately after 3 daily massed trials in a Y-maze for food reward, learning (Errors and trials) was significantly better than among other drug- or saline-treated rats. With mice, trained for food reinforcement on a visual discrimination task to a criterion of 9 out of 10 errorless choices, PTZ treatment resulted in decreased errors to criterion as the dose was increased to 10 mg/kg; at 10 to 20 mg/kg, i.p., an apparent maximum in the error decrement was reached (Krivanek and McGaugh, 1968). There was a somewhat lower incidence of mean errors among male mice (∼2–4) than among females (∼3–7) for the drug-treated animals, but these errors were appreciably less than those of saline-treated controls (18–20). Whereas this drug effect was achieved when the mice were PTZ-treated daily following the last of 3 trials, facilitation was reported if drug treatment was initiated within 15 minutes posttraining, but at longer intervals there was no apparent effect. The pretraining injection of PTZ (30 and 60 minutes) was less effective than posttraining treatment, and this has been viewed in terms of an electrocortical effect of the drug being less than 45 minutes in duration. Why a specific locus of electrical activity and a specific time course thereof should have relevance to memory processing or storage is hardly clear, nor is it apparent in what manner cortical excitability is related to a time-dependent process of memory storage. The time dependency of the process in relation to PTZ does emerge somewhat more clearly in a study wherein rats, trained to a black–white discrimination, were injected with either 7.5, 10, or 15 mg/kg of PTZ or saline. Improved performance in the drug-treated groups emerged as a function of the amount of drug and the time following each daily training session at which it was administered (Hunt and Bauer, 1969). The maximum degree of facilitation of the positively reinforced discrimination task occurred when PTZ was given 10 minutes following each daily training session.

It would appear that the difference between what may constitute a facilitatory dose of PTZ and what may serve as an amnesic agent or disruptive factor in ongoing performance depends not strictly upon the actual dose, but upon the task upon which the drug is evaluated and the conditions under which the drug is given. Probably because of meager sources of ancillary central nervous system data concerning the site, nature, and duration of PTZ effects, it is difficult to deal with the validity of a given behavioral finding in terms of its possible correlates. Other factors, such as PTZ as an antifatigue agent or modifier of response habituation, cannot be simply ruled out as possibly contributing to some of those behavioral effects attributed to cognitive processes. Some potential support for such a possibility derives from actophotometric studies of mice treated with PTZ (Greenblatt and Osterberg, 1961). Whereas locomotor activity levels (exploratory behavior) in control animals decreased following exposure to the apparatus, the drug-treated mice maintained levels of activity.

VII. Picrotoxin

The overt effect of picrotoxin (PT), being quite minimal until doses approaching convulsive level are reached, and the varied physiological effects produced have made this compound one less frequently chosen for study in learning and memory experiments. Subconvulsive doses of PT act generally as a stimulant with more obvious brainstem activity probably accounting for its respiratory stimulation (Modell, 1966). Its blockade of presynaptic inhibition (Eccles *et al.*, 1963) may be related to its suggested role in regulating α-aminobutyric acid (Esplin and Zablocka, 1965). Although motor effects (coordinated walking and running) were not affected at several doses of PT in mice (Dews, 1953), the time course of central action relative to dose still requires specification, as does the relationship between central action and behavioral effect.

Facilitation of maze learning in rats has been reported when post-trial injection of PT was given (Breen and McGaugh, 1961). Following daily pretraining in a 14-unit T-maze sublines of maze-bright and maze-dull rats were treated, 30 seconds following a food-reinforced trial, with either 0.75, 1.0, or 1.25 mg/kg of PT. Although the maze-bright rats showed some reduced error incidence at the highest drug dose given, acquisition of the maze as measured by error reduction was drug-related among the maze-dull rats; in this case, the moderate and high PT dose led to fewer errors than observed among controls. Significant improvement in learning, measured from acquisition of a Hebb-Williams maze by rats, was observed when posttrial PT injections (1.0 mg/kg) followed each daily single learning trial spaced over a 10-day period (Garg and Holland, 1968a). This effect was attributed to the effect of the drug upon the consolidation of the maze learning. Other investigators, however, have failed to find any facilitation of maze learning from PT treatment (Prien *et al.*, 1963).

It appears that the biphasic effects of analeptics upon learning and memory processes suffers from the absence of a comparative hierarchy of central and behavioral correlates, considered in terms of time course of action, duration of effect, and locus. The search for central correlates of drug action and meaningful relationships thereof with behavioral processes becomes perhaps more complicated as the nature of the central stimulant action becomes more diffuse. Indirect stimulants that are relevant here to learning and memory processes are nicotine and caffeine.

VIII. Nicotine

The effects of nicotine, which appear to engage several regions of the central nervous system electrophysiologically as well as metabolically, particularly with regard to cholinergic and other aminergic systems, present several problems in evaluating its learning and memory effects. Motor effects and performance effects of this drug are often subtle, paradoxical, and time-dependent which makes their separability from the processes of learning and memory a difficult task. Another, and perhaps relevant issue, is the form in which this compound has been administered, particularly in experimental animals; the sulfate salt of this compound is usually available only in solution, the precise concentration of which can vary considerably depending upon the conditions, allowing for the hygroscopic property of the crystalline form, under which the solution was prepared. Direct preparation of such a salt from an acidified alkaloid source seems to have been an infrequently indicated alternative, as would also the more reliable use of the dipicrate salt seem to be indicated.

Whereas the drug effect upon locomotor activity would appear to constitute an important contribution to the nature of the task utilized in learning and memory studies and also the parameters of such tasks contributing to fatigue, etc., this has seldom been considered where multiple trial tasks have been employed. A dose-related increase in locomotor activity has been observed (Bonta *et al.*, 1960) with i.v. injections over a range of 0.18 to 0.43 mg/kg, whereas, with chronic treatment (0.5 to 1.0 mg/kg, i.p. or s.c.) over several months, maze running time in rats was significantly decreased (Eisenberg, 1948, 1954). Performance levels, as measured by a variety of indices, in man appear, generally, to be decreased—at least as far as the dose of nicotine made available in cigarette smoke is concerned. This dose, estimated as equivalent to 1 to 2 μg/kg, i.v. (Editorial, 1968) for a single inhaled cigarette, when given tenfold within a 6-hour period, led to increased fatigue and no change in tracking or vigilance behavior (Heimstra, 1962); whereas inhalation of four cigarettes over a more brief time course, decreased tracking performance (Wenzel and Davis, 1961). Early animal experimentation with nicotine (?) derived from tobacco smoke has led to equivocal results. Exposure to tobacco smoke fumes prior to the introduction of acquisition training trials in a maze has been indicated as accounting for an impairment of maze learning (Pechstein and Reynolds, 1937), whereas, under comparable conditions (Phillips, 1937), no effect of tobacco smoke was apparent upon the maze learning ability of rats. The effects of nicotine upon behavior appear related to inherent factors among the animals treated with this compound; rats, manifesting a relatively high level of activity, showed activity depression following 0.4 mg/kg of nicotine, whereas less active rats showed increased activity following the same dose (Morrison and Lee, 1968). This same study noted that rearing behavior of rats, at the same dosage of drug, was depressed, whereas in other studies (Garg, 1969) nicotine bitartrate (0.8 mg/kg) given over several trials led to facilitation of rearing, with more pronounced effects noted among "nonreactive" rats and males. A generalized decrement in the swimming speed of rats that were pretrained in swimming through a water alley has been noted (Bättig, 1969); at a dose of 0.1 mg/kg a performance decrement for 1 to 2 runs was apparent, whereas with 3 to 4 runs, at the same dose, the performance difference from controls was smaller. At a higher dose (0.4

mg/kg) a more uniform swimming performance decrement was observed. Other sensory- or motor-related performance effects of nicotine in rats have also been reported, such as color-discrimination performance (with doses of 0.5 to 0.75 mg/kg, s.c., given acutely); with chronic treatment (1.5–2.0 mg/kg, s.c. for 5 days or 2.5 mg/kg, s.c. for 5 weeks) performance was depressed, but returned to baseline after tolerance levels were achieved (Mercier and Dessaigne, 1960). Maze learning errors, as well as response time, used as measures of performance were shown to be significantly increased by chronic treatment (1 month) with nicotine (0.05–1.0 mg/kg, s.c. and i.p.), indicating a generally deleterious effect (Eisenberg, 1948, 1954). Facilitation of the rate at which the food–motor conditioned response was elaborated by rats of different ages has been indicated for doses of nicotine (0.1 mg/kg) given 15 minutes prior to trials in a rectangular maze (Linuchev and Michelson, 1965). Five daily trials were given at 1-minute intervals, with conditioned response elaboration taken at a criterion of a running time interval between start box and food box of less than 2 seconds for 2 successive days. Rats, 55 days of age, reached criterion by the eighth day with nicotine treatment, as compared with 14 days to reach the same criterion for controls. In 61-day-old rats, 4 days were required for nicotine-treated rats to reach criterion, as compared with 11 days for controls. The running time of older rats (131 and 158 days of age) was not accelerated by nicotine and criterion was not reached earlier than controls; in fact, the older rats required longer (19 days) to reach criterion than the average time required by control, younger rats (12.5 days) to achieve the same rapid running time. These observations suggest that younger rats, which acquire criterion maze performance sooner than older rats, show facilitation of such acquisition when treated with nicotine, unlike any facilitative effect among the older animals. One problem with this interpretation is that the achievement of criterion would determine the duration of treatment, also, the time course of drug effect could easily be changed by age, especially if hepatic metabolism of the drug can contribute to its behavioral effects. Differences in the effect of nicotine (0.5 mg/kg given 15 minutes prior to testing) have also been further related to strain differences in avoidance conditioning among mice (Bovet *et al.*, 1966), where for two strains showing initially better performance, the drug impaired avoidance conditioning, and for four strains where initially poor performance was indicated, avoidance conditioning was facilitated by the drug. Facilitation of avoidance learning has also been reported in rats, with a greater facilitative effect among younger rats (Robustelli, 1966), and mice (Oliverio, 1967). Among rats, nicotine treatment (0.2 mg/kg, s.c.) given 15 minutes pretrial led to facilitation of a two -and five-choice visual discrimination response; the degree of facilitation was related to the difficulty of the task (Bovet-Nitti, 1966).

Another variable potentially contributing to the effect of nicotine upon learning is the time of day when treatment is initiated; at two dose levels (0.2 and 1.0 mg/kg), nicotine exerted stimulantlike action when given in the morning, whereas, when given at night, only the higher dose produced a sedative like effect, and lower dose had no effect (Bovet *et al.*, 1967). Among nine inbred strains of mice trained to an avoidance response in a shuttle box, and given nicotine sulfate (0.5 mg/kg, i.p.) 15 minutes prior to the training session, a facilitatory effect was observed in six of the strains. The number of conditioned responses among these mice was significantly increased following nicotine treatment, whereas already established conditioned behavior was not affected. In two strains of mice the same dose of nicotine led to impairment of performance. The basal activity level of strains of mice and the complexity of the task required of them to learn appear to constitute determinants of the degree to which the facilitative effects of nicotine appear; of four inbred strains of mice trained to acquire a five-choice visual discrimination response, the facilitative effects of the drug were reported in three of the strains (Bovet-Nitti, 1969).

Dose and time as well as strain differences, activity level, and daily periodicities, appear also relevant to the conditions under which nicotine appears to affect learning. With reinforcement on a variable-interval schedule, low doses of nicotine (0.05–0.1 mg/kg) given immediately before the response session led to an increased rate of responding, whereas, at a higher dose (0.4 mg/kg), lever-pressing was reduced for the first 20 minutes of the session, following which response rate was increased (Morrison and Armitage, 1967). The ability of nicotine, within a specified dose range, to augment response rates among rats learning to lever-press for water reinforcement appears to be indicated (Morrison, 1967) for variable-interval reinforcement schedules (0.65–0.4 mg/kg) as well as for differential reinforcement responses based upon low rates of response (Morrison, 1968). When rats were treated with physostigmine prior to nicotine, the facilitative effect of the latter was abolished.

Of perhaps more direct bearing upon memory processes is the consideration of posttrial administration of nicotine (Garg and Holland, 1968c). Maze learning was facilitated under such conditions, suggesting that the drug acts upon postexperiential neural activity coincident with the process by which the memory trace is fixated. A reactive strain of rats showed more facilitation of maze learning under these conditions than did a nonreactive strain, further suggesting the possibility that the facilitative effects of this drug are related to inherent differences in the rate at which memory fixation occurs; i.e., the more rapid such a process (e.g., younger rats or reactive rats), the greater the likelihood of a facilitative effect. This premise, however, is not consistent with some observations; i.e., initially poor avoidance learners (strain-specific), which might be expected to require longer rates for memory fixation, are facilitated preferentially to good avoidance learners (Bovet *et al.*, 1966). In this same study Swiss mice given nicotine (0.5 mg/kg) 15 minutes prior to avoidance training showed a significant increase in avoidance responding, and yet within a memory-process context, Swiss mice given nicotine sulfate 15 minutes before passive avoidance conditioning showed a potentiation of the amnesic effect of ECS for that response (Essman, 1969b). In mice treated with nicotine sulfate (1.0 mg/kg) 60 minutes prior to being trained, in a single conditioning trial, for acquisition of a passive avoidance response, the amnesic effect of posttraining ECS (measured on a retention trial 24 hours later) was significantly attenuated (Essman *et al.*, 1968). The effect, in part, was attributed to the ability of nicotine to prevent or reduce the ECS-induced elevation of brain 5-hydroxytryptamine (5-HT), where the latter and its partial central consequences may account for the amnesic effect (Essman, 1969a). This relationship between indolealkamines and the process of memory fixation will be treated in more detail in a later section, when other compounds of a more direct interactive role will also be considered.

In a series of studies concerned with nicotine and some of its metabolites upon the memory fixation process in mice, several biochemical parameters were also included for consideration. In these experiments, from our laboratory, CF-1 strain mice were given nicotine sulfate (1.0 mg/kg, i.p.) either 15, 30, 45, or 60 minutes prior to a single training trial to establish a passive avoidance response. The training trial was followed at either 10, 20, 30, or 60 seconds by a single transcorneal ECS, leading, in saline-treated control animals, to a retrograde amnesia for the passive avoidance response, as measured by a retention trial given 24 hours later. The incidence of retrograde amnesia among the saline-treated mice was 70, 40, 35, and 20%, respectively, for ECS given 10, 20, 30, or 60 seconds after the training trial. For those mice treated with nicotine 15 minutes preceding the training trial the incidence of ECS-induced retrograde amnesia was 90, 85, 85, and 85%, respectively, as a function of the training–ECS interval, suggesting that, as compared with controls (*1*) nicotine sulfate (1.0 mg/kg) 15 minutes prior to training–ECS potentiates the retrograde amnesic effect of ECS, and (*2*) serves to eliminate a temporal gradient for ECS-induced amnesia. For nicotine treatment given 45 or 60 minutes before the training–ECS sequence the time-related incidence of retrograde amnesia was 25, 25, 40, and 45%, suggesting that, whereas significant antagonism of the amnesic effect of ECS was brought about by nicotine treatment 45 minutes preceding the training–ECS sequence, the protective effect was not temporally distributed. The potentiation or antagonism of the ECS-induced amnesia could not be accounted for by either the effect of the drug on conditioning shock threshold or ECS threshold. The difference in effect relating to the temporal contiguity of the drug with either training or ECS suggested that the effect could be mediated by an active metabolite of nicotine, which could occur as a consequence of partial hepatic metabolism of the parenterally administered compound. In a further study, two such potential candidates for the effect observed, (−)cotinine and 3-pyridyl acetic acid were administered (0.25 mg/kg) in parallel to groups of mice, either 15 or 45 minutes before a training–ECS sequence as previously considered. Again, nicotine sulfate-treated (1.0 mg/kg) mice injected 15 minutes pretraining showed an increased incidence of ECS-induced amnesia (90% as compared with 25% for saline-treated controls), whereas when treated 45 minutes prior to training, the nicotine led to only 25% retrograde amnesia (as compared with 85% for saline-treated controls). Since (−)cotinine would be expected to have effects before 3-pyridylacetic acid because of its relative position in the pathway within which nicotine is metabolized, one could predict a greater effect of the former, earlier, than for the latter; with the 15-minute treatment–training interval the incidence of ECS-induced retrograde amnesia was 70 and 60%, respectively for (−)cotinine and 3-pyridylacetic acid, whereas for the 45-minute interval the respective amnesic incidence was 85–70%. It would appear, therefore, that whereas the antagonism of ECS-induced retrograde amnesia in mice may be partially accounted for by at least two active peripheral metabolites of nicotine, capable of exerting central effects, the potentiating effect of nicotine upon ECS-induced amnesia appears primarily related to direct effects of nicotine itself. It seems quite possible that the biphasic nature of nicotine action may be related to central mediation of biochemical changes that interact with ECS. For example, with nicotine sulfate (1.0 mg/kg) given to mice 45 minutes prior to a training–ECS sequence, by 15 minutes following ECS, 5-HT levels in whole brain, normally elevated in controls [0.67(±0.05) to 0.76(±0.06) μg/gm], was actually decreased [0.65(±0.07) to 0.61(±0.04) μg/gm] but not significantly so. Brain 5-HT turnover, which for saline treatment followed by ECS, was changed (turnover rate increased by approximately 33%) was still further altered in the nicotine-treated mice given ECS (turnover rate increased by 200%) and turnover time (3 times that of saline controls) decreased by 37%. The apparent indication for a cholinergic role of nicotine is perhaps amplified in its relevance for memory fixation by several further findings. Electrocovulsive shock produces a sequence of time-related changes in acetylcholine (ACh) levels, as measured in the cerebral cortex of mice. Within 10 minutes of ECS, whole-cortex ACh level was reduced from 16.43 ($\pm$2.30) to 7.26 ($\pm$2.40) nM/gm. The corresponding effect in tissue homogenate (bound ACh) was a reduction from 10.0 ($\pm$0.6) to 2.0 ($\pm$1.4) nM/gm, and in cortical synaptosomes from 1.3 ($\pm$0.16) to 0.90 ($\pm$0.30) nM/gm. By 120 minutes following ECS, whole-tissue levels were within pre-ECS baseline limits (16.53 $\pm$ 2.20 nM/gm), whereas bound and synaptosomal levels were still depressed (4.0 $\pm$ 0.8 and 0.53 $\pm$ 0.10 nM/gm, respectively). This might suggest that following a decrease in bound ACh after, ECS, an increase in "free" molecules occurs. Electroconvulsive shock given 45 minutes after saline treatment reduced bound and vesicular ACh (1130 $\pm$ 158.20 to 900 $\pm$ 297.00 pM/gm). Nicotine alone (no ECS) led to an appreciable decrease in vesicular ACh level (370 $\pm$ 22.20 pM/gm), but with ECS given 45 minutes following the drug, vesicular ACh levels were elevated (610 $\pm$ 36.60 pM/gm). Again, it appears that, whereas ECS can account for a time-related increase in free cortical ACh levels, this phenomenon is not modified by nicotine treatment; it is rather the existing levels of endogenous vesicular ACh that are decreased by nicotine and then increased when such drug treatment is followed 45 minutes later by ECS. If the labile phase of the memory process is regulated by central cholinergic changes the present findings may bear upon such an hypothesis. This issue, however, will be more generally treated in a later section.

IX. Caffeine

Caffeine serves to increase the locomotor activity of rats (Dews, 1953), although it appears that this property resides within the baseline activity levels of the animal; for example, animals with predrug activity levels that were high were not significantly stimulated to elevated locomotor activity levels (Greenblatt and Osterberg, 1961). The effect of caffeine upon activity level, which is probably an important component of those responses within which learning and memory are methodologically defined, appears to be even more directly related, not only to basal levels, but also to cyclical variations of such baselines. Studies from our laboratory with male mice have indicated that, whereas troughs in locomotor periodicty, occurring at approximately 4 P.M., are increased significantly by caffeine (25 mg/kg) treatment during the preceding 4-hour period, comparable treatment preceding locomotor activity peaks (between 4 and 8 A.M.) produce locomotor activity depression. There are also differences in the degree to which such caffeine treatment alters brain serotonin level; the latter is decreased when the drug stimulates locomotor activity increments. These findings may possibly have some bearing upon learning and memory processes inasmuch as factors such as circadian variations and contributions of baseline periodicities have seldom been accounted for in behavioral paradigms from which inferences regarding cognitive processes have emerged.

An early investigation of caffeine effects upon learning in the rat (Lashley, 1917) indicated that the drug provided for a dose-dependent retardation of circular maze learning. Chains of alimentary reflexes in dogs have been inhibited by caffeine (Voronin and Napalkov, 1963), and conditional reflexes have been differentially affected by the drug, depending upon whether they were negative or positive; the former were impaired, whereas the latter were enhanced, providing an apparent basis for the suggestion that "internal inhibition" is decreased by caffeine (Pavlov, 1927). Dogs given caffeine [16 mg/kg, intramuscularly (i.m.)] showed decreased latencies for the appearance of conditional responses, an increase in the effect of reinforced stimuli, and a decreased efficacy of nonreinforced stimuli (Wolff and Gantt, 1935). An apparently facilitative effect of caffeine has also been reported in man, where the drug (1.5 gr.) given $2\frac{1}{2}$ to 3 hours before the learning of lists of nonsense syllables provided for reduced "reactive inhibition" in the learning of lists comprised of stimuli judged to have pleasant associations. The number of consonants learned was also greater for the drug-treated as compared with a placebo-treated group (Tolman, 1917). It is, of course, inevitable that at some point generalizations regarding caffeine will apply to beverages containing this drug, or that such beverages, in turn, may be the generality from which inferences regarding caffeine will derive. Although this realm of inquiry is perhaps best left to individual, subjective evaluation for the coffee or tea drinker, one must in passing note that coffee has been reported to increase functions such as adding and memory span in man (administered 20, 100, or 140 minutes pretesting), but not with intraindividual consistency (Gililand and Nelson, 1939). Just as subjective differences and individual variations in the physiological consequences of coffee upon wakefulness and gastrointestinal functions occur, one might expect even greater variability, subjectivity, and dosage variations from the caffeine contents of coffee, when considered with a view toward learning and memory.

In rats, the running speed down a straight alley under conditions of hunger, satiation, or frustration was considered in terms of caffeine effects. It was concluded that the drug minimized the contribution to the learning of the response of nonreinforced trials (Miller and Miles, 1935). It apparently required some 20 years for an alternative explanation to emerge, when in a study of rats trained in a food–shock (approach–avoiddance) situation, the running speed was increased by caffeine under shock-escape conditions (Barry and Miller, 1965). It would appear that if the effect of caffeine were considered in terms of the motivating con-conditions used in learning paradigms, then perhaps the strength of the motive state might determine the extent and direction of drug effects. It has been reliably established that locomotor activity levels are increased as a function of the magnitude of the drive state, as is exploratory behavior. If caffeine itself can afford contributions to ongoing drive states (i.e., modification of appetitive behavior, shock escape, etc.), then its unique contributions to components of the learning process would indeed become still more difficult to assess. A stimulant effect of caffeine [4 mg/kg, p.o.)] has been observed in mice (maximal effects achieved in a range of 8 to 32 mg/kg), whereby exploratory behavior was decreased; it was only with appreciably higher doses (128 mg/kg) that exploratory behavior was increased (Boissier and Simon, 1967). It seems that conditions which mediate activity, dependent upon or independent from operationally defined drive states, can also regulate the degree to which caffeine, as a function of dose, can affect the learning of various responses. For rats not initially showing an escape response to auditory stress, after having been isolated, caffeine treatment led to enhancement of such escape behavior (Plotnikoff, 1962). Studies in our laboratory have indicated that isolated mice, although showing a somewhat higher activity level than group-housed animals, do not show the expected activity increase from caffeine treatment (25 mg/kg) given prior to the trough of their locomotor activity. In fact, the drug under these conditions appears to reduce activity. The character of the stimuli (positive or aversive), the appropriate response (active or passive), and the relative importance of activity to such behavioral contingencies seem to constitute considerations relevant to the nature of caffeine effects. The increase of response rates of rats operating on a lever-pressing task, following caffeine administration (Skinner and Heron, 1937), appears to anticipate subsequent findings that performance level in rats trained to suppress reinforcement was increased by caffeine but, further, that this effect was more pronounced among animals which showed poorer learning results (Tonini, 1961). The hypothesis that the drug effect might be altered by changing the motivation level has been explored in rats trained in an approach–avoidance conflict situation. Under these conditions, caffeine (20–40 mg/kg) reduced approach performance (Barry and Miller, 1962). If one were to again superimpose a relationship between drive strength and activity upon the predictive index for caffeine effect, then lowered drive strength might increase, rather than decrease the performance effects of caffeine. Unfortunately, resolution of these hypotheses appears to depend upon the biphasic nature of the drug action depending upon dose and dose–response time intervals; these issues have not been sufficiently clarified to allow for adequate hypothesis testing.

The effects of caffeine in experiments designed to test its contribution to memory processes have been determined in only a limited way. The posttrial administration of the drug appears to be a favored method by which drug effects are separated from acquisition, performance, or activity variables, and relegated to postexperiential processes by which memory is presumably brought about. Rats were trained to a criterion of avoidance responding to a black–white and horizontal–vertical discrimination. Caffeine (30 mg/kg) was given either 5 seconds, 2 minutes, or 60 minutes after the criterion had been achieved with massed training trials. When tested for retention of the avoidance discrimination response 2 days after injection, significantly few discrimination errors were made by the animals that had been given caffeine 2 seconds after achieving acquisition criterion; no effect was observed among those rats that were caffeine-treated at later postcriterion times (Pare, 1961). This result, although apparently supporting the role of caffeine in conferring a time-dependent facilitative effect upon memory fixation of a discriminative avoidance response, also rests upon the assumption that the central effects of caffeine are temporally separable and rapid in onset following parenteral administration of the drug. Such an effect might also be viewed in terms of the drug's effect upon the autonomic sequelae of avoidance conditioning and what potential contribution this could make to retention (criterion performance of a discrimination response appropriate to avoidance but in the absence of aversive stimulation) of such a response.

Other akaloids of the xanthine group have been given little consideration in terms of what contribution they could make to either learning or memory processes or what learning or memory experiments might contribute to our understanding of the cognitive or central action of compounds of this class. A notable exception to this is uric acid, which is also an endogenous intermediary or end product of purine degredation. Several experimental studies have suggested a potential relationship between this drug as a central nervous system stimulant, as an endogenous metabolite, and as a metabolic stimulant to structure–activity properties in the pharmacological realm and to molecular mechanisms to which learning and memory processes have been related.

X. Uric Acid

As an endogenous central nervous system stimulant, uric acid has been accorded a potential role in intellectual and cognitive functions (Orowan, 1955), intelligence test performance (Stetten and Heron, 1959), and achievement (Brooks and Mueller, 1966). The posible contribution of this compound to memory functions has remained largely inferential. An examination of serum uric acid level in relation to memory function in senile and senescent patients indicated that oral RNA administration (6 mg/day for 7 days) led to elevation of serum uric acid, and this rise was greater for subjects with higher memory scale scores (Kral *et al.*, 1967).

Studies with exogenous uric acid have been concerned with its relationship to RNA and learning and memory. Since base ratio changes in the RNA molecule in brain, having apparent bearing upon learning, appear consistently to involve the purine bases (Hyden and Egyhazi, 1963), and these, in turn, contribute, following deamination and oxidation, to uric acid availability, it is not surprising to find that systemic administration of RNA (100 mg/kg) to mice, led to graded increases in serum uric acid levels. The magnitude of the increase was related to the purine richness of the RNA, which derived from different sources. By 4 hours following injection, these increments ranged from 5% (yeast RNA) to 274% (brain RNA). In further studies (Essman, 1970c), uric acid injection in mice (75 mg/kg, i.p.) 60 minutes prior to water maze training led to reduction of response times and errors during both the acquisition of an escape response as well as for the reversal of that response. Treatment, under comparable conditions with uricase (1.65 mg/kg), sufficient to reduce endogenous urate levels by conversion to allantoin, led to the occurrence of increased response times and significantly more errors. Changes in whole-brain RNA level for the above treatment conditions also occurred, with a 9% increase in the former case, and a 3% decrease in the latter.

Memory processes have been viewed in terms of a possible contribution toward an understanding of their more fundamental mechanisms through the use of uric acid (Essman, 1970c). The ability of a posttraining ECS to produce a retrograde amnesia for a passive avoidance response was reduced when mice were pretreated with uric acid (0.5–20.0 mg/kg, i.p. Whereas control animals, pretreated with saline preceding the training–

ECS sequence, showed an 80% incidence of ECS-induced amnesia, the drug-treated animals, depending upon dose, showed from 27 to 53% ECS-induced amnesia, without any drug effect upon unconditioned responses, foot-shock threshold, or seizure incidence. With uric acid treatment, brain RNA levels were significantly elevated (at 1, 10, or 20 mg/kg), and in interaction with ECS, the RNA change (40% decrement among controls) did not follow significantly with doses up to 5 mg/kg, but, with 10 or 20 mg/kg, brain levels were elevated by 24 to 28%.

There are three additional avenues through which the potential relationship between uric acid treatment and memory processes has been explored.

1. The interactive effects of RNA and brain 5-HT in ECS-amnesia and antiamnesia effects of urate. These (Essman, 1970c) have essentially confirmed the correlate of ECS-induced retrograde amnesia found in brain 5-HT turnover changes, and the extent to which such changes are attenuated by uric acid reverses the amnesic effect. The inherent mechanisms operative within such a system will be discussed in more detail in a later section.

2. The effects of uric acid upon retrograde amnesia induced by other events; in this instance, some consideration is given to the amnesic properties of intracranial 5-HT injection and their modification with uric acid.

3. The effects of a synthetic analog of uric acid possessing structural resemblance to at least two behaviorally active members of the xanthine group—uric acid and caffeine. This compound, trimethyluric acid (TMUA; 1, 3, 7-trimethylxanthine), synthesized in our laboratory, has been systematically employed in a series of learning and memory tasks where its effect appears to emerge as a facilitator of the processes that underlie such responses.

First, with regard to uric acid and 5-HT-induced retrograde amnesia, several experiments in our laboratory (in collaboration with E. Heldman) have indicated that an acquisition deficit induced by 5-HT (intracranially administered in doses from 1.0 to 2.0 μg/adult mouse) before training, or a retention deficit induced by such posttraining treatment can be markedly reduced by uric acid. When uric acid (10 mg/kg, i.p.) preceded i.c. 5-HT by 20 minutes, where the latter was followed by a single passive avoidance conditioning trial, the incidence of conditioned passive avoidance behavior in evidence 24 hours later was the same (100%) as for i.c. injected, saline-treated controls. Mice given pretrial 5-HT alone showed only a 30% incidence of conditioned response retention when tested 24 hours later. The effect of pretraining 5-HT injection upon active avoidance response acquisition following passive avoidance training—avoidance of foot shock by jumping out of the box in which shock was given within 10 seconds preceding shock onset—was to reduce the number of trials upon which the criterion for active avoidance was met. Control, saline-treated mice showed an aggregate of active avoidance of 80%, whereas 5-HT-treated mice showed only 42% criterion active avoidance. When 5-HT treatment was preceded by uric acid injection the incidence of active avoidance behavior was 67%. Thus, it would appear that the impairment of both passive and active avoidance acquisition produced by intracranial 5-HT injection was appreciably reduced when prior uric acid treatment was given. In further studies, it has been established that i.c. 5-HT given 30 minutes prior to passive avoidance training in mice significantly reduced the acquisition of conditioned avoidance behavior, and prior uric acid treatment led to only slight, but not statistically significant reduction in the incidence of impaired acquisition. 5-Hydroxytryptamine given immediately following passive avoidance training, with concurrent uric acid treatment, did not alter the 40% incidence of 5-HT-induced retrograde amnesia. When uric acid injection was given 60 minutes before i.c. 5-HT, then there was some degree of attenuation of the 5-HT-induced retrograde amnesia for passive avoidance behavior. It is possible that a molecular basis for these observations may reside in a uric acid-mediated reduction in tRNA binding by 5-HT, a potential mechanism which will be treated in more detail in a later section of this survey.

The use of TMUA in a comprehensive series of behavioral and biochemical studies has suggested that this compound exerts a number of rather interesting effects on tasks requiring learning and/or retention. In mice, doses of from 10 to 50 mg/kg did not lead to any statistically significant increases in locomotor activity within 2 hours of i.p. injection. Mice were given either 10, 20, or 30 mg/kg of TMUA or saline 60 minutes prior to being trained in a water maze to escape by swimming to an escape ramp positioned so that one-directional choice was required. Response latency and incidence of incorrect choices were measured on each of the 4 training trials. Both the reduction in number of maze errors and an increased incidence of errorless performance was observed among these mice treated with 10 or 20 mg/kg of TMUA prior to training, with the latter dose leading to the maximum significant incidence of errorless performance. Mice given 30 mg/kg of drug showed almost half the maze errors committed by controls, twice the number of errorless criterion trials, but not at the same level of accelerated acquisition shown by mice receiving lower drug doses; this may, in part, be accounted for by initially high response latencies among mice treated with 30 mg/kg of drug. When pre-training motor learning experience was given in the maze situation in order to minimize any potential contribution of the drug to motor cues during maze acquisition, then acquisition trials following TMUA treatment again indicated a significant incidence of errorless maze performance at the 20-mg/kg dose. In order to assess prior cognitive learning and the effect of the drug on the acquisition of a reversal response in the maze, acquisition to a criterion was provided, followed 60 minutes later by TMUA injection (10, 20, or 30 mg/kg). Reversal trials were given 60 minutes following drug or saline injection. Although there were fewer maze errors and more errorless maze reversal trials performed by TMUA-treated mice than among saline controls, only at the 10-mg/kg dose of the drug did statistical significance emerge for this apparently facilitative effect.

In another series of experiments the effect of TMUA (10 mg/kg, i.p.) upon memory fixation was determined. Here drug treatment prior to training (15–60 minutes) was titrated against the retrograde amnesic effect upon the response produced by posttraining ECS (given at either 10, 30, or 60 seconds following the single passive avoidance conditioning trial). The posttraining interval where, among control animals, ECS led to a maximum incidence of retrograde amnesia, as determined by a 24-hour posttraining retention trial, was 10 seconds (70%); it was also at this training–ECS interval that TMUA appeared to confer the maximum degree of antagonism for the amnesia. The most marked antagonism occurred when drug treatment preceded the training–ECS sequence by 45 minutes (100% retention), with 70 to 80% retention observed at the other drug–training times. Reduced antagonism of the ECS-induced retrograde amnesia occurred at higher doses of TMUA, suggesting that its apparent memory effect was dose-specific. Several experiments have taken into account factors such as shock threshold, ECS-convulsive threshold, unconditioned response performance, and conditioned response acquisition, and in none of these cases did TMUA, within the dose range utilized, contribute any effect.

In consideration of the possibility that the central effect(s) of ECS leading to the production of retrograde amnesia might be altered by TMUA treatment after ECS, 10 or 15 mg/kg, i.p. of the drug was given at either 10 seconds or 15, 45, or 60 minutes following ECS. A retention trial for testing of the passive avoidance response was given 24 hours following the training trial. The incidence of ECS-induced retrograde manesia (90%) for a 10-second training–ECS interval was in no way altered by post-ECS TMUA neither as a function of the ECS–drug interval nor the dose.

With doses of 10, 20, or 30 mg/kg TMUA, brain tissue obtained from mice 60 minutes following injection was assayed for nucleic acid concentration and for several biogenic amines. There was a dose-related increase in brain RNA level with statistically significant increments for mice treated with 10 and 20 mg/kg of TMUA (2.86 and 2.72 mg/gm) as compared with saline-treated controls (0.94 mg/gm); adjusted DNA levels were unchanged by drug treatment. With increasing drug dose, whole-brain 5-HT levels were reduced, with a parallel, dose-related reduction in its major metabolite, 5-hydroxyindoleacetic acid. Brain norepinephrine level was slightly but not significantly reduced at the highest TMUA dose, and monoamine oxidase activity appeared unaltered for all the drug treatment conditions. Some preliminary evidence has supported the possibility that TMUA leads to an increase in brain RNA synthesis (measured by incorporation of orotic acid-^{14}C into brain RNA) and that this effect appears specific, *in vivo*, to a 10-mg/kg dose (increased incorporation rate), rather than to a dose at 30 mg/kg, where no such effect was apparent.

It is apparent that there are some, perhaps as yet incompletely defined and unexplored relationships between the effects of several central nervous system stimulants upon brain RNA content, synthesis or turnover and the potentially positive effects observed in learning and memory studies. Because of their more direct bearing upon the issue of brain RNA, learning, and memory, several other compounds have been considered as potentially facilitative agents. Two of these to be considered are the malanonitrile derivatives and magnesium pemoline.

XI. Malononitrile Derivatives

Some degree of controversy surrounds the issue of brain RNA changes resulting from pharamcological mediation which apparently confers effect on learning or memory. Apparent mediation of such effects upon the RNA content of the brain without changes in the action of DNA-dependent RNA polymerase have been reported for derivatives of malononitrile. In early studies with this parent compound, evidence was provided to suggest the stimulation of large central nervous system neurons and led to increases in their production of nucleic acid and protein. Among psychiatric patients treated with malononitrile prior to a frontal lobotomy, their tissue samples were compared with regional controls obtained from accident victims following death. Studies also concerned chronic treatment with malononitrile in psychiatric patients, wherein some improvement was shown (Hydén and Hartelius, 1948; Hartelius, 1950). The active constituent of this somewhat gross compound was a dimer characterized as 1,1,3-tricyano-2-amino-1-propene or tricyanoaminopropene (TCAP), which was shown to increase the RNA and nucleoprotein content of single neurons in the rabbit brain (Eghyazi and Hydén, 1961). This same compound was used in studies of maze learning and avoidance conditioning (Chamberlain *et al.*, 1963), where the retention of avoidance responses was apparently enhanced without any contribution of the drug toward the effects of emotionality or arousal; maze learning was not modified by the drug.

The suggestion that RNA production by the neuron is accelerated by TCAP treatment, whereas RNA level can be decreased by an amnesic event (ECS), has led to several studies concerned with the temporal character of this interaction and its relationship to the memory consolidation process (Essman, 1965). It was shown that elevation of whole-brain RNA level following TCAP treatment (20 mg/kg/day, i.p., for 3 days) in mice led to antagonism of the brain RNA decrease resulting from ECS; furthermore, the amnesic effect of the ECS was significantly reduced. In subsequent studies (Essman, 1966) similar results were obtained. Whereas ECS given within 10 seconds after a passive avoidance conditioning trial produced a retrograde amnesia for the conditioned passive avoidance response in 72% of saline-treated control mice, only 27% of the TCAP-treated mice showed a retrograde amnesia. The two brain areas showing the greatest ECS-induced RNA decrements were the corpus callossum and limbic system, whereas TCAP-treated mice showed no obvious change in the RNA level of these structures after ECS.

In a double crossover study comparing the effects of TCAP (600 mg/day, p.o. for periods of 2 weeks) with that of placebo in 23 senile patients evaluated on a series of tests for learning capacity and memory function (Talland *et al.*, 1965), it was shown that there were no statistically significant differences between drug and placebo treatments on performance; the latter as rated for all tasks, was not modified by TCAP, but rather was initially reduced by a delayed practice effect shown among the placebo-treated subjects. The state of deterioration of the subject population chosen in this study, and the possible confounding of results contributed by the interaction of practice effect with drug, render the results difficult to interpret. The absence of any motor task or motor component in either the acquisition trials or memory tasks introduces the problem of baseline evaluation for purely cognitive tasks in an already cognitive-deficient population.

Whereas several studies have indicated that TCAP administration leads to enhanced acquisition of discrimination learning (Daniels, 1967; Schmidt and Davenport, 1967) in rats, chronic treatment during early postnatal development (3–16 days) mice provided for, as young adults, more rapid rates of water maze acquisition, indicated by reduced response latencies and fewer maze errors (Essman, 1967b). Other studies have failed to demonstrate any TCAP effect on active avoidance and water maze learning (Brush *et al.*, 1966), the acquisition and extinction of a conditioned emotional response (Solyom and Gallay, 1966), maze learning (McNutt, 1967), or passive avoidance learning (Gurowitz *et al.*, 1967). Similarly, acute treatment of rats with TCAP given pretraining had no effect on the acquisition of a double-alternation sequence in adult rats. Acquisition performance on a double-alternation problem was not affected by 40 days of chronic pretreatment with TCAP (15 mg/kg/day), and chronic TCAP treatment (1.5 gm TCAP/1000 gm mash in the diet) to pregnant rats negatively influenced double-alternation acquisition in adult offspring rats (Stern and Heise, 1970). Response rates of rats in a continuous avoidance task were also not altered by TCAP. The effect of TCAP, in multiple injection upon brain RNA synthesis, brain RNA level, or antagonism of ECS-induced retrograde amnesia in mice was not demonstrated in a series of experiments (Buckholtz and Bowman, 1970). A consideration of the possible contribution of time course and the biochemical consequences of the drug–ECS interaction was not specifically considered, nor was the antithyroid property of this compound, although cited, given any relevant role in accounting for the results. One problem in comparing those studies yielding positive TCAP effects with those showing negative results are differences in dosage and the chronicity of administration. There is little evidence, for example, of a direct relationship between TCAP treatment, brain RNA effects, and changes in learning and/or memory. It has been shown that chronic TCAP treatment in adult mice (10–60 mg/kg) led to increases in whole-brain RNA level as a function of dose but did not produce any consistent change in locomotor activity nor affect the rate of water maze acquisition or error incidence (Lewis, 1967). In that study it was suggested that water maze acquisition by mice, involving motor learning, could affect the extent to which the drug interacts with cognitive cues in maze learning. Mice were, therefore, given motor training in the maze, without any opportunity for a choice discrimination or escape response. Chronic TCAP treatment (10–60 mg/kg/day, i.p., for 3 days) led to dose-related response to maze learning on subsequent trials. These findings argue against a strictly motor stimulation or antifatigue role for TCAP, since by limiting the contribution of motor learning involved in maze acquisition through prior motor training, the effects of TCAP on maze response acquisition would be expected to be chiefly nonmotor.

A trimer of malononitrile, tetracyanopropene (T4CAP), administered to mice (10–30 mg/kg) accelerated the rate of maze acquisition and habit reversal in a water maze. Higher doses of this compound were shown to be toxic (Lewis and Essman, 1967). In a more extensive series of studies with T4CAP (2-cyanomethyl-1,1,3,3-tetracyanopropene), mice given 20 mg/kg/day, i.p., for either 1,2, or 3 days prior to being trained to acquire a passive avoidance response in a single training trial, showed 35, 60, and 76% retention, respectively, of that response, when the training trial had been followed within 10 seconds by ECS; saline-treated control animals showed a 10% incidence response retention. A statistically significant increase in the RNA content of the cerebral cortex was noted (Essman and Esman, 1969). These findings have been interpreted as a drug-induced enhancement of memory consolidation through its action upon a molecular complex (RNA–5-HT) modified by the amnesic properties of ECS; such enhancement may be viewed as either an acceleration of the rate at which the memory fixation process occurs, or the ability of the drug to attenuate the central changes attending ECS that usually account for memory disruption.

Whereas it has been previously indicated that compounds such as the malononitrile derivatives affect brain RNA level without altering the activity of DNA-dependent RNA polymerase, there is some question as to the role this relationship may play in learning and memory; agents that decrease DNA-dependent RNA polymerase in brain, e.g., actinomycin D, presumably have no obvious effect upon memory (Barondes and Jarvik, 1964), whereas other compounds, notably magnesium pemoline, which increase brain RNA polymerase, have generated a rather controversial literature in regard to their merits as facilitators of learning and memory.

XII. Magnesium Pemoline

The equimolar combination of pemoline (2-imino-5-phenyl-4-oxozolidinone), a mild stimulant, and magnesium hydroxide has provided for a compound employed in studies concerned with learning and memory. In initial reports on this compound (magnesium pemoline; MP), it (20 mg/kg) was reputed to stimulate RNA polymerase activity in rat brain (Glasky and Simon, 1966), both *in vivo* and *in vitro*, with selective stimulation of the enzyme which was not observed with other central nervous system stimulants or psychotropic agents. Coincident with this report was another (Plotnikoff, 1966a) in which MP (10 mg/kg) was reported to enhance the acquisition and retention of a conditioned response in rats; the conditioning situation consisted of a 15-second buzzer, with 5 seconds overlapping foot shock in which avoidance was achieved by jumping from a box to a platform to avoid shock. The increased rate of learning observed following drug treatment was not changed when trials were given, in the absence of the drug, on the following day. The proximity of these reports suggested that MP, by its apparent RNA polymerase effect, also served to facilitate learning and memory. The theoretical or logical basis for this inference, which apparently served as a basis for generating a considerable number of subsequent studies, is extremely vague and probably unfounded, and since subsequent attempts to replicate the biochemical observations have not yielded positive results (Morris *et al.*, 1967; Stein and Yellin, 1967) the entire issue still remains in question.

In subsequent behavioral studies (Plotnikoff, 1966b,c), rats classified as "fast-learners" on an avoidance task, which were pretreated with MP (5, 10, 20 mg/kg, p.o.), showed a more rapid relearning of avoidance responding after memory disruptive ECS was given. The return to the pre-ECS level of avoidance responding was not achieved by the control group (not identified as a treatment conditions), whereas there was a dose-dependent return to pre-ECS levels in the MP-treated rats—20-mg/kg group by 60 minutes after ECS, 10-mg/kg group by 4 hours after ECS, and 5-mg/kg group within 6 to 24 hours after ECS.

Early reports of the efficacy of MP in human subjects (Cameron, 1966) included data from a geriatric population with signs of intellectual deterioration in whom improvement was shown in memory functions after treatment. In patients with clearly established memory defects of an organic origin, 25–125 mg/day of MP was given over a 2-month period with a battery of memory tests given before, during, and after treatment. By the end of 1 month of treatment, there were statistically significant differences between drug- and placebo-treated groups on the Wechsler Memory Quotient, the former group showing a point gain of approximately 10% above their initial scores.

Essentially negative results have been reported in other studies where MP has been investigated in learning and memory tasks. In a double-blind study with normal adult men given 25 and 37.5 mg, p.o., of MP 3 hours before verbal and motor learning tasks, it was shown that the drug treatment did not facilitate learning, memory, or performance (Smith, 1967). When tested among a group of college students in a double-blind study, a single oral dose (6.25, 12.5, or 25 mg) of MP 2.5 hours before a learning task had no facilitary effect upon acquisition (Burns *et al.*, 1967); the response, a discrimination to light cues, by key-pressing, was actually acquired at a faster rate by placebo-treated subjects than among those subjects given

MP. The effect could relate to either excitation as well as possibly increased reactivity to shock. Although this latter possibility represents an excellent alternative to an explanation of facilitated avoidance learning, it is unfortunate that the suggestion has not been experimentally tested. An alternative explanation has been suggested (Beach and Kimble, 1967), wherein MP-injected rats showed shorter latencies in and responded more frequently to a buzzer followed by shock. Buzzer-avoidance prevailed over shock-avoidance. However, an increased responsivity to auditory stimuli could possibly explain the apparently enhancing effect of MP under these circumstances; i.e., the CS actually acquires aversive properties. This proposal was not supported in another study (Ritzmann *et al.*, 1969) in which rats given MP (5 or 20 mg/kg, p.o.) either 30 or 60 minutes before conditioning with either a buzzer or light CS showed a greater number of avoidance responses and faster running times; this effect was neither dose nor CS-dependent. This finding, however, still does not exclude the possibility that there is a threshold change to foot shock, which, if in effect during conditioning, could easily account for the finding.

When MP was tested in two different strains of rats conditioned to a pole-climbing response (Corson, 1969), it was shown that Long-Evans strain rats tended toward a drug-induced transient interference with acquisition, whereas Sprague-Dawley rats showed prolonged extinction. Perhaps such strain differences reflect variations in "emotionality" and its interaction with the drug in acquisition tasks that are dependent upon avoidance behiavior. When a rate discrimination was imposed upon trained rats (schedule of differential reinforcement of low rates of response), MP significantly impaired such behavior (Thompson and Meyer, 1969).

In some studies using positive reinforcement, MP has been suggested as mediating enhanced performance or learning. When MP was administered (5, 10, 15, or 20 mg/kg, i.p.) 30 minutes prior to T-maze acquisition trials with light cues reinforced by goal box food reinforcement, rats given 10 mg/kg reached criterion (9 out of 10 correct responses) significantly faster than controls (Cooper *et al.*, 1969). The possibility of drug–appetitive behavior interaction was not studied or considered; since the interaction between a wide range of central nervous system stimulants and appetitive behavior is well known, it seems that this should constitute a relevant consideration. The specificity of a 10-mg/kg dose, without observed effects of lower or higher doses, would seem to suggest that the 30-minute drug training interval is perhaps too short to adequately test differences in dosage. The effect of MP studied in repeated acquisition and extinction of a bar-pressing response by rats on schedules of water reinforcement (Adams *et al.*, 1969) indicated that with 20 mg/kg, i.p.

resistance to extinction, as measured by response rate, was somewhat better maintained. Repeated exposure to the acquisition–extinction sequence reduced the possibly facilitative effects of MP. For rats treated with MP (20 mg/kg) and trained to acquire a Y-maze brightness discrimination response reinforced with sucrose, a significantly better performance was obtained (Bright and Hatton, 1969). Significant differences from controls were obtained for running speed, response latency, trials to criterion, reinforcements to criterion, and the percent of correct choices.

The administration of MP to rats prior to training on a passive-avoidance task was effective in attenuating the amnesic effect usually attending ECS (Stein and Brink, 1969). This finding bears several similarities with previous studies cited (Plotnikoff, 1966b,c), in that it may be partially explained by the anticonvulsant action of MP; this raises the question of whether an anticonvulsive effect alone is sufficient to reduce the amnesic effect of ECS. A partial answer to this question is that (*1*) anticonvulsive effects do not reduce amnesic effects (Essman, 1968b) and (*2*) reduction of the RNA-depleting effect in brain by a convulsant, through anticonvulsant action, does not necessarily reduce the amnesic effect (Essman, 1968a). In human patients, learning and memory after electroconvulsive therapy was somewhat facilitated by MP treatment (Small and Small, 1967; Small *et al.*, 1968). The apparently facilitative effect of MP upon learning and memory is difficult to reconcile with the alternative suggestions that the compound acts as a nonspecific central nervous system stimulant or as an antifatigue agent. The nature of the motivation underlying the learning task and the contribution of the task to performance variability constitute basic steps toward the evaluation of the cognitive processes affected by MP. Another consideration is the extent to which this compound proves to be more efficient as a possible "learning and memory drug" than other stimulants; for example, it has been shown that subjects required to perform a nonmotivated continuous attention task showed an increase in errors under placebo conditions (Orzack *et al.*, 1968), whereas there was no such increase with MP (50 mg), caffeine (200 mg), or methyl phenidate (15 mg).

Since behavioral and biochemical studies with MP have rarely been run in parallel, therefore only a questionable support is provided for the hypothesis that this compound exerts a facilitative effect upon learning and memory through its brain RNA effect. It is unfortunate that replicability of both behavioral methods as well as results from studies of drug dose, frequency of dosage and time course, and of biochemical effects, central uptake and time course of central action, and central locus of any presumed chemical change, have all not emerged in the literature, probably either because such studies have not been done or because of too many unfounded assumptions, or empirical results that appear to justify such assumptions.

There have been several suggested bases for increases in neural RNA level that have subsequently been followed by studies relating such effect to behavior. Aside from the pharmacological agents previously discussed, there are others which, as well as their macromolecular effects also modify other chemical and electrophysiological parameters in the brain. An increase in nucleic acid, nucleotide, or nucleoprotein level in brain can be brought about in several ways; sometimes by endogenous means and, perhaps, more indirectly by drug action. It is perhaps relevant to consider what RNA's, which proteins, and at what regional, cellular, subcellular, and organelle site, such changes become relevant to the processes of learning or memory. Unfortunately, such considerations in combined pharamacological and behavioral studies as appropriate to learning and/or memory have seldom emerged on the scientific horizon. But, it is of interest to take notice of the fact that other "systems" within which specific drug effects can be accounted for can also be dealt with in terms of a more general basis for the interaction of centrally active drug effects and learning and memory mechanisms.

XIII. Cholinergic Mechanisms

Pharmacological agents that change the transmission process involving cholinergic synapses, presumably through modification of the ratio of acetylcholine to its hydrolyzing enzyme, acetylcholinesterase, have sometimes been suggested as a means of providing for alterations in mechanisms concerned with learning and memory. It has never been perfectly clear from such hypotheses what specific brain storage pool of acetylcholine might require alteration or what degree of effect is required to result in behavioral changes. One means by which a presumed end point of optimized cholinergic transmission may be accomplished has been the use of what purports to be an efficient precursor of acetylcholine that penetrates the blood–brain barrier more effectively than choline; a compound suggested in this regard has been deanol (2-dimethylaminolethanol). There is, however, no evidence for any change in brain acetylcholine levels after administration of this compound (Pepeu *et al.*, 1960), and its stimulantlike effects upon the reticular system, in bringing about EEG and behavioral arousal (Goldstein, 1960), resemble closely effects observed with other compounds that stimulate the adrenergic system. In rats trained to respond to light on an elevated T-maze, discrimination learning, zero delay responding, and delay tasks were measured. Deanol (100 mg/kg) given 2 hours prior to training had no effect on any of the tasks measured. When retraining was given with the drug administered during the tasks, a significant increase in performance occurred during the initial stages of each task, with correspondingly longer response latencies (Karoly and Hunt, 1965).

Another approach to the concept that cholinergic mediation of learning and/or memory has been based upon the view that these processes may be responsive to pharmacological agents that combine with cholinesterase to reduce the rate of acetylcholine destruction. One such agent, physostigmine (eserine), reversibly competes with acetylcholine for cholinesterase; thereby, it may predictably prolong the effect of acetylcholine liberated at cholinergic nerve endings. The acquisition of simple discriminative avoidance learnings was reported to be facilitated with administration of eserine (Cardo, 1961), and in two strains or rats (maze-bright and maze-dull) given daily training trials in a Lashley III maze and followed by posttrial eserine, facilitation of maze acquisition was produced at lower doses (0.50–0.75 mg/kg), whereas performance disrupted at higher doses (0.75–1.00 mg/kg). A higher dose within each dose range was required to produce facilitation or disruption, respectively, in the maze-dull rats (Stratton and Petrinovich, 1963). In rats trained to learn a simple discriminative avoidance response, posttrial eserine treatment led to facilitation of response acquisition as a function of age and difficulty of the task (Doty and Johnston, 1966).

The enhancement of discrimination learning by physostigmine has been reported for rats treated (0.1 and 0.5 mg/kg, i.p.) before training in a modified T-maze with auditory stimuli. In cats trained on a Wisconsin General Test Apparatus for two discrimination problems, 0.50 mg/kg of physostigmine provided for significantly more rapid learning and, at 0.025 mg/kg, the cats showed a significant increase in the rate at which the second problem was learned. These studies have arrived at the conclusion that any apparently facilitative effect of physostigmine in these learning situations is confined to a limited dose range and may be dose-specific (Whitehouse, 1966). Maze learning in mice (Stratton and Petrinovich, 1967) has also been reported to be facilitated by physostigmine treatment.

Physostigmine (eserine) was compared with other anticholinesterase agents in rats trained on a discrete avoidance task. Given in a dose range of 0.16 to 1.28 mg/kg (eserine) and of 1.25 to 10 mg/kg (carbaryl), the dose required to suppress avoidance responding to 50% efficiency, or to reduce brain cholinesterase to 50% of normal was determined. It was determined that eserine was 9 times as active as carbaryl in disrupting avoidance behavior and also 9 times as effective as a cholinesterase inhibitor. The behavioral effects produced by cholinesterase inhibitors were interfered with by atropine (Goldberg *et al.*, 1965). The behavioral effects and central actions of atropine and related anticholinergic compounds in animals and man have been rather extensively reviewed (Longo, 1966). It has been suggested that in animals there is a drug-mediated interference with evoked motor patterns, unlearned behavior, acquisition and retention of conditioned responses, and it also provides for dissociation. In man there is evidence for a central cholinergic syndrome effected through atropine, scopolamine, and related anticholinergic compounds; this consists of diminished concentration, memory disturbances, drowsiness, ataxia, etc. Rats were trained to bar-press when a compound stimulus of light and tone signaled the delivery of a sucrose solution as reinforcement. The probability of reinforcement following a reinforced trial was 0.5, independent of response. After a response to a nonreinforced trial, nonreinforcement was continued until responses to such trials ceased, following which reinforcement probability was readjusted to 0.5. The animals were injected (either i.p. or via canula unilaterally or bilaterally into dorsal hippocampus) with either atropine sulfate or its quaternary salt, atropine methyl bromide. Saline controls were also provided, and all treatments were initiated immediately prior to the behavioral sequence. A behavioral deficit, in the form of an inability to withhold responding after bar-pressing on a nonreinforced trial, was produced by i.p. atropine or by direct central administration of these anticholinergics; but i.p. atropine methyl bromide, which does not cross the blood–brain barrier, was without effect (Khavari and Maickel, 1967). It may be noteworthy that both atropine sulfate (10–20 mg/kg) and scopolamine hydrobromide (5–10 mg/kg) produce significant anorexic effects in rats (Cohen, 1966). This observation could have particular relevance for studies in which appetitive stimuli are utilized to motivate learned behavior. In monkeys, when atropine and scopolamine were compared on a visual discrimination and active avoidance task, the latter compound was from 3 to 32 times more potent than the former drug in disrupting learned behavior (Samuel *et al.*, 1965).

The effects of scopolamine have been considered with regard to learning and memory methodologies, but rarely have the effects been related either quantitatively or with temporal regard to the anticholinergic action of the drug. Groups of rats were treated with either saline (0.1 ml, s.c.), scopolamine (0.1 and 1.0 mg/kg, s.c.), or atropine methyl nitrate (1.0 mg/kg, s.c.) during exposure to a nociceptive stimulus. This stimulation was again used, 2 weeks later, when an operant response, continuously reinforced with food and secondary light reinforcement, was followed after

10 to 12 days, by a 0.2 mA, 0.5-second shock, added to the operant task. A single scopolamine treatment without prior aversive stimulation, led to interruption of the operant behavior, even after the drug had been eliminated. With a single scopolamine treatment, with the prior aversive stimulation, there was a more prolonged disruption of the operant behavior (Berry and Stark, 1965). With scopolamine or methylscopolamine (0.1–0.8 mg/kg), severe disruption of a passive avoidance response by rats was brought about by the former drug (0.2–0.8 mg/kg) but without any such effect of the latter. Retention of the passive avoidance response after 10 days of training, with an intervening 2-day rest period, indicated a scopolamine-induced disruption of retention without any similar effect produced by methylscopolamine. The effects observed (Meyers, 1965) cannot be attributed to a drug-dissociation effect or to the development of drug tolerance. The effects of scopolamine on operant avoidance acquisition and retention in rats has also been investigated (Leaf and Muller, 1965, 1966). There was an appreciable increase in the response rates on a Sidman avoidance task at lower shock rates at a dose of 0.1 mg/kg. Drug treatment was given either immediately prior to the eleventh training session or just prior to the first training session, and the same stimulant effect upon acquisition of the Sidman-avoidance response was observed for both treatments. Methylscopolamine did not provide for the same effect, pointing toward the central rather than peripheral effects of the drug. After avoidance responding was well-learned, the same dose was ineffective in producing a comparable effect. The suggested mode of drug action, in this case, was that the inhibitory system of the central nervous system was blocked by scopolamine and physostigmine on the acquisition of a 1-trial passive avoidance response in mice; the quaternary nitrogen compounds, scopolamine methylbromide and neostigmine were administered as controls. Scopolamine (1 mg/kg) given prior to training led to a reduced incidence of avoidance learning, as indicated on a testing session given 24 hours later. Combined treatment with scopolamine and physostigmine provided for better learning in these mice than was observed for animals treated separately with each compound, and the quaternary compounds had no effect (Bohdanecky and Jarvik, 1967). These findings point even more definitively toward central cholinergic mechanisms, the alteration of which can lead to modified efficiency of learning or memory. State dependency apparently does not constitute a strong argument for cholinergic modification, such as that, for example, brought about by scopolamine. Passive avoidance behavior of mice the acquisition of which was disrupted by scopolamine, could not be convincingly used to account for any drug state-dependency effect (Stark, 1967). The irreversible com-

bination with cholinesterase by diisopropyl fluorophosphonate (DFP) has been indicated, in at least two studies as providing for enhancement of learning; this phenomenon, however appears to be highly specific to the nature of the initial learning and the time course over which the direct central effect of DFP occurs. On one hand, it was shown that direct injection of DFP into the hyppocampus can produce amnesia for a learned habit, whereas when the same habit is forgotten, DFP injection can lead to enhancement of memory (Deutsch and Leibowitz, 1966). The apparent rationale of this approach and the resolution of this finding is housed in the concept that by drug-induced prevention of acetylcholine destruction, the depolarization of the postsynaptic membrane will be promoted for those conditions wherein low levels of synaptic conductance prevail. If, as has been assumed, synaptic conductance is increased after training, increased with learning, and decreased with forgetting, then the enhancement of memory for a forgotten habit by DFP further rests upon the assumption that increased acetylcholine levels superimposed upon hypothetically low synaptic conductance becomes facilitative. In a further study (Deutsch and Lutzky, 1967) the injection of DFP resulted in enhancement of the recall of a partially learned habit, also possibly lending some support to the premise that synaptic transmission has been altered to account for facilitation.

An interesting use of DFP has been made in an investigation of cholinergic mechanisms related to the extinction of a conditioned response in rats (Glow and Rose, 1965). The combined use of DFP, i.m.), and *N,N*-trimethylene (1:3)-bis (pyridinium-4-aldoxime) bromide, i.p. which provides for reactivation of peripheral acetylcholinesterase (AChE) activity were injected selectively to provide for reduced brain AChE activity. The rate at which rats extinguished a lever-pressing response under DFP alone was characteristically different from the rate for combined DFP and *N,N*-trimethylene-treated or control rats. These findings point toward the potential requirement of a peripheral cholinergic component required for extinction behavior.

Some attention has already been given to nicotine concerning its possible cholinergic contribution through its capacity to effect the release of ACh. What appear to be considerations relevant to the effects of nicotine upon learning and memory are factors such as dose, treatment–behavior time, the age of the animal, chronicity of treatment, and strain. The points and the central mechanisms related to the behavioral role of nicotine, its metabolites, and analogs have been reviewed (Essman, 1971c), and in some instances relevant findings have been treated in an earlier section of this review.

It may be appropriate to point out that whereas nicotine involves, within a relatively short time course, a decrease in total tissue (51%), bound (87%), and vesicular (67%) ACh in the cerebral cortex of mice, there is a temporally contingent elevation of 5-HT level in the cerebral cortex, mesencephalon, and diencephalon. It is at this time (15 minutes following 1.0 mg/kg injection) that the amnesic effect of posttraining ECS is potentiated; but, at a later posttreatment time (45 minutes), when at least two metabolites of this drug have occurred and are active, the amnesic effect of ECS is antagonized and the magnitude of the brain 5-HT elevation is appreciably less. Since the effects of nicotine on cholinergic mechanisms cannot clearly be isolated from its related but, perhaps, secondary effects upon other brain biogenic amines, the relevance of this compound for learning or memory mechanisms requires some additional information and considerably more understanding of the interrelationships between the interrelationships between the brain biogenic amines that serve the mechanisms underlying the processes of learning and memory.

XIV. Catecholamines

There have only been a limited number of investigations wherein a direct relationship between brain catecholamine change and learning or memory tasks have been considered. Of course, there are several indirect sources for such a relationship which may be derived from those findings, for example the results of studies, previously considered, with the amphetamines, drugs affecting brain 5-HT, etc. An interesting proposal concerning release or enhancement of brain norepinephrine (NE) and facilitation of learning and memory has summarized some of the indirect evidence in support of such a view (Kety, 1971).

The use of α-methyltyrosine (α-MT), an inhibitor of tyrosine hydroxylase—the enzyme involved in the rate-limiting formation of 3,4-dihydroxyphenylalanine, from which dopamine an NE are formed—has found some use in behavioral studies. A dose-dependent (100–200 mg/kg, i.p.) increase in responding by rats in an operant shock-avoidance situation was observed within 2 to 5 hours after treatment (Carlton, 1963), whereas behavioral deficits have been related to the extent of α-MT-induced brain catecholamine depletion in rats (Rech *et al.*, 1966). In a rather comprehensive investigation (Hanson, 1965), conditioned avoidance behavior in cats and rats was studied in response to brain catecholamine depletion by α-MT. In cats trained to 100% conditioned avoidance responding in a shuttle box, the drug (150 and 200 mg/kg), by 12 hours postinjection, disrupted avoidance behavior; this disruption was completely reversed by L-dopa (7.5 and 10 mg/kg) given 15 hours after α-MT. The decreased dopamine and norepinephrine levels in brain brought about following α-MT treatment were again elevated by 1 hour after L-dopa treatment. Similar results were obtained for rats trained to 75% conditioned avoidance responding and given α-MT (125 or 250 mg/kg); the disrupted avoidance behavior was reversed by L-dopa (50 mg/kg) given 18 hours after α-MT.

In studies from our laboratory, several rather interesting findings concerning some of those issues previously considered have emerged. Mice, given α-MT (100 mg/kg, i.p.) between 0 and 8 hours before training on a 1-trial passive avoidance task, showed impaired acquisition that was consistent with reduced catecholamine levels; i.e., at 4 hours after treatment when dopamine and norepinephrine were maximally depleted (56 and 63%, respectively) the incidence of avoidance acquisition was maximally reduced (20%). The degree of impaired acquisition was directly related to the magnitude of the catecholamine depletion. A related finding is that in the presence of depleted brain catecholamines, the amnesic effect of posttraining ECS was attenuated; i.e., at 4 hours postdrug there was only 35% incidence of ECS-induced amnesia, as compared with 90% among controls, or 75% among animals treated 8 hours postdrug. This finding may possibly be related to the observation that, whereas ECS led to the usually noted elevation in brain 5-HT level among those animals where ECS-induced amnesia was noted, in the presence of depleted catecholamines, ECS did not lead to 5-HT elevation. α-Methyltyrosine treatment had no effect on brain 5-HT level, alone.

Pharmacological effects which in the course of affecting some aspect of learning or memory have well correlated effects upon the content or turnover of brain catecholamines probably have not been considered with the same effort or to the same depth as have other putative transmitter molecules in brain. Such effects and the role of brain catecholamines in learning and memory appear to hold considerable future promise as a means of further elucidating the basic mechanisms by which such processes are operative.

XV. Indole Amines and Molecular Interactions

Many of the drug-mediated learning or memory effects previously considered have employed either pharamacological or physiological treatment conditions involving, either directly or indirectly, some effect upon brain 5-HT content or metabolism. It is not our purpose to detail the specific interrelationships between behaviorally active drugs, their central site and mode of action, and their effect upon brain 5-HT. Such relationships have been described in several reviews and monographs (Garattini and Valzelli, 1965; Page, 1968). There is, in addition, the functional role played by 5-HT, in the presence of macromolecules which bind it, for learning and memory mechanisms. This concept of a 5-HT–nucleic acid complex or receptor has been independently proposed (Smythies *et al.*, 1969; Bittman *et al.*, 1969) and will be considered more fully later.

An early series of experiments suggesting that the level of brain 5-HT was the critical determinant of learning efficiency in mice made use of a T-maze where the sole apparent motivational basis for learning was the opportunity to hide from view (Woolley, 1965). It was determined that, out of 10 acquisition trials, normal mice showed an average of 7.4 trials on which correct maze responding was shown. In general, the results indicated that drug-mediated elevation of brain 5-HT level resulted in decreased learning ability, and reduced brain 5-HT level provided for an increased rate of learning. Increases or decreases in brain catecholamine level, in this study, did not point toward any apparent effect upon learning efficiency. When brain 5-HT level was elevated by treating mice with 5-hydroxytryptophan (5-HTP) (60 mg/kg) and 1-benzyl-2-methyl-5-methoxytryptamine hydrochloride (BAS) (15 mg/kg), the number of correct response trials was reduced from an average of 7.4 to an average of 6.1. With further elevation of brain 5-HT (300 mg/kg 5-HTP + 15 mg/kg BAS) the number of correct response trials was reduced to 5.1. Elevation of brain 5-HT through another mode (monoamine oxidase inhibition with iproniazid, 3 mg/kg) led to a maze score of 6.1. With a decreased brain 5-HT level brought about by treatment with either reserpine (1.2 mg/kg) or a combination of DL-phenylalanine and L-tyrosine, (p.o.), the maze score was increased to 8.1 and 8.3, respectively. Similarly, when increases in brain 5-HT level of approximately 35% in mice were brought about through large systemic doses, an effect upon conditioned avoidance response acquisition was noted (Essman, 1971b). There was a 10% reduction in the rate of 1-trial passive avoidance conditioning when the training foot shock was 6.0 mA. With a weaker conditioning shock (3.0 mA), there was a 25% reduction in acquisition. These results obtained with a 75-mg/kg dose of 5-HT. At a higher dose (100 mg/kg), there was no further reduction in acquisition at the higher shock level, but at the lower one, acquisition was reduced by 60%. When 5-HTP was given avoidance acquisition was only slightly impaired at the two highest doses of 75 mg/kg (20% reduction) and 100 mg/kg (25% reduction). It is of further interest to note that there was an inverse dose relationship to the amnesic effect of a posttraining ECS within the dose range where neither response acquisition nor ECS-induced convulsion were affected by 5-HTP. For example, whereas animals pretreated with saline and given a single posttraining ECS showed a 90% incidence of retrograde amnesia on a 24-hour testing trial, mice given 5-HTP (3.12 mg/kg, i.p.) 60 minutes before the training ECS series showed only a 15% incidence of retrograde amnesia.

The depletion of brain 5-HT through the use of *p*-chlorophenylalanine (PCPA), an inhibitor of tryptophan hydroxylation (Koe and Weissman, 1966) has been employed in several studies of learning and memory. It has been shown (Tenen, 1967) that PCPA in rats led to decreased emotional reactivity, an increased reactivity to painful stimuli, and an increased incidence of conditioned avoidance response acquisition. Another case of apparently facilitated learning after PCPA treatment has been reported (Stevens *et al.*, 1967) for rats; two brightness discrimination tasks were acquired with fewer errors than for controls, although position discrimination and reversal were not affected. In mice the effects of PCPA on either depletion of brain 5-HT or conditioned avoidance learning has not been quite so obvious. Studies from our laboratory in which PCPA treatment (100, 200, or 300 mg/kg, i.p.) preceded a training trial by 72 hours, indicated that the incidence of conditioned avoidance response learning and the susceptibility to posttraining ECS amnesic effects were not altered by the treatments. Moreover, whereas there was a dose-related decrease in brain 5-HT (16, 28, and 39%, respectively) this neither approximated the degree of brain 5-HT reduction reported in rats nor resulted in any appreciable learning advantage. In cats the performance of a long-term conditioned avoidance response was facilitated under conditions whereby brain 5-HT was decreased and brain norepinephrine was increased (Wada *et al.*, 1963).

We have previously indicated that intracranial administration of 5-HT to mice, following either passive or active conditioned avoidance training can serve as an extremely effective amnesic agent. Furthermore, this effect follows a well-defined temporal gradient; i.e., when given within 10 seconds of a training trial, there was a 90% incidence of retrograde amnesia but at 2, 4, 8, 16, and 32 minutes posttraining the incidence of amnesia was 85, 60, 30, 10, and 0%, respectively. We have also previously indicated (Essman, 1968c, 1969a, 1970a, 1971b) that aside from the increase in 5-HT level as an apparent requisite for disruption of a postexperiential memory consolidation process, that a 5-HT turnover change is also an apparently necessary condition. Increases in 5-HT level have accounted for inhibition of protein synthesis, measured by reduced leucine-^{14}C incorporation by isolated presynaptic nerve endings (synaptosomes) from mouse cerebral cortex (24%) and limbic system (32%). The onset of this effect has been determined at approximately 10 minutes (15%) and remains at about that level for total brain protein for at least 30 minutes (Essman *et al.*, 1971).

The interaction of 5-HT with nucleic acids in brain has been an hypothesis derived from several previous studies (Essman, 1967a, 1968d; Essman and Essman, 1969) in which a high negative correlation between brain 5-HT levels and brain RNA content for several regions of the mouse brain were apparent. In several further studies (Bittman *et al.*, 1969; Bittman and Essman, 1970; Essman *et al.*, 1971) the specific interaction of 5-HT with nucleic acids in brain was proposed as a model which might serve to generate the hypotheses concerning molecular mechanisms by which learning, memory, and amnesia are regulated. On the basis of several physical studies, we have concluded that 5-HT binds to nucleic acids, including RNA, tRNA, DNA, and polynucleotides, and it is bound by Coulombic interaction with contributions from hydrogen bonding. The contribution of ionic strength to the 5-HT–RNA binding suggests an electrostatic interaction, whereby the approach of the 5-HT molecule to RNA is enhanced by ionic forces; when within short distances, then specific hydrogen bond, charge transfer, and van der Waals forces are capable of contributing effect. On the basis of circular dichroism spectroscopy studies, we have concluded that 5-HT forms a complex with the nucleic acid between the aralkylammonium moiety of the former and the negatively charged phosphate groups of the latter, with no significant helix distortion. Our evidence sharply contradicts model-building studies suggesting that 5-HT interacts with nucleic acids by intercalation (Smythies and Antun, 1969). Conclusions regarding the interaction by hydrogen bonding (donation of a proton to the O of 5-HT, indole NH to the phosphodiester O) and electrostatic interaction ($-NH_3^+$ near phosphates or phosphodiester O) have been further supported by studies in which 5-HT derivatives and various solvent systems have altered the binding constants consistent with predictions generated by the proposed binding mechanisms (Essman *et al.*, 1971).

The nature of 5-HT-induced amnesia, disruption of learning, etc. and its molecular interaction with RNA, its contribution to brain protein synthesis, and the dependence for its binding with nucleic acids upon ionic strength and the nature of the ionic conditions regulating the interaction, have all pointed toward the need for further investigation in this area. In several further studies in our laboratory, the effect of elevated brain 5-HT in the guinea pig, upon RNA levels associated with subcellular fractions from several areas of the brain, was investigated. Whereas synaptosomes from limbic cortex and cerebellar cortex showed no appreciable change in associated RNA level, the mitochondrial fraction from cerebellar cortex showed a 5-HT-induced RNA elevation. Only in the synaptosome fraction from cerebral cortex was there a 5-HT-induced RNA decrement (from 3.58 to 0.32 μg/mg protein) by 60 minutes following treatment. Significant decrements in RNA associated with soluble cytoplasm, small external synaptic membrane fragments, large membrane fragments, and intraterminal mitochondria also followed 5-HT treatment. We have further observed that increased 5-HT levels in mouse brain lead to the most marked inhibition of protein synthesis in both the microsomes (26%) and synaptosomes (20%) from the basal ganglia and diencephalon.

It appears that relevant consideration for the molecular events discussed above focuses upon those pharmacological agents, which, in contributing to such an interaction, can have considerable importance for those mechanisms by which the processes of learning and memory can be facilitated or disrupted.

XVI. Electrolyte Effects

There has been only limited attention given to the effects of specific electrolytes on the processes of learning and memory, and still less consideration afforded drug-induced brain electrolyte alterations and the behavioral consequences thereof. There has been some attention given to potassium and calcium effects on conditioned avoidance behavior in cats (Sachs, 1961). Intraventricular K (25–37.5 μeq) given 10 minutes prior to avoidance training led to an alerting effect and rapid conditioned response acquisition. When intraventricular Ca (22.5–33.75 μeq) was given to cats, they showed what was interpreted as slowed, retarded learning of the conditioned avoidance response. Conditioned responses in cats, already well-established, were severely disrupted when either KCl or $CaCl_2$ were given intraventricularly (John *et al.*, 1959). There is some indirect evidence which may have possible relevance to alterations in avoidance learning or the performance of learned avoidance behavior as related to altered brain electrolyte concentration. These findings derive from studies of steroid hormones and learning—the relevant feature of which is that K^+ concentration in brain has been indicated as increased as a consequence of a steroid shift (Woodbury, 1954). If, therefore the increased K^+ is consistent with improved avoidance learning, then one might expect a steroid change to provide similar effects. In a passive-avoidance conditioning paradigm, where rats were trained to suppress bar-pressing for water reinforcement by shock, adrenocorticotropin (ACTH) injection (12 injections of 8 units/day) decreased responding to a mean of 0.6 response as compared with 92.4 for controls, suggesting that passive avoidance was facilitated (Levine and Jones, 1965). The maintenance of high levels of shuttle-box avoidance learning was highly correlated with high corticosteroid levels, either endogenously maintained, or provided through ACTH administration or hydrocortisone placement (Levine and Brush, 1967). One problem that arises with ACTH use in studies concerned with food or water reinforcement is the increased sodium retention provided by ACTH release; such a change in water balance may well alter appetitively based motive states.

Of recent interest because of its therapeutic application is the issue of lithium salts and the potential contribution thereof to cognitive functions. A series of experiments (Essman, 1970b) have concerned the effects of lithium salts on learning and memory in mice and the possible central effects that are mediated through the action of lithium. Brain uptake of lithium was determined, and doses of 1.18 and 2.35 meq/kg brain provided for maximum levels within 15 minutes following parenteral injection. Also, there were significant increases in brain magnesium levels, highly correlated (0.89) with the uptake of lithium. This latter finding may be of interest because Mg^{++}-induced activation of cerebral AChE (Shitov, 1965), its role as a cofactor in cellular enzyme reactions, its mediation of junctional ACh release (del Castillo and Engbaek, 1954), its effect in alteration of acidic lipid distribution in brain and reversibly displacing other ions in brain lipids (Folch *et al.*, 1957), and the regulation of brain adenosine triphosphatase (ATPase) activity (Palladin, 1961). The action of several tranquilizers has been potentiated by Mg (Shitov, 1965), but this interaction remains to be explored on a behavioral level.

Our behavioral findings have indicated that lithium carbonate (2.35 meq/kg, i.p.), 30 or 60 minutes prior to passive avoidance training, led to (*1*) reinstatement of avoidance behavior by 48 hours after posttraining ECS, where this response, when tested at 24 hours, was not in evidence; (*2*) a lithium-related decrease in turnover of brain 5-HT; and (*3*) lithium-induced reduction in the 5-HT alterations produced by ECS. The possibility of lithium-induced increases in norepinephrine deamination (Schildkraut *et al.*, 1966a,b, 1969) or related facilitation of *O*-methylated norepinephrine products provided through elevated brain Mg^{++} (LaBrosse *et al.*, 1958) remains an uninvestigated issue to which the possibility of electrolytes playing a role in learning or memory may be related and certainly bear consideration for further study.

Those molecules which, as putative transmitters, have been considered in view of their functional role in mechanisms related to learning and memory also exert effects upon and are affected by electrolyte distribution and electrolyte effects on related events such as molecular binding, threshold to the cellular effects of drugs, and duration of lipid binding of drugs. In a similar regard, there are drugs that in their own right can contribute to brain electrolyte changes and thereby mediate not only direct effects of such changes upon events relevant to learning and memory, but also provide secondary effects, such as those referred to above. A large body of such active pharmacological agents include barbiturates, sedatives, and several classes of mood stabilizers—including tranquilizers, antianxiety agents, and antidepressants. The individual contribution of these compounds to changes in brain electrolytes and the relevance of such ionic shifts for learning and memory processes remain issues beyond the scope of present consideration, but are, perhaps, a point of departure for future investigation.

XVII. Barbiturates, Sedatives, and Mood Stabilizers

Although the barbiturates have not found the same degree of attention in learning and memory studies, their effect can hardly be ignored. Perhaps, because the effects of these compounds concerning pharmacology, electrophysiology, and biochemistry have been extensively covered, their behavioral effect might be designated by hypotheses generated from such physiological data. However, this has not always been the case or the apparent intent of the limited behavioral studies which have concerned learning or memory. Also, because of differences in time course of effect, degree of sedation or anesthesia produced, etc., intercomparisons between specific barbiturates, having designated effects upon either learning or memory have been difficult to make.

Sodium barbital appears to be one of the least behaviorally investigated of the barbiturates, probably because of its long duration of sedative and hypnotic effect, as well as side effects and withdrawal effects having potential behavioral contributions which render the primary effect of the drug more difficult to assess behaviorally. Chronic treatment of rats with barbital sodium (100 mg/kg/day, increased at weekly increments by 100 100 mg/kg/day over 5 weeks, p.o.) until drug habituation had occurred, were either trained in a T-maze or a shuttle box, either following drug habituation or prior to drug habituation. The number of errors, response times, and failure to respond during acquisition of the T-maze increased significantly during the time wherein barbital was being chronically administered, but control levels were achieved by 5 days after drug withdrawal. During habituation there was a significant rise in food intake, which fell below control shortly after withdrawal, and rose again to control level by about 1 week following withdrawal. The acquisition of the avoidance response in the shuttle box was not affected by the barbiturate, but avoidance responses were significantly decreased by 24 to 48 hours after withdrawal and then reinstated to control level by 3 to 4 days after withdrawal (Leonard, 1967). Rats chronically treated with sodium barbital showed an increase in the running time in response to a food-motivated multiple-T-maze situation. Food intake, as well as body weight were increased in the drug-treated animals (Leonard, 1969). The observed effect was partially antagonized by ACTH, but not by amphetamine. The same investigator (Leonard, 1966a) has previously indicated common features of sodium barbital habituation include decreased brain ATP and creatine phosphate and increased ammonia. It has also been shown (Leonard, 1966b) that drug withdrawal after habituation results in increased central nervous system excitability, possibly linked to adrenocortical hyperactivity.

A possibly relevant point around which studies of learning or memory may relate is the blocking effect of another barbiturate, amobarbital, on ACh in peripheral cholinergic junctions—an effect which might be viewed as reduced responsivity in a postjunctional effector cell. When rats were given amobarbital sodium (20 mg/kg) in order to reduce fear in an avoidance task, performance of the response was increased, but in a nondrug state there was no transfer of this effect (Miller, 1961). The possible state dependency of this effect might be suggested by such an observation; however, the possible interaction of the drug with the situation-derived motivational factors could present another consideration. Under conditions of varied reinforcement incidence, rats given 100% reinforcement showed a greater drug-induced (20 mg/kg) running time than did 50% reinforced animals (Wagner, 1963). With a smaller amobarbital dose (5 mg/kg), social factors offering a potential contribution to the motivational state of the animal, such as exploration, mating response, submission, and escape behavior, were reduced (Chance and Silverman, 1964).

In pigeons, amobarbital (6 to 60 mg/kg, i.m.) treatment following training to key-peck on a positive reinforcement schedule led to predrug-related response rate effects (Dews, 1964) wherein an inhibitory stimulus did not find drug-imposed modification of its effect on response rate. A drug-related (0.1 and 0.3 gm, p.o.) reduction in positive conditioned reflexes has been reported (Guseva, 1964), and this may perhaps be related to the observation (Sofronov and Tsobkallo, 1959) that dogs in a conditioning situation showed increased internal inhibition where small doses were chronically administered, but with chronic treatment at larger doses, internal inhibition was weakened.

Training of rats in a conflict situation, either under placebo or amobarbital sodium (20 mg/kg, i.p.) conditions led to an increase in approach performance under drug treatment, independent of the conditions of the conflict training conditions (Barry *et al.*, 1962). During extinction of a response, the characteristic decrement in running speed was attenuated when rats were treated with amobarbital (15 mg/kg), suggesting that the rate of extinction could be slowed (Stretch *et al.*, 1964). Through the use of a potentiated startle response, used in rats as an index of conditioned fear, amobarbital sodium (10, 20, or 40 mg/kg) was given 10 minutes pretesting to obtain a startle score. The startle score was proportionate to the force of the startle response; the latter was decreased as a function of increased drug dosage (Chi, 1965). A differential effect of amobarbital on running speed of rats, depending upon the motivational conditions providing for running, has been considered (Barry and Miller, 1965). Food-motivated approach and shock-motivated escape and avoidance were compared in animals equalized during 6 days of predrug training. A decrease in running speed following amobarbital treatment was observed for avoidance escape and approach conditions in a descending degree of magnitude. This result may also suggest that amobarbital has different effects depending upon whether the stimuli motivating learning or performance are appetitive or aversive and how thresholds for each condition may be preferentially modified by the barbiturate. Under aversive stimulus conditions providing for conditioned avoidance acquisition in a jump box, three light-intensity levels were used (CS) with 15 CS-UCS pairings (5-second interval) for 6 days, with amobarbital sodium (20 mg/kg) given 20 minutes pretraining. There was generally improved performance, with the greatest difference between the intermediate- and high-intensity CS (Powell *et al.*, 1966). In a hurdle-crossing avoidance conditioning situation, amobarbital (5–40 mg/kg) was given 20 minutes prior to the conditioning session. An increase in the rate of avoidance conditioning was observed, with optimal efficiency at 20 to 30 mg/kg, and a reduced efficiency at 40 mg/kg. One explanation for these results is that the drug may provide for attentuation of freezing behavior (Kamano *et al.*, 1966a). When a conditioned emotional response and conditioned avoidance response (hurdle-crossing) were considered with amobarbital treatment (20 mg/kg, i.p.), the former was not significantly affected, whereas acquisition of the latter was facilitated (Kamano *et al.*, 1966b). It would seem that a highly relevant consideration involved in assessing the effects of amobarbital on learning is the time course of its action for stimulus-specific response contingencies. This could, as suggested, also be dose-linked and task-dependent.

The use of pentobarbital in several studies has suggested a variety of effects—again, as its previously considered structural relative, highly related to dose, time course, and the nature of the behavioral task. It has been shown, for example, that diffuse, conditioned motor reflexes, which included several parts of the body and also involved the forelimbs, could be developed in dogs under pentobarbital anesthesia (Teitelbaum *et al.*, 1961). This drug, administered to the rhesus monkey abolished lever-pressing for the reduction of painful stimuli (Malis, 1962). Rats given pentobarbital sodium (13 mg/kg) showed acquisition of a conditioned avoidance response comparable to that occurring among control animals; however, when drug treatment was continued following avoidance acquisition the incidence of avoidance behavior was reduced in the absence of reinforcement. In the absence of the barbiturate, following relearning of the response, the conditioned avoidance behavior became independent of the presence or absence of the drug (Holmgren and Condi, 1964). When rats, given pentobarbital sodium (25 mg/kg), relearned a response, this was not transferred to a nondrug state, and relearning under the nondrug state was similarly not transferred to the drug state (Overton, 1964). Such apparent evidence favoring a barbiturate-induced state-specificity of state dependency for learning allows wide speculation as to mechanisms of drug action. The apparent involvement of the reticular system of the brain and thalamic relay nuclei might suggest that alternate input and integration pathways are related to a drug-mediated specificity for learning. However, maintained behavior does not seem to follow the same pattern as temporally (and drug-related) separated learning situations. A considerable drug-related accuracy decrement was initially observed in pigeons trained to press a color-illuminated response key when pentobarbital sodium (5 or 10 mg/kg) was given. A relatively rapid recovery of the response occurred thereafter, and normal levels of response accuracy were then recorded (Berryman *et al.*, 1962).

Rats trained to press one of two bars for water and then required to reverse the procedure were given either placebo or pentobarbital sodium (1 mg/kg) before both training and/or reversal, 20 minutes prior to the session. For the response learned under the barbiturate, a change to the undrugged state resulted in a reduced strength. The view was taken that barbiturate treatment during escape extinction may provide a basis for facilitated extinction of the escape response (Meltzer *et al.*, 1966).

In man, pentobarbital has found some attention in tasks wherein running memory span was considered among several other tasks (Quarton and Talland, 1962). Pentobarbital (100 mg/150 lb of body weight, i.v.) led to reduced memory span. When running memory span was evaluated under pentobarbital treatment (100 mg/68 kg, i.v.) or placebo in a double-blind investigation, there was a drug-related narrowing effect (Talland and Quarton, 1965). Strings of digits from 8 to 20 items in length were presented as one item, either every second or every 4 seconds with the task requiring the reproduction of the last five digits in the correct sequence. At the slow rate of item presentation, there was an impairment, related to the barbiturate, of organization and rehearsal for storage.

In at least one study (Garg and Holland, 1968b) pentobarbital sodium was administered to rats immediately after training, with a view toward relating the postexperiential drug effects to the consolidation of the memory trace for that experience. A daily trial, followed either by barbiturate or by distilled water control injection, was given on problem 4 of the Hebb-Williams maze. Significantly more errors were made by the rats given posttraining barbiturate treatment than occurred among controls, and the inferred drug-related disruption of learning was attributed to a decreased rate of consolidation.

Of the other barbiturates, phenobarbital and thiopental have also been employed in studies of learning or memory and their choice has probably resided in diversities of duration—the former being long-acting, whereas the latter has an ultrashort duration of action. In response to foot shock, there was a tendency for phenobarbital (45 mg/kg) to provide for habituation to arousal from such stimulation (Kelleher *et al.*, 1961), but this may also reflect a depression of motor activity resulting from a relatively high drug dose. In a situation wherein rats were trained to press a disc or a lever for food reinforcement, phenobarbital treatment led to increased response rates (Kelleher *et al.*, 1961). A dose-related enhacement of response rates of pigeons trained on a multiple fixed ratio (33), fixed interval (5-minute) schedule has been also observed (Bignami and Gatti, 1969).

Thiopental sedation in human subjects given a series of simple tests for recognition memory of pictures and recall memory of associated pairs of letters and words led to amnesic effects that were judged not to be retroactive. Memory loss, as apparently brought about by intermittent thiopental treatment was correlated with drug levels in the venous blood. When items were learned under thiopental sedation and then tested either 30 minutes or 24 hours later, there was better item recognition at the latter time interval. Better performance was in evidence on associative learning tests when testing was given 30 minutes after learning (sedation period) than 24 hours after learning (waking). Drug administration prior to testing at 24 hours after learning did not improve memory (Osborn *et al.*, 1967). These findings suggest that both short- and long-term memory processes can be affected by thiopental sedation and that such learning–memory relationships are not drug state-dependent.

Barbiturates as tools for basic investigation of learning and memory processes carry with them a large repertoire of central effects which may account for alterations in these behavioral events. Aside from a series of diverse electrophysiological alterations, there are also the effects upon putative transmitter molecules, such as 5-HT (elevated during barbiturate sedation or anesthesia) and ACh (altered storage pools); these molecules hold a special interest for specific events by which the processes of learning and memory are regulated and have been considered in previous discussion.

Among the classic sedative agents, there has been very limited application to behavioral investigation, particularly with regard to learning or memory. One compound for which some limited exploration has been made is bromide; in dogs where an "experimental neurosis" rendered them incapable of demonstrating stimulus selectivity and discriminative conditioned responding, potassium bromide (2 gm/day) resulted in restoration of negative conditional reflexes. This finding was used as support for the conclusion (Pavlov, 1927, 1941) that bromides should not be regarded as central nervous system activity-reducing sedatives; their action resides in regulation of central nervous system activity through strengthening the intensity of internal inhibition. Among "normal" dogs similar results with this drug were also obtained (Wolff and Gantt, 1935).

Aside from those agents previously considered, which might be considered either by virtue of their central actions or in terms of their therapeutic direction of action to be potential stabilizers of mood, affect, or arousal level, there are, of course, the more classic psychoactive agents which have been rather extensively treated in studies using various methods to assess their effects upon learning or memory. It is not our purpose to summarize again the many studies that have already been sufficiently reviewed, summarized, and criticized, but, rather to select from several classes of such agents the representative effects that have been reported in studies of learning and memory and consider these in the light of their overall significance for either the pharmacology of the class of compounds or the mechanisms relevant to learning and memory processes.

Among the phenothiazines, chlorpromazine (CPZ) has probably been the most extensively studied representative of this class. Among those tasks which have been behaviorally utilized, maze performance among rodents has been given considerable attention. In general and very likely related to its locomotor activity effects, CPZ treatment leads to increases in maze response time and task time and holds consistently so both for positively and negatively reinforced maze responses (Courvoisier *et al.*, 1958; Herr *et al.*, 1961; Latz, 1964). Low doses of CPZ (1.0–6.0 mg/kg) did not alter the frequency of errors in the acquisition of a multiple T-maze (Domer and Schueler, 1960), but at higher doses (10–20 mg kg, s.c. and p.o.) the incidence of maze errors was increased (Courvoisier *et al.*, 1958). The water maze has been used to test the hypothesis that CPZ could reduce motivational strength and thereby eliminate stereotyped behavior. The results (Mitchell and King, 1960) indicated that both acquisition and retention of stereotyped and nonstereotyped responses occurred. One problem facing the generality of such findings is that, whereas water temperature, under usual circumstances, may serve as a basis for defining different motivational levels providing for graded degrees of acquisition for such a maze, the thermolytic properties of CPZ pose a special problem. Drug-induced impairment of thermoregulation in rodents provided for impaired maze performance as a function of hypothermia induced by lowered ambient temperature (Essman and Sudak, 1962). It has been indicated that CPZ-induced changes in susceptibility to core-temperature change by cold exposure is different depending upon that temperature; for rats given CPZ and forced to swim in 19°C water there was a slower rate of body temperature loss than for CPZ-treated rats forced to swim in 32°C water (LeBlanc, 1958). The effect of CPZ in graduated doses (1–8 mg/kg) on Y-maze exploratory behavior by rats has been investigated (Shilleto, 1967). Activity was initially depressed at lower doses, but then maze arm entries became normal; at higher doses (4–8 mg/kg) the number of maze arm entries was significantly depressed during acquisition training, and subsequent maze testing suggested that acquisition had not occurred. In the guppy, CPZ (0.0005 mg/ml) led to some increase in the number of trials required to achieve a criterion for T-maze learning (Woodruff and Faltz, 1965). As compared with controls (freshwater), the drug-treated fish showed an average of 44% more trials required to reach the learning criterion.

For rats tested on operant conditioning tasks, with food and water as well as aversive stimuli as reinforcement, CPZ has generally led to a reduction in response rate, which appears to be a dose-dependent phenomenon. Acquisition of a discriminative response in pigeons, based upon stimulus-specific fixed-ratio or fixed-interval training was unaffected at relatively low CPZ doses (1.7–3.0 mg/kg, i.m., wherein response rate effects seemed dose-related (Dews, 1956). Chronic drug treatment appeared to alter escape and avoidance behavior acquired under a temporal schedule of negative reinforcement (Sidley and Schoenfeld, 1963) in rats. In rats and monkeys, CPZ (1.25–5 mg/kg, p.o.) led to a loss of avoidance responding at moderate doses, the animals having been trained on a Sidman avoidance schedule; at the highest dose, avoidance responding was decreased (Hanson, 1961).

A positive effect of CPZ has been reported for the reversal of discrimination learning by the rat (Gonzales and Ross, 1961). Animals given either 1, 2, or 5 mg/kg/day of CPZ and trained for the reversal of a visual or spatial discrimination response showed significantly greater reversal than controls with greater drug effect being apparent for the visual discrimination than for the spatial problem. The spatial discrimination required more than 1 trial for reversal. In a 1-trial discriminated avoidance response, rats treated with either 1, 5, or 10 mg/kg of CPZ showed no effect on the avoidance, but at the highest dose there was evidence of motor impairment without any effect on response latency (White and Suborski, 1969). A passive and active avoidance conditioning task was utilized to compare the effects of CPZ in four strains of mice. In a two-compartment cage, active avoidance consisted of frequency in crossing to avoid shock, whereas passive avoidance consisted of remaining in one compartment in order to avoid being shocked in the other. Those mice that learned the active task well did poorly on the passive task, and those animals that showed poor learning of the active task showed superior learning of the passive task. The effect of CPZ was apparent for both tasks; the drug decreased the number of crossing on the active task and increased the crossings on the passive task (Fuller, 1970). These findings would suggest a learning impairment that cannot be simply attributed to a locomotor effect of the drug or to a specific type of avoidance for which the drug exerts selective effects. In an active avoidance conditioning situation wherein conditioned avoidance was based upon a hurdle-jump response within a 10-second period followed by foot shock, mice trained following CPZ treatment (6 mg/kg, i.p.) showed no single-trial avoidance learning (as compared with a 35% 1-trial acquisition for saline-treated controls), but there was a statistically significant reduction in the time required to show an escape response to foot shock (Essman, 1970b).

There has been some evidence to suggest that CPZ may contribute to states of learning dissociation, especially with regard to avoidance learning. This has been shown in drug-treated rats under saline-treatment conditions or when the training–testing treatment conditions were reversed (Otis, 1964). Rats trained under CPZ (1.25 mg/kg) and tested in an avoidance situation under saline or visa versa, showed appreciably less avoidance response recovery than did rats trained and tested under CPZ or saline throughout. A CPZ-induced internal state has been suggested, which serving as a stimulus in a learning situation, may acquire associative connections with a response. The more exact nature of such an "internal state" has not been further elaborated upon, and, in view of the multiple central effects of this drug, one could find several sources from which a dissociative learning state might be inferred. Alterations in membrane permeability by CPZ leading to change in electrolyte distribution, putative transmitter storage, or amino acid transport could provide some basis for the concept of state-dependent learning. However, one must temper such suggestions with more sobering evidence of tissue binding of CPZ, prolonged degredation and excretion, and additive effects—all of which make the separation of drug- and nondrug-specific states rather difficult and designation of drug-induced dissociative learning still more of a problem. At somewhat higher doses of CPZ (3–4 mg/kg, i.p.), animals trained to choose one colored goal box differed from saline-treatment conditions when tested under nondrug conditions with a different colored goal box (Stewart, 1962); this finding is strong support for a state dependency of learning induced by CPZ. Viewing extinction of a conditioned response as a special case of learning, it has been shown that rats trained to acquire a conditioned emotional response in a shuttle box and then given extinction trials under saline had appreciably weaker conditioned emotional responses than saline-treated controls and extinguished the response more rapidly. For rats given the same avoidance training under saline and extinction trials under CPZ, there was a persistence of the conditioned response for 2 days after the completion of the extinction series (Hunt, 1956). The effect of CPZ on extinction of learned behaviors appears related to task complexity, acquisition conditions, motivating stimuli, and the strength of the response established. Particularly in conditions of avoidance conditioning, fear acquisition, or behaviors contingent upon learning involved with the reduction, prevention, or abolition of aversive stimuli the issue of drug-induced analgesia presents itself. Chlorpromazine-induced analgesia has been reported (Maxwell *et al.*, 1961; Barkov, 1961a), and the effect has been considered in view of a spinal cord locus of drug action. It is of interest to note in this regard that rats treated with 5 mg/kg of CPZ showed analgesic effects equivalent to those conferred by an equivalent dose of morphine; combined CPZ (5 mg/kg) and morphine (5 mg/kg) treatment exceeded the analgesic potency of 10 mg/kg of morphine (Barkov, 1961b). If the concept of analgesic effects of CPZ is extended into the interpretation of findings on avoidance conditioning, one would not be terribly surprised to expect a reduced degree of avoidance response acquisition where stimulus aversive properties are reduced through an analgesic effect. Similarly, one might also be willing to accept somewhat less esoteric alternatives to the notion of state-dependent learning or response dissociation if, depending upon the drug state, one were dealing with stimuli of divergent magnitude or aversive properties. It seems that one necessary control that most of the studies considered lack is a careful assessment of stimulus efficacy titrated against the potential analgesia contributed by CPZ treatment. A dose–effect relationship and time course study of the latter also seems highly warranted.

The issue of CPZ effects upon the short-term fixation of memory has been explored in mice trained in a 1-trial passive-avoidance conditioning situation. Chlorpromazine was administered either 10 minutes before, or 0.5, 2, or 10 minutes posttraining. Acquisition of the passive-avoidance response was blocked by pretraining CPZ treatment, whereas posttraining treatment (which would satisfy any criticism previously posed regarding analgesic effects of CPZ on acquisition) led to a reduced expression of avoidance responding and rapid extinction (Johnson, 1969).

Reserpine (RP), which is probably the best representative of the *Rauwolfia* alkaloids has been used to a limited degree in studies of learning of memory. A number of considerations probably account for such caution; primarily, the long-term behavioral effects of RP, which persist beyond the period within which systemic elimination has accounted for the drug, make separation of drug and nondrug states and drug-task times extrememly difficult. When RP (1.3 and 1.5 mg/kg, i.p.) was given to mice prior to testing on a buzzer shock contingency for conditioned avoidance behavior, there was a 9–10 day period within which avoidance responding was abolished. Since the RP injected was eliminated by 2 hours following treatment the persisting behavioral effect was far in excess of the presence of the drug (Shugayev, 1965). The prolonged effect was attributed to an RP-initiated disruption of brain 5-HT metabolism. Some potential support for such an hypothesis derives from data indicating RP-induced reduction of brain 5-HT levels (Pletscher *et al.*, 1955). Further studies have also provided evidence for persistent RP-induced behavioral effects; semichronic RP treatment (0.1 mg/kg/day, i.p., from 11 to 30 days of age) in rats led to a significant deficit in discriminative response learning as adult animals (Kulkarni *et al.*, 1966).

The exploratory behavior of rats was impaired by RP (0.4 mg/kg), although avoidance learning was facilitated by the drug at considerably lower doses (0.05 mg/kg) under conditions where a short treatment–testing interval was utilized. When the dose was slightly increased (0.25 mg/kg), patterned discrimination learning was reduced (Walk *et al.*, 1961), and observation possibly accounted for by the strabismatogenic effects of CPZ at this dose in the rat.

Reserpine appears to exert differential effects upon escape and avoidance behavior, as suggested by findings on the drug's effect on pole-climbing in rats. Escape behavior to shock onset was not affected by CPZ (25 mg/kg, p.o.) when given in two doses, 17 hours apart, when the behavior was tested 3 hours after treatment. Avoidance behavior, under the same con-conditions, was blocked to a significant degree (Cook and Weidley, 1957; Cook *et al.*, 1953). Whereas RP (0.5 mg/kg) did not impair the conditioning of an emotional response in rats (Stein, 1956), an already established conditioned emotional response could be eliminated through RP treatment (Brady, 1956b). Conditioned emotional response performance was decreased by RP (0.2 mg/kg) given chronically, when this performance was assessed by variable-interval response rates and suppression ratios at a low shock intensity (Appel, 1963).

More complex behaviors, such as chains of alimentary reflexes, were not altered by RP (0.08–0.09 mg/kg), but chains of defensive reflexes and efferent generalization were inhibited and depressed, respectively (Voronin and Napalkov, 1963). Conditioned food reflexes were inhibited (positive reactions and differentiation) by RP (0.1 mg/kg), but conditioned escape responses were not altered by the drug at this dose and there was an intensification of differentiation inhibition (Hecht, 1963).

For conditioned emotional responding established with a noise-shock contingency in the monkey, RP (0.7 mg/kg) increased the number of trials required to reach criterion. When RP (0.75 mg/kg) was given during extinction the number of criterion level extinction trials were increased (Weiskrantz and Wilson, 1956). A deficit in auditory discrimination, not accounted for by an increased latency period, was observed in monkeys given RP (0.2–0.5 mg/kg, i.m.), and under these same conditions there was no change in the performance of a spatial delayed response (Gross and Weiskrantz, 1961).

The analgesic properties considered for CPZ do not appear to constitute any serious problem for RP, so far as the results of tasks involving aversive stimuli are concerned. At unusually high doses (2.5 mg/kg) of RP, mice were capable of escaping a 3-mA foot shock in a grid box, even though torpor and ataxia were in evidence. As compared with saline-treated control animals, the latency to escape from the onset of foot shock was not elevated. The incidence of acquisition and retention of a conditioned avoidance response established with 1 training trial did not differ from controls (testing was done 24 hours after training with drug treatment 60 minutes prior to the training trial). Reserpine treatment, similarly, neither modified the unconditioned response, in the absence of foot shock, nor the response to foot shock in the conditioning situation (Essman, 1967a). When saline-treated mice were given ECS within 10 seconds following a passive-avoidance response training trial, a retrograde amnesia for the avoidance response was produced for 78% of the animals; RP treatment (2.5 mg/kg) 60 minutes prior to training reduced ECS-induced amnesia to 50%. In an active avoidance procedure, there was no essential difference between RP-treated mice (5 mg/kg) and saline-treated animals in the acquisition of active avoidance after a single training trial, and the drug-treated mice were equally capable of reducing their latency response to escape shock as were controls (Essman, 1970b).

Among the tricyclic compounds, imipramine (IM) has found some application in learning and memory studies, as has its structural relative, amitriptyline (AM). The behavior of normal animals does not appear to be modified by IM (Domenjoz and Theobald, 1959) nor has this compound been found to affect conditioned escape behavior in the rat (Gatti, 1961). Lever-pressing for maintenance of avoidance behavior was somewhat stimulated by IM, yet slight indications of behavioral sedation have also been reported in several studies (Bättig, 1961; Hanson, 1961; Herr *et al.*, 1961; Maxwell and Palmer, 1961; Sulser *et al.*, 1962; Vernier, 1961). Imipramine (10 mg/kg, i.p.) has also been shown to potentiate the stimulant effect of amphetamine (1 mg/kg, i.p.) among rats performing a nondiscriminative avoidance response (Weissman, 1961). In a lever-pressing avoidance conditioning task, rats given IM (25 or 50 mg/kg) 90 minutes prior to testing showed a reduction in the response times and in the number of punishments sustained during the course of avoidance performance (Gatti and Bovet, 1963). Imipramine and AM were both evaluated in a study wherein cats were trained to elaborate defensive motor-conditioned responses to stereotypes of sequential auditory and visual stimuli reinforced with electric shock, as the unconditioned stimulus. Within a dose range of 0.1 to 1 mg/kg of AM and 0.05 to 3 mg/kg of IM, the elaboration of the conditioned responses was unaffected. At higher doses (2.0 and 0.1 mg/kg, respectively) there was an increase of responding between stimulus intervals with no loss of differentiation. At doses of 3 to 10 mg/kg, there was an appreciable decrease in conditioned as well as unconditioned responses (Vinogradov, 1969).

Studies using IM have also been carried out in mice, where the antagonism of this drug toward the retrograde amnesic effects of ECS were investigated (Essman, 1970b). Imipramine (20 mg/kg) given to mice 60 minutes prior to a 1-trial passive-avoidance training trial, followed within 10 seconds by a single ECS, succeeded in reducing the amnesic effect by 14%, without altering conditioned avoidance behavior under non-ECS conditions or susceptibility to ECS-induced convulsions. Amitriptyline (10 mg/kg, i.p.) resulted in a similar mode of antagonism toward the amnesic effects of ECS in a passive-avoidance situation with mice (Essman, 1968d). In an active-avoidance conditioning task, wherein mice were given a single avoidance training trial and a single active-avoidance testing trial, IM (10 mg/kg, i.p.) 60 minutes prior to training led to a significant reduction in escape latency after a single trial and an increase (10%) over control (saline) levels of 1-trial active-avoidance acquisition. Amitriptyline (10 mg/kg) neither provided for escape latency reduction nor increased active-avoidance behavior; in fact, active-avoidance acquisition was significantly reduced to 30% below that of saline-treated controls (Essman, 1970b). It was further demonstrated in these studies that at least one correlate of ECS-induced retrograde amnesia, an elevation of brain 5-HT level, was either prevented or attenuated in animals that had been previously treated with IM.

Although previous reviews and surveys have treated other classes of psychoactive agents, there are perhaps several additional comments that may be made in order to include meprobamate and the benzodiazepines, since these may have relevance to the processes of learning or memory. Probably because of difficulties in specifying modes and sites of action, the basic mechanisms relating to learning and memory processes have not easily relied upon meprobamate as an investigative tool. In another context the behavioral effects of this compound have been diverse and not always simple to deal with. The operant behavior of rats has been used as a means of assessing the effects of meprobamate (Kelleher *et al.*, 1961). Animals trained to press either a disc or lever for food reinforcement showed an increase in response rate when they were treated with the drug. The question of state-specificity for learning and meprobamate has also been raised. Rats trained to acquire a conditioned avoidance response, either while treated with meprobamate or saline, were tested either under drug or control conditions. A decrement in the latency to perform a conditioned avoidance response and also a reduced incidence of avoidance responses were observed for those rats having been trained while drug-treated and tested without it. Animals trained on saline and tested on drug, or trained and tested on either both drug or both saline conditions did not show any such comparable learning deficit (Barnhart and Abbott, 1967). The concept of a drug-specific learning state is not clearly indicated for meprobamate, but what findings such as these could suggest is the dependence of the acquisition phase of avoidance learning upon the somatic and visceral effects of aversive stimuli, as modifiable through peripheral and central effects of drugs such as meprobamate.

What appears to have considerably more favor as a candidate for induced dissociative state in learning is chlordiazepoxide (CDP). When this compound was administered to rats (5–10 mg/kg, i.p.) at either 10 or 60 minutes prior to training on a conditioned escape task, the lower dose had no effect, but the higher dose retarded learning. The interval between drug treatment and training did not contribute significantly to the effects. When the drug was administered both before training and before testing, animals treated under these conditions performed the conditioned escape response less well than rats given a placebo–drug or placebo–placebo training–testing sequence. When a drug–placebo sequence was used, evidence for learning during the placebo phase suggested a drug-induced acquisition deficit, not a performance effect (Cicala and Hartley, 1965). A possible specificity for the central locus of benzodiazepine action may be suggested by the finding that CDP and diazepam (5 mg/kg, i.p.) administered to rats with electrodes implanted in anterior and posterior-lateral hypothalamus, where pedal-pressing provided for either stimulation or escape from stimulation, respectively, to these areas, altered the behavior. The rate of pedal-pressing for electrical stimulation to the posterior hypothalamus was increased by the drugs. Chlordiazepoxide led to decreased rates of pedal-pressing for stimulation to the anterior hypothalamus, and diazepam produced equivocal results (Olds, 1966). The acquisition of avoidance learning in the rat is another paradigm within which CDP has found favor as mediating a drug-specific learning state. Animals were trained in a hurdle-jump apparatus to acquire a conditioned avoidance response after being given either CDP (15 mg/kg), CPZ (0.25–2 mg/kg), or saline. The rats were tested for transfer of training with 20 trials (1/minute), 4 days apart under either the same or different treatment conditions from those used at training. The CPZ-treated animals could not reach the same criterion (20/20) achieved by other drug-treated rats, but the CDP–saline treatment conditions suggested that there was no retention (Sachs *et al.*, 1966). These findings would offer strong support for a drug dissociation hypothesis except for several points. Lack of transfer of the avoidance behavior from the drug to a nondrug state has implied drug-state-specificity without regard to more parsimonious explanations such as a drug-induced acceleration of response to foot shock that may not be reflected in a stable acquisition of conditioned avoidance learning, as defined for this situation. This same general view has been presented in another study, wherein drug-produced internal cues serving as discriminative stimuli have been proposed to account for an apparent dissociative effect. Unfortunately, it seems impossible to verify or reject such an hypothesis with measurement or specificity of an "internal cue." Treatment of rats with either CDP (15 mg/kg) or saline during acquisition of a conditioned response, based upon a brightness discrimination, provided for learning, and alteration of the drug state from that employed during training resulted in only a slight and transitory decrement in performance (Brown *et al.*, 1968). In rabbits, a decrement in the acquisition of a two-way shuttle-box avoidance response occurred at various doses of CDP (Chisholm and Moore, 1970), being inconsistent with the view that CDP reduced fear, and also raising questions as to the efficiency with which avoidance acquisition under CDP treatment occurs. Serious methodological issues remain to be considered with greater care than the literature would indicate has been afforded them. These include basic questions concerned with benzodiazepine metabolism and particularly the relevance of a single, acute dose of drugs of this family to the more general question of a drug state and its bearing upon learning or memory.

XVIII. Present Indications and New Research Directions

The effects of several varieties of pharmacological agents upon the processes of learning or memory may be considered in view of the behavioral consequences of drug action viewed methodologically be several techniques from which learning or memory, as dynamic events, may be inferred. As such, the observed effects may be considered positive (to exert some degree of facilitation), negative (to induce impairment), or without effect. It appears as though a critical determinant of such outcome resides in the behavioral technique employed (i.e., appetitive reinforcement, avoidance behavior, etc.), the measure of behavior utilized as a "process" index (i.e., response rate, response errors, response latency, etc.), and some implicit hypothesis concerning the relationship between drug action and the process being acted upon. Although phenomenological studies probably have some place in the relationship between drug action and the processes of learning and memory, they seldom offer much in the way of understanding mechanisms of drug action or mechanisms involved with the learning or memory process. If we pause to consider what form of investigation can potentially contribute to our understanding of one or both of the above-stated issues of mechanism, then one also must take into account the questions of acute versus chronic treatment conditions and their respective effects, the nature of the possible contributions to drug effect provided by variables such as species, strain, and sex differences, population density, and age, and potential applicability to and value for a human population. This, of course, raises and even more fundamental question concerning the relative generality of the cognitive processes studied in animals and the comparable events in man, particularly insofar as drug action providing for alterations in these processes are concerned. It would appear that the therapeutic goals in man might be the alleviation of learning or memory defects, selective disruption of acquired habits or memories that represent possibly poor adaptive behavior or connote negative affect, or screening for therapeutic agents which have unwanted side effects. Unfortunately, neither experiments in animals nor man have provided for any compounds which improve poor learning, increase re-retentive ability or capacity, selectively erase learned information, or serve a purpose in relating learning or memory effects to therapeutic efficacy. What appears to be a more promising avenue for future studies to follow is the mutual consideration of neuropharmacological effect and the learning and memory processes; i.e., common denominators of both seem to provide a sound basis for generating hypothesis from data obtained in animal investigation and testing such hypothesis in man. Perhaps a useful context within which such mutual accord may be reached in the acceptance of a basic premise that the events regulating learning or memory also have in common their regulation of synaptic processes. One can then proceed with the basic requirements which synaptic events dictate for efficiency—synthesis, storage, release, and degredation of molecules having a putative transmitter role. Since most of these pharmacological agents previously discussed do, in one way or other, affect one or more putative transmitter substances—their content, turnover, availability, or removal—then this would seem a logical course on which to proceed. It also seems apparent that drugs exerting negative effects upon learned behavior, i.e., disruption of learned performance, or compounds assigned a dissociative or state-dependent role, have in common the ability to disrupt synaptic events with the ultimate result that one is merely evaluating the consequences or brain functions that survive either selective, regional, or diffuse synaptic loss. In most instances the synaptic effect is reversible, as is the behavioral effect. There are a number of specific cases in which this may, however, not occur. The administration of behaviorally active compounds prenatally or during early postnatal development superimposes the metabolic effects of the drug upon a novel metabolic environment within which synapses may not have completely developed, or wherein their transmitter requirements are quite different from those of the organism with a more completely developed nervous system. Under these circumstances a new area of investigation begins to emerge—pharmacosynaptogenesis and the ultimate behavioral correlates which emerge from such developmental changes.

Considering the potential contributions of synaptology to the understanding of drug action and learning and memory processes, one may also view this relationship in terms of the subsynaptic site and time course of drug effect. It seems obvious from such an approach that drug-induced facilitation cannot be considered as a simple opposite of impairment of learning or memory events induced by other drugs. Even for a single drug exerting biphasic, time-dependent effects on learning or memory, the biphasic synaptic countercorrelate probably defies identification. A further point is that most of the attention thus far accorded putative transmitters, synaptic events, and learning and memory has concerned molecules of the excitatory type, whereas the mediation of inhibitory transmission by molecules such as γ-aminobutyric acid and glycine has not really been given any attention, even though several of those drugs which affect the behavioral events considered can alter molecular events related to inhibitory synaptic transmission.

It is obvious that reliance upon a single molecular event as a model for learning and memory processing imposes severe limitation upon the ultimate utility of such a model or the scientific rationale of applied studies which derive from such a scheme. Perhaps examples of this may be found in RNA-based drug-learning hypotheses or cholinergic-memory investigations with drugs that affect such a molecular event.

There are potentially a large number of compounds which, by virtue of their effect upon putative transmitter molecular metabolism or upon events that regulate such molecular interactions at subcellular sites, would find an ideal place in relating drug action to the mechanisms by which learning and memory are regulated. There are, also, on the behavioral side of this issue, several approaches which remain to be taken in order, perhaps, to approach more meaningfully some of the relevant questions, for example, tasks that provide for multiple drive states or contingent reinforcement for a single drive, multiple response hierarchies that are based on stimulus specificity or reinforcement probability, or learning tasks based upon units of increasing difficulty. It would appear that data from animal studies derived from behavioral tasks of this type could relate in a more obvious way to comparable tasks which, in man, have been used to evaluate drug effects upon learning and memory.

On pharmacological as well as behavioral grounds, there is room for warranted additional investigation and further confirmation of generality of existing data. The neurobiological substrates of learning and memory processes still provide a rich ground upon which several drugs may be utilized as tools for the study of centrally active drugs. Behavioral techniques from which learning or memory are inferred or operationally defined impose the limitations of the methods themselves. These limitations might be exceeded through better standardization of existing methods, more accurate definition of variables contributing to a drug's effect on these behaviors, or use of a battery of tasks which approximate a behavioral repertoire within which ongoing events critical to learning and memory may be more globally defined.

Acknowledgments

The author's research findings reported here were supported, in part, by Grants HD 03493 from the National Institutes of Health, 623B from the Council for Tobacco Research–U.S.A., and 5-SO5-FR-07064-05 from NIH Biomedical Science Support. The author wishes to express his appreciation to S. G. Essman for assistance with the literature search and to C. Watkins for aid in the preparation of the manuscript.

References

Adám, G., ed. (1970). "Biology of Memory." Akademiai Kiado, Budapest.

Adams, P. M., Crawford, F. T., and Lee, W. G. (1969). *Psychon. Sci*, **14**, 101.

Agranoff, B. W. (1969). *In* "Progress in Molecular and Subcellular Biology" (F. E. Hahn, ed.), p. 203–212. Springer-Verlag, Berlin and New York.

Aird, R. B., Strait, L. A., Pace, J. W., Hrenoff, M. K., and Bowditch, S. C. (1956). *AMA Arch. Neurol. Psychiat.* **75**, 371.

Appel, J. B. (1963). *Psychopharmacologia* **4**, 148.

Bättig, K. (1961). *Pfluegers Arch. Gesamte Physiol. Menschen Tiere* **274**, 59.

Bättig, K. (1969). *Psychopharmacologia* **15**, 19.

Barkov, N. K. (1961a). *Bull. Exp. Biol. Med.* (*USSR*) **50**, 950.

Barkov, N. K. (1961b). *Bull Exp. Biol. Med.* (*USSR*) **51**, 185.

Barnhart, S., and Abbott, D. W. (1967). *Psychol. Rep.* **20**, 520.

Barondes, S. H., and Cohen, H. D. (1966). *Science* **151**, 594.

Barondes, S. H., and Cohen, H. D. (1968). *Science* **160**, 556.

Barondes, S. H., and Jarvik, M. E. (1964). *J. Neurochem.* **11**, 187.

Barry, H., III., and Miller, N. E. (1962). *J. Comp. Physiol. Psychol.* **55**, 201.

Barry, H., III., and Miller, N. E. (1965) *J. Comp. Physiol. Psychol.* **59**, 18.

Barry, H., III., Miller, N. E., and Tidd, G. E. (1962). *J. Comp. Physiol. Psychol.* **55**, 1071.

Beach, G., and Kimble, D. P. (1967). *Science* **155**, 698.

Berry, C. A., and Stark, L. G. (1965). *Psychopharmacologia* **7**, 409.

Berryman, R., Jarvik, M. E., and Nevin, J. A. (1962). *Psychopharmacologia* **3**, 60.

Bignami, G., and Gatti, G. L. (1969). *Psychopharmacologia* **15**, 310.

Bittman, R., and Essman, W. B. (1970). *Abstr. Pap., 3rd Annu. Winter Conf. Brain Res., Snowmass-at-Aspen, Col.*

Bittman, R., Essman, W. B., and Golod, M. I. (1969). *Abstr. Amer. Chem. Soc.* p. 330.

Bivens, L. W., and Ray, O. S. (1966). Paper presented at the meeting of the Midwest. Psychol. Ass., Chicago, Illinois. Abstracts published in *Amer. Psychol.*, 1966.

Bösser, T. H., Joyce, D., and Summerfield, A. (1970). *Brit. J. Pharmacol.* **38**, 459P.

Bohdanecky, Z., and Jarvik, M. E. (1967). *Int. J. Neuropharmacol.* **7**, 217.

Boissier, J. R., and Simon, P. (1967). *Arch Int. Pharmacodyn. Ther.* **166**, 362.

Boissier, J. R., Simon, P., and Lwoff, J. M. (1966). *J. Pharm. Pharmacol.* **18**, 687.

Bonta, I. L., Dlever, A., Simons, L., and deVos, C. J. (1960). *Arch Int. Pharmacodyn. Ther.* **129**, 381.

Bovet, D., and Gatti, G. L. (1965). *In* "Pharmacology of Conditioning, Learning and Retention" (M. Y. Mikhel'son, and V. G. Longo, eds.), p. 75–89. Pergamon, Oxford.
Bovet, D., McGaugh, J. L., and Oliverio, A. (1966). *Life Sci.* **5,** 1309.
Bovet, D., Bovet-Nitti, F., and Oliverio, A. (1967). *Ann. N. Y. Acad. Sci.* **142,** 261.
Bovet-Nitti, F. (1966). *Psychopharmacologia* **10,** 59.
Bovet-Nitti, F. (1969). *Psychopharmacologia* **14,** 193–199.
Brady, J. V. (1956a). *Science* **123,** 1033.
Brady, J. V. (1956b). *Ann. N. Y. Acad. Sci.* **64,** 632.
Breen, R. A., and McGaugh, J. L. (1961). *J. Comp. Physiol. Psychol.* **54,** 498.
Bright, J. G., and Hatton, G. I. (1969). *Psychon. Sci.* **15,** 52.
Brooks, G. W., and Mueller, E. (1966). *J. Amer. Med. Ass.* **195,** 415.
Brown, H. (1966). *Psychol. Rec.* **16,** 173–176.
Brown, A., Feldman, R. S., and Moore, J. W. (1968). *J. Comp. Physiol. Psychol.* **66,** 211.
Brush, F. R., Davenport, J. W., and Polidora, V. J. (1966). *Psychon. Sci.* **4,** 183.
Buckholtz, N. S., and Bowman, R. E. (1970). *Physiol. Behav.* **5,** 911.
Bunch, M. E., and Mueller, C. G. (1941). *J. Comp. Psychol.* **32,** 569.
Burns, J. T., House, R. F., Fensch, F. C., and Miller, J. G. (1967). *Science* **155,** 849.
Byrne, W. L., ed. (1970). "Molecular Approaches to Learning and Memory." Academic Press, New York.
Calhoun, W. H. (1965). *Psychopharmacologia* **8,** 227.
Calhoun, W. H. (1966). *Psychol. Rep.* **18,** 715.
Cameron, D. E. (1966). Presidential address. Soc. of Biol. Psychiat. Meeting, Washington, D.C. (Unpublished.)
Cameron, D. E., and Solyom, L. (1961). *Geriatrics* **16,** 74.
Cardo, B. (1961). *J. Physiol. (Paris)* **53,** 1.
Carlini, G. R. S., and Carlini, E. A. (1965). *Med. Pharmacol. Exp.* **12,** 21.
Carlton, P. L. (1963). *Nature (London)* **200,** 586.
Chamberlain, T. J., Rothschild, G. H., and Gerard, R. W. (1963). *Proc. Nat. Acad. Sci. U.S.* **52,** 918.
Chance, M. R. A., and Silverman, A. P. (1964). *In* "Animal Behavior and Drug Action" (H. Steinberg, A. V. S. de Reuck, and J. Knight, eds.), p. 65–82. Little, Brown, Boston, Massachusetts.
Chi, C. C. (1965). *Psychopharmacologia* **7,** 115.
Chisholm, D. C., and Moore, J. W. (1970). *Psychon. Sci.* **19,** 21.
Cholewiak, R. W., Hammond, R., Seigler, I. C., and Papsdorf, J. D. (1968). *J. Comp. Physiol. Psychol.* **66,** 77.
Cicala, G. A., and Hartley, D. L. (1965). *Psychol. Rec.* **15,** 435.
Cohen, M. (1966). *Arch. Int. Pharmacodyn. Ther.* **16,** 120.
Coker, D. L., and Abbott, D. W. (1967). *Psychon. Sci.* **9,** 607.
Cole, S. O. (1968). *Psychon. Sci.* **10,** 19.
Cook, L. (1964). *In* "Animal Behavior and Drug Action" (H. Steinberg, ed.), p. 23–43. Little, Brown, Boston, Massachusetts.
Cook, L., and Davidson, A. B. (1968). *In* "Psychopharmacology. A Review of Progress, 1957–1967" (D.H. Efron, ed.), pp. 931–946. US Govt. Printing Office, Washington, D.C.
Cook, L., and Kelleher, R. T. (1963). *Annu. Rev. Pharmacol.* **3,** 205.
Cook, L., and Weidley, E. (1957). *Ann. N. Y. Acad. Sci.* **66,** 740.
Cook, L., Weidley, E., Morris, R. W., and Mattis, P. A. (1953). *J. Pharmacol. Exp. Ther.* **113,** 11.
Cook, L., Davidson, A. B., Davis, D. J., Green, H., and Fellows, E. J. (1963). *Science* **141,** 268.

Cooper, B. R., Potts, W., Morse, D. L., and Black, W. C. (1969). *Psychon. Sci.* **14,** 225.

Cooper, R. M., and Krass, M. (1963). **4,** 472.

Corning, W. C., and John, E. R. (1961). *Science* **134,** 1363.

Corson, J. A. (1969). *Psychon. Sci.* **17,** 45.

Corson, J. A., and Enesco, H. E. (1966). *Psychon. Sci.* **5,** 217.

Costa, E., and Garattini, S. eds. (1970). *Int. Symp. Amphetamines Relat. Compounds, Proc. Mario Negri Inst. Pharmacol. Res. Milan.* Raven Press, New York.

Courvoisier, S., Ducrot, R., and Julou, L. (1958). *In* "Psychotropic Drugs" (S. Garattini and V. Ghetti, eds.), p. 373. Elsevier, Amsterdam.

Daniels, D. (1967). *Psychon. Sci.* **7,** 5.

Davis, R. E. (1968). *J. Comp. Physiol. Psychol.* **65,** 72.

del Castillo, J., and Engbaek, L. (1954). *J. Physiol.* (*London*) **124,** 370.

Del Rio, J. (1970). *Abstr. Pap., Colleg. Int. Neuro-Psychopharmacol., 7th Cong.* **1,** 111.

Dergachey, V. V. (1970). *Abstr. Pap., Colleg. Int. Neuro. Psychopharmacol., 7th Cong.* **1,** 115.

Deutsch, J. A., and Leibowitz, S. F. (1966). *Science* **153,** 1017.

Deutsch, J. A., and Lutzky, H. (1967). *Nature* (*London*) **213,** 742.

Dews, P. B. (1953). *Brit. J. Pharmacol. Chemoth.* **8,** 46.

Dews, P. B. (1956). *J. Pharmacol. Exp. Ther.* **116,** 16.

Dews, P. B. (1964). *Naunyn-Schmiedeberg's Arch. Exp. Pathol. Pharmakol.* **248,** 296.

Dews, P. B., and Morse, W. H. (1961). *Annu. Rev. Pharmacol.* **1,** 145.

DiCarlo, R., Edel, S., Randrianarisoa, H., and Mandel, P. (1970). *Abstr. Pap., Colleg. Int. Neuro-Psychopharmacol., 7th Congr.* **1,** 117.

Dingman, N., and Sporn, M. B. (1961). *J. Psychiat. Res.* **1,** 1–11.

Domenjoz, R., and Theobàld, W. (1959). *Arch. Int. Pharmacodyn. Ther.* **120,** 450.

Domer, F. R., and Schueler, F. W. (1960). *Arch. Int. Pharmacodyn. Ther.* **127,** 449–458.

Doty, B. A., and Doty, L. A. (1966). *Psychopharmacologia* **9,** 234.

Doty, B. A., and Johnston, M. M. (1966). *Psychon. Sci.* **6,** 101.

Dusewicz, R. A., and Livecchi, S. G. (1969). *Psychol. Rec.* **19,** 461.

Eccles, J. C., Schmidt, R. F., and Willis, W. D. (1963). *J. Physiol.* (*London*) **168,** 500.

Editorial (1968). *Brit. Med. J.* **1,** 73.

Egyhazi, E., and Hydén, H. (1961). *J. Biophys. Biochem. Cytol.* **10,** 403.

Eisenberg, J. M. (1948). *Fed Proc. Fed. Amer. Soc. Exp. Biol.* **7,** 31.

Eisenberg, J. M. (1954). *J. Psychol.* **37,** 291.

Esplin, D. W., and Zablocka, B. (1965). *In* "The Pharmacological Basis of Therapeutics" (L. S. Goodman and A. Gilman, eds.), Ch. 18. Macmillan, New York.

Essman, W. B. (1965) *Int. Congr. Physiol. Sci., Lect. Symp., 23rd, Tokyo* p. 470.

Essman, W. B. (1966). *Psychopharmacologia* **9,** 426.

Essman, W. B. (1967a). *Proc. Colleg. Int. Neuro-Psychopharmacol.* pp. 108–113.

Essman, W. B. (1967b). *Psychon. Sci.* **9,** 51.

Essman, W. B. (1968a). *Physiol. Behav.* **3,** 549.

Essman, W. B. (1968b). *Psychol. Rep.* **22,** 929.

Essman, W. B. (1968c). *Physiol. Behav.* **3,** 527.

Essman, W. B. (1968d). *Psychopharmacologia* **13,** 258.

Essman, W. B. (1969a). *In* "The Present Status of Psychotropic Drugs" (A. Cerletti and F. J. Bové, eds), p. 305–306. Excerpta Med. Found., Amsterdam.

Essman, W. B. (1969b). *Proc. 4th Int. Congr. Pharmacol., Basel* p. 289.

Essman, W. B. (1970a). *In* "The Biology of Memory" (G. Adám, ed.), p. 213–238. Akademiai Kiado, Budapest.

Essman, W. B. (1970b). *In* "Drugs and Cerebral Function" (W. L. Smith, ed.), p. 151–175. Thomas, Springfield, Illinois.
Essman, W. B. (1970c). *In* "Molecular Approaches to Learning and Memory" (W. Byrne, ed.), p. 307–323. Academic Press, New York.
Essman, W. B. (1971a). *In* "Handbook of Abnormal Psychology" (H. J. Eysenck), 2nd Ed. Pitman, London. In press.
Essman, W. B. (1971b). *Trans. N. Y. Acad. Sci.* **32,** 948–973.
Essman, W. B. (1971c). *In* "Cerebral Function Development and Drug Action" (W. L. Smith, ed.). Thomas, Springfield, Illinois. In press.
Essman, W. B. (1971d). *In* "The Search for New Drugs" (A. L. Rubin, ed.). Decker, New York. In press.
Essman, W. B., and Essman, S. G. (1969). *Pharmako-Psychiat. Neuropsychopharmacol.* **2,** 28.
Essman, W. B., and Sudak, F. N. (1962). *J. Appl. Physiol.* **17,** 113.
Essman, W. B., Steinberg, M. I., and Golod, M. I. (1968). *Psychon. Sci.* **12,** 107.
Essman, W. B., Bittman, R., and Heldman, E. (1971). *Proc. IV Annu. Winter Conf. Brain Res., Snowmass-at-Aspen, Col.*
Evans, W. O., and Jewett, A. (1962). *Psychopharmacologia* **3,** 124.
Fink, M., and Green, M. A. (1958). *Dis. Nerv. Syst.* **19,** 227.
Flexner, L. B., and Flexner, J. A. (1966). *Proc. Nat. Acad. Sci. U.S.* **55,** 396.
Flexner, L. B., and Flexner, J. A. (1968). *Science* **159,** 330.
Folch, J., Lees, M., and Sloane-Stanley, G. H. (1957). *In* "Metabolism of the Nervous System" (D. Richter, ed.), p. 174. Pergamon, Oxford.
Franks, C. M., and Trouton, D. (1958). *J. Comp. Physiol. Psychol.* **51,** 220.
Fuller, J. L. (1970). *Psychopharmacologia* **16,** 261.
Garattini, S., and Sigg, E. B., eds. (1969). "Aggressive Behavior." Excerpta Med. Found., Amsterdam.
Garattini, S., and Valzelli, L. (1957). *In* "Psychotropic Drugs" (S. Garattini and V. Ghetti, eds.), p. 428–436. Elsevier, Amsterdam.
Garattini, S., and Valzelli, L. (1965). "Serotonin." Elsevier, Amsterdam.
Garg, M. (1969). *Psychopharmacologia* **15,** 408.
Garg, M., and Holland, H. C. (1968a). *Psychopharmacologia* **12,** 96.
Garg, M., and Holland, H. C. (1968b). *Psychopharmacologia* **12,** 127
Garg, M., and Holland, H. C. (1968c). *Int. J. Neuropharmacol.* **7,** 55.
Gatti, G. L. (1961). *Riv. Sper. Freniat. Med. Leg. Alienazioni Met.* **85,** 1.
Gatti, G. L., and Bovet, D. (1963). *In* "Psychopharmacological Methods" (Z. Votava, M. Harváth, and O. Vinar, eds.), p. 50–57. Pergamon, Oxford.
Gellhorn, E. (1943). *Lancet* **63,** 307.
Gibby, R. G., Sr., Gibby, R. G., Jr., Kish, G. B., and Theologus, G. C. (1965). *Psychol. Rep.* **17,** 123.
Gililand, A. R., and Nelson, D. (1939). *J. Gen. Psychol.* **21,** 339.
Glasky, A. J., and Simon, L. N. (1966). *Science* **151,** 702.
Glow, P. H., and Rose, S. (1965). *Nature (London)* **206,** 475.
Goldberg, M. E., Johnson, H. E., and Knaak, J. B (1965). *Psychopharmacologia* **7,** 72.
Goldstein, L. (1960). *J. Pharmacol. Exp. Ther.* **128,** 392.
Golob, L. R., and Brady, J. V. (1965). *Annu. Rev. Pharmacol.* **5,** 235.
Gonzales, R. C., and Ross, S. (1961). *J. Comp. Physiol. Psychol.* **54,** 645.
Goodhart, R. S., and Helenore, J. C., eds. (1963). "Modern Drug Encyclopedia and Therapeutic Index," 9th Ed. Rueben H. Donnelley, New York.
Greenblatt, E. N., and Osterberg, A. V. (1961). *Fed. Proc. Fed. Amer. Soc. Exp. Biol.* **20,** 397.

Greenough, W. T., and McGaugh, J. L. (1965). *Psychopharmacologia* **8,** 290.
Gross, C. G., and Weiskrantz, L. A. (1961). *Quart. J. Exp. Psychol.* **13,** 34.
Gunn, J. A., and Gurd, J (1940). *J. Physiol. (London)* **7,** 463.
Gurowitz, E. M., Lubar, J. F., Ain, B. R., and Gross, D. A. (1967). *Psychon. Sci.* **8,** 19.
Guseva, Y. G. (1964). *Zh. Vyssh. Nerv. Deyatel im. I. P. Pavlova* **14,** 480. (Abstr.)
Hanson, H. M. (1961). *Fed. Proc. Fed. Amer. Soc. Exp. Biol.* **20,** 396.
Hanson, L. C. F. (1965). *Psychopharmacologia* **8,** 110.
Hartelius, H. (1950). *Amer. J. Psychiat.* **107,** 95.
Hearst, E., and Whalen, R. E. (1963). *J. Comp. Physiol. Psychol.* **56,** 124.
Hecht, K. (1963). *In* "Psychoparmacological Methods" (Z. Votava, M. Horváth, and O. Vinar, eds.), p. 58. Macmillan, New York.
Heimstra, N. W. (1962). *Psychopharmacologia* **3,** 72.
Heron, W. T., and Carlson, W. S. (1941). *J. Comp. Physiol. Psychol.* **32,** 307.
Herr, F., Stewart, J., and Charest, M. P. (1961). *Arch. Int. Pharmacodyn. Ther.* **134,** 328.
Holliday, A. R. (1965). *Fed. Proc. Fed. Amer. Soc. Exp. Biol.* **24,** 328.
Holmgren, B., and Condi, C. (1964). *Bol. Inst. Estud. Med. Biol. (Univ. Nac. Auton. Mex.)* **22,** 21.
Hunt, E. B., and Bauer, R. H. (1969). *Psychopharmacologia* **16,** 139.
Hunt, E. B., and Krivanek, J. (1966). *Psychopharmacologia* **9,** 1.
Hunt, H. F. (1956). *Ann. N. Y. Acad. Sci.* **65,** 258, 267.
Hurst, P. M., Radlov, R., Chubb, N., and Bagley, S. K. (1969). *Amer. J. Psychol.* **82,** 307.
Hydén, H. (1959). *Proc. 4th Int. Congr. Biochem., Vienna, 1958* **3,** 64.
Hydén, H., and Egyhazi, E. (1963). *Proc. Nat. Acad. Sci. U.S.* **49,** 618.
Hydén, H., and Hartelius, H. (1948). *Acta Psychiat. Neurol. Suppl.* **48,** 117 p.
Irwin, S., and Benuazizi, A. (1966). *Science* **152,** 100.
Jewett, R. E., Prich, J. H., and Norton, S. (1965). *Nature (London)* **207,** 277.
John E. R., Tschirgi, R., and Wenzel, B. M. (1959). *J. Physiol (London)* **146,** 550.
Johnson, F. N. (1969). *Psychopharmacologia* **16,** 105.
Kahan, S. A. (1966). *Physiol. Behav.* **1,** 117.
Kamano, D. K., Martin, L. K., and Powell, B. J. (1966a). *Psychopharmacologia* **8,** 319.
Kamano, D. K., Martin, L. K., Ogle, M. E., and Powell, B. J. (1966b). *Psychol. Rec.* **16,** 13.
Karoly, A. J., and Hunt, L. J. (1965). *Fed. Proc. Fed. Amer. Soc. Exp. Biol* **24,** 196
Katz, J. J., and Halstead, W. C. (1960). *Comp. Pyschol. Monogr.* **20,** 1.
Keleman, K., and Bovet, D. (1961a). *Acta Physiol.* **19,** 143.
Keleman, K., and Bovet, D. (1961b). *Kiserl. Orvostud.* **13,** 419.
Keleman, K., and Bovet, D. (1961c). *Acta Physiol.* **1,** 333.
Kelleher, R. T., Fry, W., Deegan, J., and Cook, L. (1961). *J. Pharmacol. Exp. Ther.,* **133,** 271.
Kety, S. S. (1971). *In* "The Neurosicences: Second Study Program" (F. O. Schmitt, ed.), p. 324–336. Rockerfeller Univ. Press, New York.
Khavari, K. A., and Maickel, R. P. (1967). *Int. J. Neuropharmacol.* **6,** 301.
Koe, B. K., and Weissman, A. (1966). *J. Pharmacol. Exp. Ther.* **154,** 499.
Kral, V. A., Solyom, L., and Enesco, H. E. (1967). *J. Amer. Geriat. Soc.* **15,** 364.
Krivanek, J., and Hunt, E. (1967). *Psychopharmacologia* **10,** 189.
Krivanek, J., and McGaugh, J. L. (1968). *Psychopharmacologia* **12,** 303.

Kulkarni, A. S., Thompson, T., and Shideman, F. E. (1966). *J. Neurochem.* **13,** 1143.
LaBrosse, E. H., Axelrod, J., and Kety, S.S. (1958). *Science* **128,** 593.
Lashley, K. S. (1917). *Psychobiology* **1,** 141.
Latz, A. (1964). *Fed. Proc. Fed. Amer. Soc. Exp. Biol.* **22,** 509.
Leaf, R. C., and Muller, S. A. (1965). *Fed. Proc. Fed. Amer. Soc. Exp. Biol.* **24,** 196.
Leaf, R. C., and Muller, S. A. (1966). *Psychopharmacologia* **9,** 101.
LeBlanc, J. (1958). *Proc. Soc. Exp. Biol. Med.* **98,** 648.
Leonard, B. E. (1966a). *Biochem. Pharmacol.* **15,** 255.
Leonard, B. E. (1966b). *Biochem. Pharmacol.* **15,** 263.
Leonard, B. E. (1967). *Int. J. Neuropharmacol.* **6,** 63.
Leonard, B. E. (1969). *Int. J. Neuropharmacol.* **8,** 427.
Levine, S., and Brush, F. (1967). *Physiol. Behav.* **2,** 385.
Levine, S., and Jones, L. E. (1965). *J. Comp. Physiol. Psychol.* **59,** 357.
Lewis, S. (1967). Paper presented at the meeting of the East. Psychol. Ass., Boston, April, 1967. (Unpublished.)
Lewis, S., and Essman, W. B. (1967). Unpublished observations.
Linuchev, M. N., and Michelson, M. J. (1965). *Activ. Nerv. Super.* **7,** 25.
Livecchi, S. G., and Dusewicz, R. A. (1969). *Psychol. Rep.* **24,** 735.
Loken, R. D. (1940). *Psychol. Bull.* **37,** 592.
Loken, R. D. (1941). *J. Comp. Psychol.* **32,** 11.
Longo, V. G. (1966). *Pharmacol. Rev.* **18,** 965.
Longo, V. G., and Silvestrini, B. (1957). *J. Pharmacol. Exp. Ther.* **120,** 160.
Loutit, R. T. (1965). *Psychol. Rec.* **15,** 97.
Luco, J. V., Martorell, R., and Reid, A. (1949). *J. Pharmacol. Exp. Ther.* **97,** 171.
McGaugh, J. L. (1961). *Psychol. Rep.* **8,** 99.
McGaugh, J. L. (1966). *Science* **153,** 1351.
McGaugh, J. L. (1968). *In* "Psychopharmacology: A Review of Progress, 1957–1967" (D. H. Efron, ed.), pp. 891–904. US Govt. Printing Office, Washington, D.C.
McGaugh, J. L., and Petrinovich, L. (1965). *Int. Rev. Neurobiol.* **8,** 139.
McGaugh, J. L., and Thomson, C. W. (1962). *Psychopharmacologia* **3,** 166.
McGaugh, J. L., Westbrook, W. H., and Burt, S. (1961). *J. Comp. Physiol. Psychol.* **54,** 501.
McGaugh, J. L., Thomson, C. W., Westbrook, W. H., and Hudspeth, W. J. (1962). *Psychopharmacologia* **3,** 352.
McNutt, L. (1967). *Proc. 75th Annu. Conv. Amer. Psychol. Ass.* **2,** 77.
Malis, J. L. (1962). *Fed. Proc. Fed. Amer. Soc. Exp. Biol.* **2,** 327.
Marazzi, A. (1953). *Science,* **118,** 367.
Maxwell, D. R., and Palmer, H. T. (1961). *Nature* (*London*) **191,** 84.
Maxwell, D. R., Palmer, H. T., and Ryall, R. W. (1961). *Arch. Int. Pharmacodyn. Ther.* **132,** 60.
Meltzer, D., Merkler, N. L., and Maxey, G. C. (1966). *Psychon. Sci.* **11,** 413.
Mercier, J., and Dessaigne, S. (1960). *Ann. Pharm. Fr.,* **18,** 502.
Meyers, B. (1965). *Psychopharmacologia* **8,** 111.
Mihailović, L., Janković, B. D., Petrović, M., and Isaković, K. (1958). *Experientia* **14,** 144.
Miller, N. E. (1961). *Amer. Psychol.* **16,** 12.
Miller, N. E., and Miles, W. R. (1935). *J. Comp. Psychol.* **20,** 397.
Mitchell, J. C., and King, F. A. (1960). *Psychopharmacologia* **1,** 463.
Modell, W. (1966) "Drugs of Choice," Ch. 12, Mosby, St. Louis, Missouri.

Moriguchi, N. (1963) *Ann. Anim. Psychol.* **13,** 49.
Morris, N. R., Aghajanian, G. K., and Bloom, F. E. (1967). *Science* **155,** 1225.
Morrison, C. F., (1967). *Int. J. Neuropharmacol.* **6,** 229.
Morrison, C. F. (1968). *Psychopharmacologia* **12,** 176.
Morrison, C. F., and Armitage, A. K. (1967). *Ann. N. Y. Acad. Sci.* **142,** 268.
Morrison, C. F., and Lee, P. N. (1968). *Psychopharmacologia* **13,** 210.
Müller, G. E., and Pilzecker, A. (1900). *Z. Psychol.* **1,** 1.
Nachmansohn, D. (1938). *C. R. Soc. Biol.* **129,** 941.
Nash, H. (1962). *J. Nerv. Ment. Dis.* **134,** 203.
Olds, M. E. (1966). *J. Comp. Physiol. Psychol.* **62,** 136.
Oliverio, A. (1967). *Il Farmaco* **6,** 441–449.
Orowan, E. (1955). *Nature (London)* **175,** 683.
Orzack, M. H., Taylor, C. L., and Kornetsky, C. (1968). *Psychopharmacologia* **13,** 413.
Osborn, A. G., Bunker, J. P., Cooper, L. M., Frank, G. S., and Hildgard, E. P. *Science* **157,** 574.
Otis, L. S. (1964). *Science* **143,** 1347.
Overton, D. A. (1964). *J. Comp. Physiol. Psychol.* **57,** 3.
Page, I. H. (1968). "Serotonin." Yearbook Publ., Chicago, Illinois.
Palladin, A. V. (1961). *In* "Regional Neurochemistry" (S. S. Kety and J. Elkes, eds.), p. 8. Pergamon, Oxford.
Pare, W. (1961). *J. Comp. Physiol. Psychol.* **54,** 506.
Pavlov, I. P. (1927). "Conditioned Reflexes." Oxford Univ. Press, London and New York.
Pavlov, I. P. (1941). "Conditioned Reflexes and Psychiatry." Int. Publ., New York.
Pearl, S., and McKean, D. B. (1967). *Science* **157,** 220.
Pearlman, C. A., Jr., Sharpless, S. K., and Jarvik, M. E. (1961). *J. Comp. Physiol. Psychol.* **54,** 109.
Pechstein, L. A., and Reynolds, W. R. (1937). *J. Comp. Psychol.* **24,** 459.
Pepeu, G., Freedman, D. X., and Giarman, N. J. (1960). *J. Pharmacol. Exp. Ther.* **129,** 291.
Petrinovich, L. (1963). *Psychopharmacologia* **4,** 103.
Petrinovich, L. (1967). *Psychopharmacologia* **5,** 375.
Petrinovich, L., Bradford, D., and McGaugh, J. L. (1965). *Psychon. Sci.* **2,** 191.
Phillips, H. C. (1937). *J. Comp. Psychol.* **24,** 471.
Pletscher, A., Shore, P. A., and Brodie, B. B. (1955). *Science* **122,** 374.
Plotnikoff, N. (1962). *Fed. Proc. Fed. Amer. Soc. Exp. Biol.* **21,** 420.
Plotnikoff, N. (1966a). *Science* **151,** 703.
Plotnikoff, N. (1966b). *Fed. Proc. Fed. Amer. Soc. Exp. Biol.* **25,** 262.
Plotnikoff, N. (1966c). *Life Sci.* **5,** 1495.
Porsolt, R. D., Joyce, D., and Summerfield, A. (1970). *Abstr. Pap., Colleg. Int. Neuro-Psychopharmacol., 7th Congr.* **2,** 349.
Powell, B. J., Martin, L. K., and Kamano, D. K. (1965). *Psychol. Rep.* **17,** 330.
Powell, B. J., Ogle, M. E., Martin, L. K., and Kamano, D. K. (1966). *Psychol. Rep.* **18,** 645.
Prien, R. F., Wagner, M. J., Jr., and Kahn, S. (1963). *Amer. J. Psychol.* **204,** 448.
Quarton, G. C., and Talland, G. A. (1962). *Psychopharmacologia* **3,** 66.
Rahmann, H. (1961). *Pfluegers Arch. Gesamte Physiol. Mencshen Tiere* **273,** 247.
Rech, R. H. (1966). *Psychopharmacologia* **9,** 110.
Rech, R. H., Borys, H. K., and Moore, K. E. (1966). *J. Pharmacol. Exp. Ther.* **153,** 412.

Rensch, R., and Rahmann, H. (1960). *Pfluegers Arch. Gesamte Physiol. Menschen Tiere* **271,** 693.
Richter, D., and Crossland, J. (1949). *Amer. J. Physiol.* **159,** 275.
Riley, H., and Spinks, A. (1958). *J. Pharmacol. Exp. Ther.* **10,** 721.
Ritzmann, R. F., Miller, L., and Bell, R. W. (1969). *Psychon. Sci.* **14,** 103.
Robustelli, F. (1966). *Atti Accad. Naz. Lincei, Cl. Sci. Fis., Mat. Natur., Rend.* **40,** 490.
Roll, R. M., Brown, G. B., DiCarlo, F. J., and Schultz, A. S. (1949). *J. Biol. Chem.* **180,** 333.
Ross, R. B. (1964). *Nature (London)* **201,** 109.
Rushton, R., and Steinberg, H. (1963). *Brit. J. Pharmacol.* **21,** 295.
Sachs, E. (1961). *Fed. Proc. Fed. Amer. Soc. Exp. Biol.* **20,** 339.
Sachs, E., Weingarten, M., and Klein, N. W., Jr. (1966). *Psychopharmacologia* **9,** 17.
Samuel, G. K., Kodama, J. K., and Menneor, J. H. (1965). *Psychopharmacologia* **8,** 259.
Schildkraut, J. J., Green, R., Gordon, E. K., and Durell, J. (1966a). *Amer. J. Psychiat.* **123,** 690.
Schildkraut, J. J., Schanberg, S. M., and Kopin, I. J. (1966b). *Life Sci.* **5,** 1479.
Schildkraut, J. J., Logue, M. A., and Dodge, G. A. (1969). *Psychopharmacologia* **14,** 135.
Schmidt, M. J., and Davenport, J. W. (1967). *Psychon. Sci.* **7,** 185.
Shillito, E. E. (1967). *Brit. J. Pharmacol. Chemother.* **32,** 258.
Shitov, Y. Y. (1965). *Farmakol. Toksikol. (Moscow)* **28,** 13.
Shugayev, V. A. (1965). *Farmakol. Toksikol. (Moscow)* **28,** 3.
Sidley, N. A., and Schoenfeld, W. N. (1963). *J. Exp. Anal. Behav.* **6,** 293.
Skinner, B. F., and Heron, W. T. (1937). *Psychol. Rec.* **1,** 340.
Small, I. F., Sharpley, P., and Small, J. G. (1968). *Amer. J. Psychiat.* **125,** 837.
Small, J. G., and Small, I. F. (1967). *Dis. Nerv. Syst.* **28,** 523.
Smith, R. G. (1967). *Science* **155,** 603.
Smythies, J. R., and Antun, F. (1969). *Nature (London)* **223,** 1061.
Smythies, J. R., Benington, F., and Morin, R. D. (1969). *Proc. 4th Int. Congr. Pharmacol., Basel,* p. 82. (Abstr.)
Sofronov, M. S., and Tsobkallo, G. I. (1959). "Physiological-Patologü Nervoy Sistemy," pp. 717–730. Acad. Sci. USSR, Moscow.
Solyom, L., and Gallay, H. M. (1966). *Int. J. Neuropsychiat.* **2,** 577.
Solyom, L., Enesco, H. E., and Beaulieu, C. (1967). *J. Gerontol.* **22,** 1.
Stark, L. G. (1967). *Proc. West. Pharmacol. Soc.* **10,** 90.
Stein, D. G., and Brink, J. J. (1969). *Psychopharmacologia* **14,** 240.
Stein, L. (1956). *Science* **124,** 1082.
Stein, L. (1964). In: Steinberg, H., deRueck, A. V. S., and Knight, J. (Eds). *Anim. Behav. Drug Action, Ciba Found. Symp. Jointly Coord. Comm. Symp. Drug Action, 1963,* pp. 91–113.
Stein, H. H., and Yellin, T. O. (1967). *Science* **157,** 96.
Stern, W. C., and Heise, G. A. (1970). *Physiol. Behav.* **5,** 449.
Stetten, D., and Heron, S. Z. (1959). *Science* **129,** 1737.
Stevens, D. A., Resnick, O., and Krus, D. M. (1967). *Life Sci.* **6,** 2215.
Stewart, J. (1962). *Psychopharmacologia* **3,** 132.
Stratton, L. O., and Petrinovich, L. (1963). *Psychopharmacologia* **5,** 47.
Stratton, L. O., and Petrinovich, L. F. (1967). *Psychopharmacologia* **10,** 204.
Stretch, R., Houston, M., and Jenkins, A. (1964). *Nature (London)* **201,** 472.
Sulser, F., Watts, J., and Brodie, B. B. (1962). *Ann. N.Y. Acad. Sci.* **96,** 279.
Sved, S. (1965). *Can. J. Biochem.* **43,** 949.
Talland, G. A., and Quarton, G. C. (1965). *Psychopharmacologiga* **7,** 379.

Talland, G. A., Mendleson, J. W., Koz, G., and Aaron, R. (1965). *J. Psychiat. Res.* **3,** 171.
Teitelbaum, H. A., Newton, J. E. O., Gliedman, L. H., and Gantt, W. H. (1961). *Psychosom. Med.* **23,** 446.
Tenen, S. S. (1967). *Psychopharmacologia* **10,** 204.
Thompson, R., and Meyer, M. E. (1969). *Psychol. Rep.* **24,** 425.
Tolman, E. C. (1917). *Psychol. Monogr.* **18,** No. 107.
Tonini, G. (1961). *Biochem. Pharmacol.* **8,** 59.
Ungar, G. (1970). *In* "Molecular Mechanisms in Memory and Learning" (G. Ungar, ed.), pp. 149–175. Plenum, New York.
Verhave, T. (1961). *Fed. Proc. Fed. Amer. Soc. Exp. Biol.* **20,** 395.
Vernier, V. G. (1961). *Dis. Nerve. Syst.* **22, 7**.
Vinogradov, V. V. (1969). *Farmakol. Toksikol.* (*Moscow*) **32,** 259.
Voronin, L. G., and Napalkov, A. V. (1963). *In* "Psychopharmacological Methods" (Z. Votava, M. Horvath, and O. Vinar, eds.), p. 182. Macmillan, New York.
Voronin, L. G., Tushmalava, N. A., and Kazënnova, I. I. (1968). *Z. Vyssheĭ Nerv. Deyat.* **18,** 3.
Wada, J. A., Wrinch, J., Hill, D., McGeer, P. L., and McGeer, E. G. (1963). *Arch. Neurol.* (*Chicago*) **9,** 69.
Wagner, A. R. (1963). *J. Exp. Psychol.* **65,** 474.
Wagner, A. R., Carder, J. B., and Beatty, W. W. (1966). *Psychon. Sci.* **4,** 33.
Walk, R. D., Owens, J. W. M., and Davidson, B. S. (1961). *Psychol. Rep.* **8,** 251.
Walsh, F. B. (1947). "Clinical Neuro-Ophthalmology," Williams and Wilkins, Baltimore, Maryland.
Weiskrantz, L., and Wilson, W. A. (1956). *Science* **123,** 1116.
Weiss, B., and Laties, V. G. (1962). *Pharmacol. Rev.* **14,** 1.
Weissman, A. (1961). *Pharmacologia* **3,** 60.
Weissman, A. (1967). *Int. Rev. Neurobiol.* **10,** 167.
Wenzel, D. C., and Davis, P. W. (1961). *Tech. Rep., Off. Nav. Res., Armed Serv. Tech. Tech. Inform. Ag.* pp. 1–11.
White, O. A., and Suborski, M. D. (1969). *Psychopharmacologia* **16,** 25.
Whitehouse, J. M. (1966). *Psychopharmacologia* **9,** 183.
Wolff, H. C., and Gantt, W. H. (1935). *Arch. Neurol. Psychiat.* **33,** 1030.
Wolff, K. (1962). *Dis. Nerv. Syst.* **23,** 199.
Woodbury, D. M. (1954). *Recent Progr. Horm. Res.* **10,** 65.
Woodruff, A. B., and Faltz, C. A. (1965) *Psychol. Rep.* **16,** 592.
Woolley, D. W. (1965). *In* "Pharmacology of Conditioning, Learning and Retention" (M. Y. Mikhel'son and V. G. Longo, eds.), pp. 231–236. Pergamon, Oxford.

AUTHOR INDEX

Numbers in italics refer to the pages on which the complete references are listed.

C

D

E

F

G

H

M

N

O

P

Q

R

S

U

V

W

Y

Z

SUBJECT INDEX